Chén Xiūyuán's 陳修園

神農本草經讀

Reading the Divine Farmer's Classic of Materia Medica

Shén Nóng Běn Cǎo Jīng Dú

Corinna Theisinger

Edited by Eran Even Dr. TCM, R.Ac.
and Jonathan Schell L.Ac.

The Chinese Medicine Database
www.cm-db.com
Portland, Oregon

Reading the Divine Farmer's Classic of Materia Medica

神農本草經讀

Shén Nóng Běn Cǎo Jīng Dú

Corinna Theisinger

Edited by Eran Even Dr. TCM, R.Ac.
and Jonathan Schell L.Ac.

Copyright © 2016 The Chinese Medicine Database

1017 SW Morrison #307A
Portland, OR 97205 USA

COMP designation original Chinese work and English translation

Cover Design by Jonathan Schell L.Ac.
Library of Congress Cataloging-in-Publication Data:

Chen, Xiuyuan, 1753-1823.
　　[Reading the Divine Farmer's Classic of Materia Medica. English]
　　Shen Nong Ben Cao Jing Du = Reading the Divine Farmer's Classic of Materia Medica
　　/ translation Corinna Theisinger
　　　　　p.　cm.
　　Includes Index.
　　ISBN 978-0-9906029-2-7　(alk. paper)
　　Medicine, Chinese　　　　　　　I. Theisinger, Corinna.　II. Title: Reading the Divine
　　Farmer's Classic of Materia Medica

International Standard Book Number (ISBN): 978-0-9906029-2-7
Printed in the United States of America

Contents

Chapter II

Medicinals of the Highest Grade

Chapter III

Medicinals of the Middle Grade

Chapter IV

Medicinals of the Middle Grade

神
農
本
草
經
讀

Indices

神
農
本
草
經
讀

The editing of Chén Xiūyuán's *Shén Nóng Běn Cǎo Jīng Dú* 《神農本草經讀》
(Reading the Divine Farmer's Classic of Materia Medica) was made possible in part
by a grant from:
The Institute of East West Medicine, New York NY 10016
www.eastwestmedicine.org

Foreword by Arnaud Versluys

Chén Xiūyuán (1753-1823) was a prominent *Qīng* dynasty medical scholar. As a classicist and purist, he is mainly known for his love of the *Hàn* dynasty medical classics in general, and the herbal classics of the *Shānghán Lùn* and *Jīnguì Yàolüè* in particular.

Using his scholarly abilities, and academic wherewithal, Chén indefatigably advocated for classical studies, explaining how the theoretical foundation of Chinese medicine originates from the *Huángdì Nèijīng,* and the practice of its herbal medicine is codified in the writings of Zhāng Zhòngjǐng. And although he is open to referencing the varied *Táng, Sòng, Jīn,* and *Yuán* dynasty medical treatises, he clearly states in his preface to the *Shénnóng Běncǎo Jīng Dú* that to understand the laws of yīn and yáng in the context of herbal medicine, and the use of specific herbs and formulas by Zhāng Zhòngjǐng, one must study the source of all herbal knowledge, which is the *Divine Farmer's Materia Medica.* Chén's *Shénnóng Běncǎo Jīng Dú* (Reading of the Diving Farmer's Materica Medica) teaches us how to interpret the difficult to decode ancient language of this herbal classic to attain a better understanding of the practice of canonical herbal medicine.

This publication is the third translation of a Chén Xiūyuán treatise, by the translation team of the Chinese Medicine Database and is an absolute blessing for all serious Chinese medicine practitioners, who do not personally possess the ability to read Chinese. By now, Chinese medicine has been taught and practiced in the West for almost 40 years, and we are finally starting to witness the publication of a series of translations of medical classics of different eras. *Qīng* dynasty texts are relatively easier to access than the almost occult *Hàn* dynasty ones, and are therefore a perfect gateway for any serious student or practitioner into the study of pre-Communist Chinese medicine. For the past ten years, the Chinese Medicine Database has been on the forefront of this important work and I cannot commend them strongly enough for their important continued contributions to the betterment of both Chinese medicine education and practice in the West!

Arnaud Versluys, Ph.D., MD (China), L.Ac.
Director, Institute of Classics in East Asian Medicine

Translator's Acknowledgments

I would like to thank my parents and the rest of my family for their support.

Translator's Preface

This text is written by the famous Confucianist and medical doctor Chén Xiūyuán 陳修園 (1753 – 1823 in Fú Jiàn), which was first printed in 1803. The original text of the *Shén Nóng Běn Cǎo Jīng* 《 神農本草經 》 (Divine Farmer's Classic of Materia Medica) was compiled in the first or second century A.D. and consists of three parts. The first part discusses high-grade medicines that can prevent illnesses and lead to longevity, the second part contains medicines to cure patients, and the third one deals with toxic medicines of the lowest grade, which cure diseases, but have side effects. There are 365 herbs described in the *Shén Nóng Běn Cǎo Jīng*, and in the following translation, there are 116 medicinals which have been excerpted from the original, and 46 from later appendices. The *Reading of the Divine Farmer's Classic of Materia Medica* includes commentaries by Chén Xiūyuán 陳修園, Zhāng Yǐn'ān[1] 張隱庵 and the scholar-physician Xú Lingtāi[2] 徐靈胎, whose commentary on the *Divine Farmer's Classic of Materia Medica* was first published in 1736.

The ancient part of the *Shén Nóng Běn Cǎo Jīng* gives the yīn and yáng qualities, the qì and flavor of each medicine, and also lists the indications. That is all. In his commentary Chén Xiūyuán explains the attributes of each herb quality according to the five elements and gives plenty of information on the Chinese understanding of physiology and pathophysiology. He tries to make clear why this or that indication is listed for a certain medicine and sometimes even includes the doctrine of signatures.

---

1. A scholar-physician and specialist on the six-levels theory (1644-1722) in Zhè Jiāng.
2. 1693-1771 in Jiāng Sū.

神農本草經讀序

Reading the Divine Farmer's Classic of Materia Medica Preface

陳修園老友，精於岐黃之朮，自負長沙後身，世醫環而姍笑之。及遇危證，繮斷桅橫，萬手齊束。修園往，脫冠幾上，探手舉脈，目霍霍上聳，良久乾笑曰：「候本不奇，治之者擾之耳。」主人曰：「某名醫。」曰：「誤矣。」曰：「法本朱、張、王、李。」曰：「更誤矣。天下豈有朱、張、王、李而能愈疾者乎！」口吃吃然罵，手仡仡然書，方具，則又自批自贊自解，自起調刀圭火齊，促服之。服之，如其言。

[My] old friend Chén Xiūyuán is refined in the arts of Qí Bó and Huáng Dì,[3] he regards himself as successor of [Zhāng] Chángshā,[4] and ridicules those hereditary[5] doctors. [When the hereditary doctors] encountered a critical pattern, [it was as if] the reins had been cut, or the masts hung crosswise—ten thousand hands were equally tied.[6] Xiúyuán went there, took off his cap and threw it onto a small table, raised his hands to feel the patient's pulses, his eyes absently gazing upwards, and [after] a good while, he gave a hollow laugh and said: "The symptoms and the cause [of this ailment] are not unusual, and it is merely harassment due to the previous doctor's [improper] cures."[7] The host said: "It was a certain famous doctor." [Xiúyuán] replied: "[He made a] mistake!" [The

---

3. The art of Qí Bó 岐伯 and Huáng Dì 黃帝 is the medicine of *Huáng Dì Nèi Jīng Sù Wèn* 《黃帝內經素問》 (Inner Canon of the Yellow Emperor Plain Questions), which is composed in the form of dialogue between the emperor Huáng Dì with and his minister Qí Bó.

4. This is another name for Zhāng Zhòngjǐng 張仲景, who was governor of the province of Chángshā. See: *Zhōng Guǒ Yī Rén Wù Cí Diǎn Zhǔ Biān Lǐ Jīng Wěi*, Shànghǎi Cí Shū Chū Bǎn Shè. 《中國醫人物詞典》主編李經緯上海辭書出版社 Lǐ Jīng Wěi (Ed.) (*Dictionary of Chinese Medical Physicians*) Shanghai Dictionary Publishing House 1985, p. 356.

5. Hereditary doctors were non-scholars who learned from their fathers and grandfathers by oral tradition and were more practically oriented. The scholar-physicians studied the Chinese philosophical classics, as well as medical books, etc., and tended to be more theorists, even though they were also clinicians.

6. This means that none amongst the hereditary doctors could help the patient.

7. According to Wiseman, harassment can be phlegm-fire harassing the heart or phlegm turbidity harassing the upper body. See: Nigel Wiseman, Feng Ye: *A Practical Dictionary of Chinese Medicine*. Brookline 1998, p. 254 "harassment."

host] said: "His method originates from Zhū, Zhāng, Wáng, and Lǐ."[8] [Xiúyuán] answered: "This is even a bigger mistake! How could there be anyone curing illnesses [like] Zhū, Zhāng, Wáng and Lǐ in the world [now]?" [Xiúyuán] prescribed a formula while continuing to scold [the family]. When he finished, he began to discuss and admire his prescription, he initiated the preparation of the medicine by taking very small amounts of it and boiling it on an even fire,[9] [then] urged the patient to take it. Once taken, it was as he had said.

嘗以李時珍《綱目》為讕陋，著有《神農本草經注》六卷，其言簡，其旨賅，其義奇而不戾於正。其鈎深索隱也，玄之又玄，如李將軍之畫，不肯使一直筆。其扃辟奧啟也，仍復明白坦易，如白香山詩句，雖竈下老嫗，亦可與知，觿解不可解而後解，及其解之了，不異人也。可謂金心在中，銀手如斷矣。

Chén tried to have some superficial knowledge of Lǐ Shízhēn's *Gāng Mù*[10] and [so Chén] wrote the *Shén Nóng Běn Cǎo Jīng Zhù* 《神農本草經注》 (Commentary on the Divine Farmer's Classic of Materia Medica)[11] in six chapters. His text was short and succinct; its meaning was surprising, but did not digress from the main points.[12] He explored it profoundly and traced out the hidden meanings, which are extremely mysterious and profound, like the paintings of Lǐ Jiāngjūn, [who was] not willing to use a straight stroke.[13] He opened closed doors with [his text],[14] and made clear and easy what was still complex, similar to the verse of the "white fragrant mountain," [which was completed by the poet] only if the elderly women in the kitchen could also understand it; he picked it to pieces,[15] [so they could understand], and what they [still] did not understand he later

---

8. Most likely, the host means the famous physicians: Zhū Dānxī 朱丹溪, also named Zhū Zhènhēng 朱震亨 (1281-1358), who is the founder of the yīn-nourishing school, see: Lǐ, 1985, p.134, Zhāng Zǐhé 張子和 (1151-1231 or 1156-1228), originator of the *gōng xià pài* 攻下派 (purgative school) see: Lǐ, 1985, p.351. Wáng Hàogǔ 王好古 (1200-1264), a famous representative of the spleen-fortifying school and successor of Lǐ Gǎo 李杲 (1180-1251), author of the *Pí Wèi Lùn* 《脾胃論》 (Treatise on the Spleen and Stomach), see: Lǐ, 1985, p. 210.

9. This means that when preparing dosages of medicine, the water should be boiled to reach a certain temperature. A *dāo guī* 刀圭 is an ancient tool for measuring tiny amounts of medicine. *Huǒ qí* 火齊 is a degree of heat, the time, and the temperature in which the medicine is prepared.

10. This is the short title of the famous *Běn Cǎo Gāng Mù* 《本草綱目》 (Compendium of the Materia Medica) (1578), which took Lǐ Shízhēn 李時珍 (1518-1593) 27 years of work.

11. This was a *Běn Cǎo* that Chén had written previous to writing the *Shén Nóng Běn Cǎo Jīng Dú* 《神農本草經讀》.

12. *Wěi* 骫 originally meant buckled bone, so literally, this passage can be translated as: does not bend around [what should be] straightforward.

13. Lǐ Jiāngjūn 李將軍, whose real name is Lǐ Sīxùn 李思訓 (651-716), was a landscape artist of the *Táng*, famous for his elaborated "green landscapes," which were partially gilded.

14. He opened closed doors: this means to open the door and enter, which is to add deeper understanding. *Jiōng* 扃 is door; *bì* 啟 is open, or to open.

15. *Xī* 觿 is a kind of tool made of bones, a bodkin for undoing knots. This means to "untwine" difficult passages and put them into an order.

explained until they could get it entirely without exception.[16] This can be called a golden heart in the center and silver hands as if cut![17]

出山後，斂抑才華。每診一病，必半日許，才出一方，有難之者，其言訥訥然如不能出。

After taking over his [governmental] office, Chén restrained his [medical] talent. For each examination of a patient, he necessarily took about half a day before he made a prescription; and in difficult cases, his speech was cautious and slow as if the words would not come out.

壬戌冬，回籍讀禮，閉門謝客，復取舊著六卷中，遴其切用者一百余種，附以《別錄》，分為四卷，俱從所以然處發揮，與舊著頗異，名曰《本草經讀》。蓋欲讀經者，讀於無字處也。修園為余言，所著尚有《傷寒論注》四卷，重訂《柯注傷寒論》八卷，重訂《活人百問》八卷，《金匱淺注》十六卷，《醫醫偶錄》二卷，《醫學從眾錄》八卷，《真方歌括》二卷，《景岳新方砭》四卷，《傷寒論讀》四卷，《金匱讀》四卷，《醫約》二卷，《醫訣》三卷。雖依類立言，義各有取要。其闡抉古經之旨，多與此書相發明。暇日予將遍讀焉。

In the winter of the eighth year of Rén Xū (1802), [Xiúyuán] returned home for mourning,[18] kept his door closed, and did not receive guests. [Xiúyuán] took out his old manuscript of six chapters, chose more than one hundred kinds [of herbs] he frequently used, made another classification appendix, and separated it into four chapters, and developed all of it further. [As such the result was] quite different from the former work, and he called it *Běn Cǎo Jīng Dú* 《本草經讀》 (Reading the Divine Farmer's Classic of Materia Medica). Maybe he wanted those who study the

---

16. *Bái Xiāng Shān Shī Jù* 《白香山詩句》 (Verse of the "White Fragrant Mountain") is a collection of verses by a group of *Táng* poets, the founder of which was the famous poet Bái Jūyì 白居易 (772-846). He lived on the Xiāng Shān 香山, a mountain in Luòyáng. He was in the habit of mock-performing his poems in front of elderly women, and would change his works until each of the women could perfectly understand him. See the expression: *Lǎo yù néng jiě* 老嫗能解, which means: "easy to comprehend." For the original text, see Huì Hóng 惠洪 (*Sòng* 宋): *Lěng Zhāi Yè Huà* 《冷齋夜話》卷一 (Nocturnal Conversations in the Cold Study), Chapter One:

"白樂天每作詩，問曰解否？嫗曰解，則录之；不解，則易之。"
Bái lè tiān měi zuò shī, wèn yuē jiě fǒu? Yù yuē jiě, zé lù zhī; bù jiě, zé yì zhī.

"Whenever Bái Lètiān (this is the style name for Bái Jūyì) composed a verse, he asked, if he could be understood. When the elderly women could comprehend his speech, he wrote it down, and if they could not, he simplified it."

17. This expresses the difference in quality between these two books. Golden refers to the *Shén Nóng Běn Cǎo Jīng* 《神農本草經》 (Divine Farmer's Classic of Materia Medica), and the inferior silver refers to the *Běn Cǎo Gāng Mù* 《本草綱目》 (Compendium of the Materia Medica).

18. In Chén Xiūyuán's biography it is mentioned that his father died early, so this time he came home from his post to mourn for his mother.

classics to read between the lines. Apart from the [book] I mentioned above, Xiúyuán also wrote the *Shāng Hán Lùn [Qiǎn] Zhù* 《傷寒論[淺]注》 ([Shallow] Commentary to the Discussion On Cold Damage) in four chapters, revised [Kē Qín's] *Kē Zhù Shāng Hán Lùn* 《柯注傷寒論》 (Commentary to the Discussion On Cold Damage) in eight chapters,[19] revised *Huó Rén Bǎi Wèn* 《活人百問》 (One Hundred Questions on How to Save Lives) in eight chapters,[20] *Jīn Guì [Yào Lüè] Qiǎn Zhù* 《金匱[要略]淺注》 (Superficial Commentary on Formulas from the Golden Cabinet) in sixteen chapters, *Yī Yī Ǒu Lù* 《醫醫偶錄》 (Medical Records in Pairs) in two chapters,[21] *Yī Xué Cóng Zhòng Lù* 《醫學從眾錄》 (A Record of Medicine by Others) in eight chapters, [*Shāng Hán*] *Zhēn Fāng Gē Kuò* 《[傷寒]真方歌括》 (True Prescriptions from On Cold Damage with Poems) in two chapters, *Jǐng Yuè Xīn Fāng Biān* 《景岳新方砭》 (A Critique of Jǐngyuè's New Prescriptions) in four chapters,[22] *Shāng Hán Lùn Dú* 《傷寒論讀》 (Reading the Discussion On Cold Damage) in four chapters,[23] *Jīn Guì Dú* 《金匱讀》 (Reading the Formulas from the Golden Cabinet) in four chapters,[24] *Yī Yuē* 《醫約》 (Outlines of Medicine) in two chapters,[25] and *Yī Jué* 《醫訣》 (Methods of Medicine) in three chapters.[26] Although the ideas he expounded are similar, and each of their meanings are important, his aim of choosing ancient texts for explanation is made clearest in this book at hand. When I have the leisure, I would like to read it over again!

---

19. The *Shāng Hán Lùn Zhù* 《傷寒論注》 (Commentary to the Discussion on Cold Damage) was written by the *Qīng* physician Kē Qín 柯琴, named Yùn Bó 韵伯, who was born in Zhèjiāng. His life dates are unknown, but from a preface written by his own hand to his commentary, it is known, that the commentary was written in 1669. See: Lǐ, 1985, p. 424.

20. This title is an abbreviation of *Shāng Hán Bái Wèn* 《傷寒百問》 (One Hundred Questions on Cold Damage), which was written in the *Sòng* dynasty by Zhū Gōng 朱肱 (1050-1125), and later simply called *Huó Rén Shū* 《活人书》 (Book on How to Save People's Lives).

21. Though signed by him, this book is no longer regarded as Chén's own work today. For further research on this topic see: *Liaoning Journal of Traditional Chinese Medicine*, 2007, 34 (12).

22. Jǐng Yuè 景岳 is the famous *Míng* dynasty physician Zhāng Jièbīn 張介賓 (1563-1640), who wrote *Xīn Fāng Bā Zhèn* 《新方八陣》 (New Prescriptions Divided into the Eight Classifications). See: *Jǐng Yuè Quán Shū* 《景岳全書》, Chapter 50-51 (Complete Works of Jǐngyuè). For biographical information see: Lǐ, 1985, p. 350.
The eight classifications of formula actions are: *bǔ* 補 (supplement), *hé* 和 (harmonize), *gōng* 攻 (attack), *sǎn* 散 (diffuse), *hán* 寒 (cool), *rè* 熱 (heat), *gù* 固 (firm), *yīn* 因 (causal).

23. This book title does not appear in any of the official accounts on Chén.

24. This title does also not appear in official accounts on Chén.

25. The actual title of this book is: *Shāng Hán Yī Yuē Lù* 《傷寒醫約錄》 (Record on the Medical Outlines of the Discussion on Cold Damage). See: *World Journal of Integrated Traditional and Western Medicine*. 2007, Vol.2, No.3, p.132.

26. This is likely to be a previous version of *Shāng Hán Yī Jué Chuàn Jiě* 《傷寒醫訣串解》 (The Medical Method of the Discussion on Cold Damage Collected and Explained), which was compiled by Chén around 1821 in six scrolls. See: Yaron Seidmann's preface in the *Jīn Guì Fāng Gē Kuò* 《金匱方歌括》 (Formulas from the Golden Cabinet with Songs Volume I-III). Chinese Medicine Database, Portland 2010, p. 29.

嘉慶八年，歲次昭陽大淵獻，皋月既望，侯官愚弟蔣慶齡小榕氏序。

Eighth year of the reign-period Jiā Qìng, the year Zhāo Yáng Dà Yuān Xiān, fifth lunar month, sixteenth day (Monday, July 4, 1803), waiting for an official post, humbly, Jiǎng Qìngling 蔣慶齡, named Xiǎo Róng 小榕, made this foreword.[27]

---

27. The translator was unable to further identify this person.

後敍

A Later Preface [by Guō Rǔcōng 郭汝聰]

上古之聖人，仰觀天之六氣，俯察地之五行，辨草木、金石、禽獸之性，而合於人之五臟、六腑、十二經脈，著有《本草經》，詞古義深，難於窺測。漢季張長沙《傷寒論》、《金匱要略》，多采中古遺方，用藥之義悉遵《本經》，應驗如響。自李唐而後，《千金》、《外臺》等書，有驗有不驗者。蓋與《本經》之旨，有合有不合也。沿及宋、元諸家，師心自用，藥品日增，經義日晦，只云某藥治某病，某病宜某藥，因陋就簡，愈趨愈下。

The sages of ancient times observed the six qì of heaven and examined the five phases of the earth; they identified the nature of the grass and trees, metal and stones, birds and quadrupeds, and associated them with the human five viscera, six bowels, and the twelve channel-vessels. [All of] this was recorded in the *Shén Nóng Běn Cǎo Jīng*, [and] the original meaning of its phrases are deep and difficult to assess. Zhāng Chángshā of the *Hàn* period gathered many ancient formulas which had been handed down in his *Shāng Hán Lùn* and *Jīn Guì Yào Lüè*. [For the] meaning and use of [these] medicinals, in all cases he followed the *Shén Nóng Běn Cǎo Jīng*, and fulfilled it like an echo. From the *Táng*[28] dynasty onwards, there are the *Qiān Jīn* and the *Wài Tái*[29] and other books; some of them examined [the ancient texts] and some not; and some of them are in conformity with the aim of the *Běn Cǎo Jīng*, some are not. Continuing with all the *Sòng* and *Yuán* dynasty doctors, [who] regarded themselves as masters, [while] the medicinals increased by the day, the meaning of the classics became [more] obscure by the day. [These physicians would] merely say: this certain medicine treats this certain illness, or this certain illness is appropriate for this certain medicine. [Their methods were] crude yet simple, and the more hurried they were, the lower [their effectiveness would be].

---

28. The surname of the imperial family at this time was Lǐ 李.

29. The *Qiān Jīn* 《千金》 is the *Bèi Jí Qiān Jīn Yào Fāng* 《備急千金要方》 (Essential Prescriptions Worth a Thousand in Gold for Every Emergency) by Sūn Sīmiǎo 孫思邈 (581-682), and the *Wài Tái* 《外臺》 is the *Wài Tái Mì Yào* 《外臺秘要》 (Essential Secrets from Outside the Metropolis): ca. 752 by Wáng Tāo 王濤 (670-755). For these persons, see: Lǐ, 1985, pp.181 and 29.

而流毒之最甚者，莫如宋之雷斆，竊古聖之名，著為《炮制》，顛倒是非，不知《本經》為何物。潔古，日華，東垣輩因之，而東垣純盜虛名，無稽臆說流傳至今，無有非之者。李瀕湖《綱目》卷帙浩繁，徒雜採世俗之說，以多為貴，不無喧客奪主之嫌。汪訒庵照《綱目》而約為《備要》，逐末忘本，不足道也。余友孝廉陳修園精通醫學，起死回生，指不勝屈。

But the worst person to spread the poison was none other than Léi Xiào of the *Sòng*, who wrote the *Pào Zhì*《炮制》(Processing of Drugs)[30] under the stolen name of an ancient sage. He reversed right and wrong and did not understand what the *Shén Nóng Běn Cǎo Jīng* was made for. The generation of [Zhāng] Jiégǔ, Rì Huà[zǐ], and [Lǐ] Dōngyuán[31] followed this [form of thought], and [Lǐ] Dōngyuán simply stole an unfounded reputation, but without examining the thoughts and theories which were handed down up to now; nobody is free of these. Lǐ Bīnhú's[32] *Gāng Mù* is vast, [but it] is merely a collection of sayings and common customs, and because it is prolific, it is precious, but it is not without suspicion that the guest is predominating the host.[33] Wāng Rèn'ān[34] reflected on the *Gāng Mù* and approximately made it into the *Běn Cǎo Bèi Yào*《本草備要》(Complete Essentials of Materia Medica), [but] in chasing the tips [he] neglected the roots, [so his] method is insufficient. My friend Chén Xiūyuán with the title *Xiào Lián*[35] is proficient in the study of medicine, and the dead which have been raised [because of him] are too many to be enumerated.

前著有《本草經注》六卷，字櫛句解，不遺剩義，繕本出，紙貴一時。茲復著《本草經讀》四卷，視前著又高一格，俱從所以然處發揮，且以《內經》之旨，《金匱》、《傷寒》之法融貫於中，一書堪為醫林之全書，洵神農之功臣也。

First he wrote the *Běn Cǎo Jīng Zhù*《本草經注》(Commentary on the Divine Farmer's Classic of Materia Medica) in six chapters, which was clearly structured,[36] without surplus meanings; it was a rare edition, and a bestseller for a while. Now, again he has written in four chapters the *Běn Cǎo Jīng Dú*《本草經讀》(Reading the Divine Farmer's Classic of Materia Medica), and in

---

30. This is the *Sòng* dynasty of the Northern and Southern Dynasties, which lasted from 420 till 479 A.D. The *Pào Zhì*《炮制》(Processing of Drugs) is an abbreviation for the *Léi Gōng Páo Zhì Lùn*《雷公炮制論》(Master Léi's Discussion on Processing of Medicinals) by Léi Xiào 雷斆 (who lived during the fifth century). See: Lǐ, 1985, p.637.

31. Zhāng Jiégǔ 張潔古 (1151-1234) was a scholar-physician of the Western *Yuán* dynasty. Concerning Rì Huàzǐ 日華子, is most likely the same person as Dà Míng 大明 (of the tenth century). There is a book with the title *Rì Huàzǐ Zhū Jiā Běn Cǎo*《日華子諸家本草》(Materia Medica of Various Schools by Rì Huàzǐ), which was compiled in the state of *Wú* (吳) during the Five dynasties and Ten States period (907-979). Lǐ Dōngyuán 李東垣 is another name for Lǐ Gǎo 李杲 (1180-1251).

32. This is another name for Lǐ Shízhēn 李時珍 (1518-1593).

33. This means, though vast, it could still be full of mistakes.

34. Wāng Rèn'ān 汪訒庵, also called Wāng Áng 汪昂 (1615-1699), from Ānhuī, was a physician who came from a poor family and had more than 30 years of textual study and clinical practice. See: Lǐ, 1985, p. 282.

35. *Xiào lián* 孝廉 (filial and upright) is a title for candidates for Imperial examinations.

36. *Zhì* 櫛 (comb): verbally this is a general designation for a comb; figuratively it means carding, clarifying.

神農本草經讀・後敘

comparison with the former, [this one] is of an even higher standard. All of them further develop the basic positions, and moreover, the purpose of the [*Huáng Dì*] *Nèi Jīng* and the methods of the *Jīn Gùi* [*Yào Lüè*] and *Shāng Hán* [*Lùn*] are well digested and completely understood[37] in it. This single book may be considered as a complete work within the medical world, and is truly a minister in service[38] to Shén Nóng!

余自齠年，以慈闈多病，矢志於醫。因本草向無繕本，集張隱庵、葉天士、陳修園三家之說，而附以管見，名為《本草經三注》，而集中唯修園之說最多。今得修園之《本草經讀》，則餘《三注》之刻，可以俟之異日矣。喜其書之成而為之序。

When I was a child, my mother was constantly ill, so I took an oath to become a physician. Because previously there had not been a fair transcription of the [*Shén Nóng*] *Běn Cǎo* [*Jīng*], I gathered the sayings from the three specialists Zhāng Yǐn'ān,[39] Yè Tiānshì[40] and I, Chén Xiūyuán, added my humble opinion, and called it *Běn Cǎo Jīng Sān Zhù* 《本草經三注》 (The Divine Farmer's Classic of Materia Medica Commented [on] by [the] Three);[41] and in this collection only Xiūyuán's sayings are the most [numerous]. Currently, Xiūyuán's *Běn Cǎo Jīng Dú* 《本草經讀》 (Reading the Divine Farmer's Classic of Materia Medica) [can] be obtained; however, for surplus printings of the *Sān Zhù* 《三注》 (Commentated on by the Three), we will have to wait until another day! [I] hope for the success of this book and have created this preface.

---

37. *Róng guàn* 融貫 is an abbreviation for *róng huì guàn tōng* 融會貫通 (well digested and completely understood, or to master the subject via a comprehensive study of surrounding areas).

38. A *gōng chén* 功臣 is one, who has made a significant contribution to a specific task.

39. Zhāng Yǐn'ān 張隱庵, also named Zhāng Zhìcōng 張志聰 (1644-1722 in Zhè Jiāng) was a scholar physician and specialist of the six-levels theory.

40. Yè Tiānshì 葉天士, also known as Yè Guì 葉桂 (1666-1745) in Jiāng Sū, was an influential person in the development of warm disease theory. He is the author of the *Wēn Rè Lùn* 《溫熱論》 (Discussion on Warm Diseases) and his disciples made the *Lín Zhèng Zhǐ Nán Yī Àn* 《臨證指南醫案》 (Guide to Clinical Practice in Cases) out of his notes. On his treatment of the eight extraordinary channels, see: Jason Blalack: *Ye Tian-Shi & the Eight Extraordinary Channels*, 2009.

41. This book is available today under the title *Běn Cǎo Sān Jiā Hé Zhù* 《本草三家合注》 (The Three Specialists' Combined Commentary on the [Divine Farmer's] Classic of Materia Medica) compiled by Guō Rǔcōng 郭汝聰 and first printed in 1803. From this passage, it also becomes clear, the introduction was written by Guō Rǔcōng.

凡例
Reader's Guide

一、明藥性者，始自神農，而伊尹配合而為湯液。仲景《傷寒》、《金匱》之方，即其遺書也。闡陰陽之秘，泄天地之藏，所以效如桴鼓。今人不敢用者，緣唐、宋以後，諸家之臆說盛行，全違聖訓，查對與經方所用之藥不合，始疑之，終且毀之也。

1. Understanding the nature of medicinals began with Shén Nóng, and he set rules for their correspondence and making of decoctions and liquids. [Zhāng] Zhòngjǐng's formulas from the *Shāng Hán* [*Lùn*] and *Jīn Gùi* [*Yào Lüè*] have come close to [Shén Nóng's] lost book. [Zhòngjǐng] explained the secrets of yīn and yáng [and] revealed the treasures of heaven and earth, and therefore [these formulas] are as effective as a drumstick which fits the drum. [But] the people of today are not courageous enough to use these formulas. The reason this is so, is because following the *Táng* and *Sòng* [dynasties], various specialists' subjective opinions [became] fashionable. [These ideas] completely violated the sage's teachings, and upon investigating, it was verified that [the specialists' opinions] did not conform to the use of herbs in the classical formulas. So, [the people] began to doubt [the classical formulas], and in the end [the specialists' opinions] further damaged [the reputation of the classical formulas].

二、《神農本草》藥止三百六十品，字字精確，遵法用之，其效如神。自陶弘景以後，藥味日多，而聖經日晦矣。張潔古、李東垣輩，分經專派。徐之才相須、相使、相惡、相反等法，皆小家伎倆，不足言也。是刻只錄一百餘種，其餘不常用與不可得之品闕之。其注解俱遵原文，逐字疏發，經中不遺一字，經外不溢一詞。

2. There are 360 medicinals in the *Shén Nóng Běn Cǎo*, every word is precise, and when one follows the methods of use, the effect is marvelous. After Táo Hóngjǐng[42] the number of medicinal flavors increased daily, and the sage's classic got darker day by day! Zhāng Jiégǔ and Lǐ Dōngyuán's generation divided the classic into specialized schools. Methods like Xú Zhīcái's[43] mutual need, mutual empowerment, mutual aversion, and mutual antagonism are all the craft of minor schools of

---

42. Táo Hóngjǐng 陶弘景 (456-536) was not only a famous Daoist, but also an outstanding physician. He called himself Huà Yáng Yǐn Jū 華陽隐居 hermit of Huà Yáng. See: Lǐ, 1985, p.541.

43. Xú Zhīcái 徐之才 (492-572 to 505-572) was a physician who learned his skills via oral tradition from his father and grandfather. See: Lǐ, 1985, p. 510. Chén seems to look down on him.

thought and not worth mentioning. This engraving[44] just records one hundred or more herbs; the rest are rarely used or cannot be obtained. The annotations entirely explain and follow the original text, the commentary occurs character by character, and within the classic, not a single character is forgotten, and not a single word is added that goes beyond the classic.

三、是刻只錄時用之藥，其品第及字樣，不盡遵舊本。考陶隱居本草，有朱書墨書之別：朱書為《 神農本經 》，墨書為《 名醫別錄 》。開寶間重定印本，易朱書為白字，茲因其近古而遵之。是刻遵古分上中下三品，《 別錄 》等本，采附於後。

3. This engraving just records medicinals that are frequently used; its quality and diction does not exhaustively follow the old book. When one examines hermit Táo's[45] *Běn Cǎo*, it is divided into red books[46] and black books: the red books were made into the *Shén Nóng Běn [Cǎo] Jīng* and the black books became the *Míng Yī Bié Lù* 《 名醫別錄 》 (Specific Recordings by Famous Physicians). The duplicate copy produced in the year 973[47] caused [some of] the red book's characters to be written incorrectly; this is the reason why the [red books] are [still relatively] close to antiquity and in accordance with it. This engraving follows the ancient divisions of the three grades of medicinals: high, middle and low; [excerpts of] the *Bié Lù* 《 別錄 》 (Supplementary Records)[48] and other books are collectively added in the rear.

四、藥性始於神農。用藥者不讀《 本草經 》，如士子進場作制藝，不知題目出於四子書也。渠輩亦云藥性，大抵系《 珍珠囊藥性賦 》、《 本草備要 》及李時珍《 本草綱目 》之類，雜收眾說，經旨反為其所掩，尚可云本草耶？

4. The [classification of the] nature of medicinals began with Shén Nóng. Those who use medicines without studying the *Běn Cǎo Jīng* are like a scholar who enters the examination room to write the essay without knowing that the subject is from the Four Classics.[49] How can it be that for generations, when [scholars] also spoke of the nature of medicinals, they also connected the main points

---

44. The original reproductions of these texts were done by block print.

45. See Footnote 42 above.

46. *Zhū shū* 朱書 literally means cinnabar book; that is, the book was written with red ink. Black books are accordingly books written with black ink.

47. There is a reprint in 20 chapters of the important *Běn Cǎo* made in the *Sòng* dynasty, called the *Kāi Bǎo Chóng Dìng Běn Cǎo* 《 開寶重定本草 》 (Kāi Bǎo Revised Materia Medica). It was produced by more than nine medical authors from the *Hàn Lín Yuàn* 翰林院 *Hàn Lín* Imperial Academy in the sixth year of the reign period of Kāi Bǎo 開寶, and, therefore, this would be 972 or 973.

48. This is the short title of *Míng Yī Bié Lù* 《 名醫別錄 》 (Supplementary Records of Famous Doctors).

49. The Four Classics are the four most influential Confucian Classics, which every student had to memorize, and then write an essay in eight parts on [them]. They are: *Dà Xué* 《 大學 》 (The Great Learning), *Zhōng Yōng* 《 中庸 》 (The Doctrine of the Mean), *Lún Yǔ* 《 論語 》 (The Analects) and *Mèng Zǐ* 《 孟子 》 (Mencius).

神農本草經讀・凡例

to the *Zhēn Zhū Náng Yào Xìng Fù* 《 珍珠囊藥性賦 》 (Poetic Essay on the Nature of Medicinals of the Bag of Pearls),[50] *Běn Cǎo Bèi Yào* 《 本草備要 》 (Complete Essentials of the Materia Medica),[51] as well as Lǐ Shízhēn's *Běn Cǎo Gāng Mù* 《 本草綱目 》 (Compendium of the Materia Medica) and [books] of this kind? [These books] miscellaneously gathered popular ideas, [but] when the purpose of the classic is on the contrary covered, can one still speak of a Materia Medica?

五、近傳《本草崇原》，越之張隱庵著也。《本草經解》，吳之葉天士著也。二書超出諸群書之上。然隱庵專言運氣，其立論多失於蹈虛。天士囿於時好，其立論多失於膚淺。而隱庵間有精實處，天士間有超脫處，則修園謝不敏矣，故茲刻多附二家之注。

5. The writing of Zhāng Yǐn'ān from [the ancient state of] Yuè[52] [was] transmitted [so that it was] easy to understand [in the] *Běn Cǎo Chóng Yuán* 《 本草崇原 》 (Honored Originals of the Materia Medica); [so too was] the writing of Yè Tiānshì from [the ancient state of] Wú[53] in the *Běn Cǎo Jīng Jiě* 《 本草經解 》 (Explaining the Materia Medica Classic) [easy to understand]. These two books far and above exceed all the other books. However successful Yǐn'ān's specialized words are, his arguments often neglect the historical facts. Tiānshì was limited to good times [for writing, so his] arguments [were] often only skin deep. But in Yǐn'ān's [book] there are refined and substantial parts, [while] in Tiānshì there are unconventional passages; however, [I] Xiūyuán, have to apologize for not being clever! Therefore, I have added many commentaries by these two specialists.

六、上古以司歲備物，謂得天地之專精。如君相二火司歲，則收取薑、桂、附子之熱類。如太陽寒水司歲，則收取黃芩、大黃之寒類。如太陰土氣司歲，則收取耆，朮、參、苓、山藥、黃精之土類。如厥陰風木司歲，則收取羌活、防風、天麻、鉤藤之風類。如陽明燥金司歲，則收取蒼朮、桑皮、半夏之燥類。蓋得主歲之氣以助之，則物之功力倍厚。中古之世，不能司歲備物，故用炮製以代天地之氣，如製附子曰「炮」，助其熱也。製蒼朮曰炒，助其燥也。製黃連以水浸，助其寒也。今人識見不及，每用相反之藥，而反製之，何異束縛手足而使之戰斗哉？《侶山堂》之說最精，故節錄之。

---

50. This book was written by the above-mentioned Zhāng Jiégǔ 張潔古, more commonly known as Zhāng Yuánsù 張元素 (1151-1234).

51. This is a book by Wāng Áng 汪昂 and was published in 1694.

52. Today this is the eastern part of Zhè Jiāng province.

53. Today this is the south of Jiāng Sū province.

神農本草經讀 · 凡例

6. In ancient times, [people] made use of the seasonal inspection [to distinguish the qì in charge of the order of the season] to prepare things[54] and called it receiving the concentrated essence of heaven and earth. For example, [when] the two fires of sovereign and minister control the [qì of the] season,[55] then harvest the hot type [of medicinals] like *jiāng* 薑, *guì* 桂, and *fù zǐ* 附子. When *tàiyáng* cold and water control the [qì of the] season, then harvest the cold type [of medicinals] like *huáng qín* 黃芩 and *dà huáng* 大黃. When *tàiyīn* earth and qì control the [qì of the] season, then harvest the earth type [of medicinals] such as *qí* 耆, *zhú* 朮, *shēn* 參, *líng* 苓, *shān yào* 山藥, or *huáng jīng* 黃精. When *juéyīn* wind and wood control the [qì of the] season, then harvest the wind type [of medicinals] like *qiāng huó* 羌活, *fáng fēng* 防風, *tiān má* 天麻, and *gōu téng* 鉤藤. When *yángmíng* dryness and metal control the [qì of the] season, then harvest the dry type [of medicinals] like *cāng zhú* 蒼朮, *sāng pí* 桑皮, and *bàn xià* 半夏. Now, when one uses the help of the qì controlling the season, then the efficacy and strength of the herbs will be twice as substantial. In the era of mid-antiquity, [people] were not able to control the [qì of the] season to prepare substances; therefore they used the processing of medicinals in order to act on behalf of the qì of heaven and earth. For example, to process *fù zǐ* it says: "blast-fry" and [this] reinforces the hot [nature of *fù zǐ*]. To process *cāng zhú* it says: "stir-fry" and [this] reinforces the dry [nature of *cāng zhú*]. To process *huáng lián*, soak it in water [in order to] reinforce the cold [nature of the *huáng lián*]. Nowadays people's knowledge and experience is inferior; whenever they use opposed herbs and prepare them in the opposite way, how is this different than messengers who are sent to the battle with [their] hands and feet bound!? What is written in the *Lǚ Shān Táng* 《侶山堂》[56] is most refined; therefore [I have] partially excerpted from it.

---

54. This is a quotation from the *Huáng Dì Nèi Jīng Sù Wèn · Zhì Zhēn Yào Dà Lùn* 《黃帝内經素問 · 至真要大論》 (Inner Canon of the Yellow Emperor Plain Questions · Great Discussion on Arriving at True Essentials), Chapter 74. This means, if medical substances are prepared in accordance to the qì controlling a certain season, they can have the most complete qì and flavor of this season. For example, when preparing sour herbs in the juéyīn season, then the sourness is complete [and most effective], because the herb receives the refined and condensed transformation from the season.

55. This is part of the *Wǔ Yùn Liù Qì Xué Shuō* 五運六氣學説 (Theory on the Five Transformations and Six Qì), in which the sequence of the natural seasonal qì is as follows:

厥陰風木（ 一陰 ）、少陰君火（ 二陰 ）、太陰溼土（ 三陰 ）、少陽相火（ 一陽 ）、陽明燥金（ 二陽 ）、太陽寒水（ 三陽 ）。
Juéyīn fēng mù (yī yīn), shàoyīn jūn huǒ (èr yīn), tàiyīn shī tǔ (sān yīn), shàoyáng xiāng huǒ (yī yáng), yángmíng zào jīn (èr yáng), tàiyáng hán shuǐ (sān yáng).

Juéyīn is wind and wood, shàoyīn is sovereign fire, tàiyīn is moisture and earth, shàoyáng is ministerial fire, yángmíng is dryness and metal, tàiyáng is coldness and water.

In this theory, the model of the five phases (fire, earth, metal, water, and wood) is combined with the six climates (wind, fire, summer-heat, dampness, dryness, and cold) and thereby one is able to deduce the relations between changes of the weather and occurrences of diseases. See: *Zhōu Yì Hán Shū Yuē Cún* 《周易函書約存》 (Stored Letters on the Book of Changes), Ch. 9.

56. The *Lǚ Shān Táng* 《侶山堂》 is the *Lǚ Shān Táng Lèi Biàn* 《侶山堂類辨》 (The Differentiation of Categories from the Lǚ Shān Hall) by Zhāng Yǐn'ān 張隱庵, who had the Lǚ Shān Hall as place for studies and discussions. It was written in 1663 or 1664.

按：製藥始於雷公，炮製荒謬，難以悉舉。要知此人名斅，宋時人，非黄帝時之雷公也。

Commentary: The processing of medicinals began with Léi Gōng,[57] [but] to process drugs is ridiculous and can hardly be entirely recommended. It is important to know that this person's name was Xiào; [he was] a person [of the] Sòng [dynasty], and not the Léi Gōng of the Yellow Emperor's time.[58]

七、熟地黄、枸杞，取其潤也。市醫炒松則上浮，燒灰則枯燥矣。附子、乾薑，取其烈也。市醫泡淡則力薄，炮黑則氣浮矣。以及竹瀝鹽、咸枳實之類，皆庸醫兩可之見，不足責也。至於棗仁生則令人不眠，熟則令人熟睡。黄耆生用則托裏發汗，炒熟則補中止汗。麥門冬不去心，令人煩躁。桑白皮不炒，大瀉肺氣之類，數百年相沿之陋，不得不急正之。

7. Shú dì huáng and gǒu qǐ [are best] picked [when] they are moist. Market-doctors stir-fry [the medicinals], release [the moisture which] floats up, [then] char them into ash, and wither [them] dry! Fù zǐ and gān jiāng [are best] picked [when] they are [at their] strongest. Market-doctors soak them [until they become] bland; then [their] strength is weak, and [when] blast-fried until black, the qì floats [to the surface]! It is [the same] as well with types of zhú lì salt and salted zhǐ shí, in view of both possibilities [of either processing the moisture away or adding saltiness to already cold medicinals]; all the vulgar healers are not responsible enough. As to [the claim that] raw [suān] zǎo rén will make people sleepless, but cooked, it will make people sleep soundly. [Or the claim that] when fresh huáng qí is used, then it supports the interior and induce sweating, but when cooked, then it supplements the center and stops sweating. [Or the claim that] when one does not remove the heart of mài mén dōng, it will cause people irritability and restlessness. [Or the last claims that], if sāng bái pí is not stir-fried, it would strongly drain the qi of the lungs [—all this] ignorance has been passed on for several hundred years and one cannot but urgently correct it.

八、本經每藥主治，不過三、四證及六、七證而止。古聖人洞悉所以然之妙，而得其專長，非若後世諸書之泛泛也。最陋是李時珍《綱目》，泛引雜說而無當。李士材、汪訒庵，每味必摘其所短，俱是臆說，反啟時輩聚訟紛紛。修園為活人計，不得不痛斥之。

8. In the Běn Jīng, each medicinal's indications do not exceed three to four patterns, or up to six or seven patterns. The ancient sages clearly understood the subtlety of the reasons and were able to foster [their] special abilities, [which] is unlike the superficiality of all the books by later generations, the most ignorant of which is Lǐ Shízhēn's Běn Cǎo Gāng Mù, as it quotes various opinions

---

57. Léi Gōng 雷公 here is the legendary physician of Chinese antiquity.

58. This means, he is not the right one to refer to.

神
農
本
草
經
讀
・
凡
例

but without taking [responsibility for the opinions]. Lǐ Shìcái[59] and Wāng Rèn'ān[60] would select every flavor [of medicinal which] lacked [thorough discussion; however] these were [merely their own] personal opinions, [and] contrary to [their] expectations [this] started numerous and disorderly discussions by the [famous doctors] of that time, which continued for a long period of time without resolution. Xiūyuán cannot avoid being scolded severely by countless numbers of people.

九、神農嘗草而作《本草經》，實無可考，其為開天明道之聖人所傳無疑也。張仲景、華元化起而述之，陶隱居之說不誣也。漢時去古未遠，二公為醫中之傑，遵所聞而記之，謂非神農所著可也，謂為神農所著亦可也。

9. Shén Nóng distinguished the tastes and flavors of the medicinals and wrote the *Běn Cǎo Jīng*, the practicality [of which] cannot be verified, [but that which] this sage, who opened up the way of the mandate of heaven, transmitted is not to be doubted. Zhāng Zhòngjǐng and Huà Yuánhuà[61] began to follow him, and Táo Yǐnjū's theories are not false. The *Hàn* period was not yet so distant from antiquity; [these] two gentlemen (Zhāng and Huà) became the heroes of Chinese medicine, they obeyed what they heard and recorded it, so it is possible to say this is not written by Shén Nóng [personally]; it is also possible to say it is written by Shén Nóng.

十、每藥注解，必透發出所以然之妙，求與《內經》、《難經》、仲景等書，字字吻合而後快。古云：群言淆亂衷於聖，願同志者取法乎上。

10. Each medicinal has been explained with notes, and will thoroughly issue forth the reason for their excellence, and seeks to be literally identical and straightforward as the *Nèi Jīng*, *Nán Jīng*,[62] and other books by Zhòngjǐng. The ancients say: The writing of the flock confused the inner feelings of the sages. I sincerely hope that the comrades will take the highest quality to serve as norm.[63]

---

59. Lǐ Shìcái 李士材 (1588-1655), also named Lǐ Zhōngzǐ 李中梓 is a physician from Jiāngsū. See: Lǐ, 1985, p. 220.

60. See Footnote 34 above.

61. Huà Yuánhuà 華元化 is the famous physician Huà Tuó 華佗 (~145-208). He was the first to apply surgical techniques. See: Mair, Victor H (Ed.): *The Columbia Anthology of Traditional Chinese Literature*, Columbia University Press 1994, pp.688-696.

62. The *Nán Jīng* 《難經》 (Classic of Difficult Issues) is the abbreviation for *Huáng Dì Bā Shí Yī Nán Jīng* 《黃帝八十一難經》 (Huáng Dì's Classic on Eighty-One Difficult Issues). It was compiled around the Western *Hàn* dynasty (206 B.C. to 23 A.D.).

63. This is a Chinese proverb: *Qǔ fǎ hū shàng, jìn dé hū zhōng.* 取法乎上，僅得乎中。 Better to take the highest quality as norm, otherwise one will merely be mediocre.

卷之一
Chapter One

閩吳航陳念祖修園甫著
男 元豹道彪古愚
元犀道照灵石 同挍字 靈

Written by Chén Niànzǔ Xiūyuán[1] from Mǐn Wúháng[2]
Revised by Yuánbào[3] Dàobiāo Gǔyú and Yuánxī[4] Dàozhào Língshí.

---

1. Chén 陳 was his family name, Niànzǔ 念祖 his birth name and Xiūyuán 修園 his courtesy name as an adult. In ancient China, people regarded their name as something private, belonging to family affairs, so they chose other names as adults by which other people could address them freely. In addition, Chinese scholars also had one or more pen names. This seal is repeated at the beginning of each chapter.

2. Mǐn 閩 is the old name for Fújiàn province, Wú Háng 吳航 is a town in the northwest of Cháng Lè 長樂 county.

3. Chén Yuánbào 陳元豹 was Chén Xiūyuán's 陳修園 eldest son.

4. Chén Yuánxī 陳元犀 was Chén Xiūyuán's 陳修園 second son.

上品
Medicinals of the Highest Grade

Rén Shēn 人參
Root of Panax ginseng

氣味甘、微寒，無毒。主補五臟，安精神，定魂魄，止驚悸，除邪氣，明目開心益智。久服輕身延年。

The qì and flavor are sweet, slightly cold, and non-toxic. [*Rén shēn*] governs and supplements the five viscera, quiets the essence and spirit, settles the *hún* (ethereal) and *pò* (corporeal souls), stops fright-palpitations, eliminates evil qì, brightens the eyes, opens the heart, and sharpens the wit. When taken over a long period of time, it lightens the body and prolongs life.

陳修園曰：《本經》止此三十七字。其提綱云：主補五臟，以五臟屬陰也。精神不安，魂魄不定，驚悸不止，目不明，心智不足，皆陰虛為亢陽所擾也。今五臟得甘寒之助，則有安之、定之、止之、明之、開之、益之之效矣。曰邪氣者，非指外邪而言，乃陰虛而壯火食氣，火即邪氣也。今五臟得甘寒之助，則邪氣除矣。余細味經文，無一字言及溫補回陽。故仲景於汗、吐、下陰傷之證，用之以救津液。而一切回陽方中，絕不加此陰柔之品，反緩薑、附之功。故四逆湯、通脈四逆湯為回陽第一方，皆不用人參。而四逆加人參湯，以其利止亡血而加之也。茯苓四逆湯用之者，以其在汗、下之後也。今人輒云：以人參回陽，此說倡自宋、元以後，而大盛於薛立齋、張景岳、李士材輩，而李時珍《本草綱目》尤為雜沓。學者必於此等書焚去，方可與言醫道。

Chén Xiūyuán said: The [*Shén Nóng] Běn [Cǎo] Jīng* stops after these thirty-seven characters. Its keypoint is that [*rén shēn*] governs and supplements the five viscera, and the five viscera belong to yīn. [If the] essence and spirit are disquieted, the *hún* and *pò* are unstable, [and there are] incessant fright-palpitations, unclear vision, and the heart and wit are insufficient: these are all [signs of] yīn vacuity being disturbed by hyperactive yáng. Now, when the five viscera are reinforced by the sweet and cold [flavor], then the effect is quieting, settling, stopping, brightening, opening, and benefitting! Speaking of evil qì does not indicate external evil, but yīn vacuity and "vigorous fire-consuming qì;"[5] the fire is then the evil qì. When the five viscera receive the assistance of sweet and cold, then the evil qì is eliminated! I [have] carefully pondered the writing of the classics, [and] there is not a single word about *rén shēn* warmly supplementing to return the yáng. Therefore, in cases of yīn-damaging patterns like sweating, vomiting, and diarrhea, [Zhāng] Zhòngjǐng used [*rén shēn*] in order to rescue the bodily fluids. Within all formulas [which] return the yáng, this yīn and soft medicinal is absolutely not added, and on the contrary, it moderates the effect of *jiāng* and *fù*. Therefore, *Sì Nì Tāng* and *Tōng Mài Sì Nì Tāng* are the best formulas for returning yáng, although neither use *rén shēn*. And in *Sì Nì Jiā Rén Shēn Tāng* it is added for blood collapse when the diarrhea stops.[6] In *Fú Líng Sì Nì Tāng*, [*rén shēn*] is used so as to [replenish fluids] after sweating or purging. The people of today always say: Take *rén shēn* to return the yáng. This theory was introduced after the *Sòng* and *Yuán* [dynasties] and was abundant among the contemporaries of Xuē Lìzhāi, Zhāng Jǐngyuè, Lǐ Shìcái,[7] and Lǐ Shízhēn's *Běn Cǎo Gāng Mù* 《本草綱目》 (Compendium of Materia Medica) is of especially small craftsmanship. Students must burn away this and other books [of this kind], and only then they can speak of the Dào of healing.

仲景一百一十三方中，用人參者祇有一十七方：新加湯、小柴胡湯、柴胡桂枝湯、半夏瀉心湯、黃連湯、生薑瀉心湯、旋覆代赭石湯、乾薑黃芩黃連人參湯、厚朴生薑半夏人參湯、桂枝人參湯、四逆加人參湯、茯苓四逆湯、吳茱萸湯、理中湯、白虎加人參湯、竹葉石膏湯、炙甘草湯，皆是因汗、吐、下之後，亡其陰津，取其救陰。如理中湯、吳茱萸湯以剛燥劑中陽藥太過，取人參甘寒之性，養陰配陽，以臻於中和之妙也。

In [Zhāng] Zhòngjǐng's one hundred and thirteen formulas[8] there are only seventeen containing *rén shēn* [and they are]: *Xīn Jiā Tāng, Xiǎo Chái Hú Tāng, Chái Hú Guì Zhī Tāng, Bàn Xià Xiè Xīn Tāng, Huáng Lián Tāng, Shēng Jiāng Xiè Xīn Tāng, Xuán Fù Dài Zhě Shí Tāng, Gān Jiāng Huáng Qín Huáng Lián Rén Shēn Tāng, Hòu Pò Shēng Jiāng Bàn Xià Rén Shēn Tāng, Guì Zhī Rén Shēn Tāng, Sì Nì Jiā Rén Shēn Tāng, Fú Líng Sì Nì Tāng, Wú Zhū Yú Tāng, Lǐ Zhōng Tāng, Bái Hǔ Jiā Rén Shēn Tāng, Zhú Yè Shí Gāo Tāng*, and *Zhì Gān Cǎo Tāng*. All of these [formulas] are [used] after sweating, vomiting or purging which cause collapse of the yīn and fluids. Take [these formulas in order to] rescue the yīn. For example, *Lǐ Zhōng Tāng* and *Wú Zhū Yú Tāng* use strongly drying preparations [which] greatly increase the yáng within the medicinal; [therefore] applying *rén shēn's* nature of sweet and cold nourishes the yīn and matches the yáng, in order to attain the wonder of harmony in the center.

---

5. *Zhuàng huǒ shí qì* 壯火食氣 is a quotation from: *Huáng Dì Nèi Jīng Sù Wèn* 《黃帝內經素問》 (Inner Canon of the Yellow Emperor, Plain Questions), Chapter 2.

6. In line 385 of the *Shāng Hán Lùn*, *Sì Nì Jiā Rén Shēn Tāng* is used, when there is aversion to cold with faint pulse and diarrhea. The commentary explains that this is due to yáng vacuity. When in this case the diarrhea ceases, this means that the body fluids are exhausted and there is blood collapse. See: Craig Mitchell et al: *Shāng Hán Lùn* 《傷寒論》 (On Cold Damage), Paradigm Publications, Brookline 1999, p. 585.

7. Xuē Lìzhāi 薛立齋, also named Xuē Jǐ 薛己 (1487-1559), was a physician from Jiāngsū. For Zhāng Jǐngyuè 張景岳 and Lǐ Shìcái 李士材 see Footnote 22 and Footnote 59 in the preface.

8. This means the *Shāng Hán Lùn* 《傷寒論》 (Discussion on Cold Damage), as it contains one hundred and thirteen formulas.

又曰：自時珍之《綱目》盛行，而神農之《本草經》遂廢。即如人參，《本經》明說微寒，時珍說生則寒，熟則溫，附會之甚。蓋藥有一定之性，除是生搗取汁冷服，與蒸曬八、九次，色味俱變者，頗有生熟之辨。若入煎劑，則生者亦熟矣。況寒熱本屬冰炭，豈一物蒸熟不蒸熟間，遂如許分別乎？嘗考古聖用參之旨，原為扶生氣安五臟起見。而為五臟之長，百脈之宗，司清濁之運化，為一身之橐籥者，肺也。人參惟微寒清肺，肺清則氣旺，氣旺則陰長而五臟安。古人所謂補陽者，即指其甘寒之用不助壯火以食氣而言，非謂其性溫補火也。

[Chén Xiūyuán] further said: After [Lǐ] Shízhēn's Compendium became prevalent, *Shén Nóng's Classic of Materia Medica* was subsequently abandoned. False conclusions were drawn, such as with *rén shēn*, [where] the *Shén Nóng Běn Cǎo Jīng* clearly says [that it is] slightly cold, [but] Shízhēn says that when it is fresh, then it is cold and when it is cooked, then it is warm. The fact is that medicinals have a certain nature. To eliminate this: [take the] fresh [medicinal], pound to obtain the juice, and take [it] cold, or steam-dry [the medicinal] in the sun eight or nine times. The color and flavor both will transform; this is rather the distinction between fresh and cooked herbs. If ingesting a decocted formula, then this is [also] the fresh [medicinal] that [has been] cooked! Moreover, cold and hot originally belong to ice and fire.[9] How can one separate substances [into] steamed and cooked or not steamed and cooked? Upon examining the aim for which the ancient sages used [*rén*] *shēn*, [it was] originally for the purpose of supporting the generation of qì and to quiet the five viscera. But, because it fosters the five viscera, is the ancestor of the hundred vessels, [and] controls the transportation and transformation of clear and turbid, it is the bellows of the entire body,[10] namely the lungs. *Rén shēn* is only slightly cold and clears the lungs. When the lungs are clear, then the qì flourishes, and when the qì flourishes, then the yīn is fostered and the five viscera are quiet. What the ancient people called "supplementing the yáng," this then refers to the use of the sweet and cold [flavors] without the assistance and invigoration of fire, [which] causes consumption of the qì and does not refer to the warm nature or supplementing fire.

陶弘景謂：功用同甘草。凡一切寒溫補瀉之劑，皆可共濟成功。然甘草功兼陰陽，故《本經》云：主五臟六腑。人參功專補陰，故《本經》云：主五臟。仲景於咳嗽病去之者，亦以形寒飲冷之傷，非此陰寒之品所宜也。

Táo Hóngjǐng said: The action is similar to that of *gān cǎo*. Generally all formulas [which are] cold, warm, supplementing, or draining can assist to accomplish the success. However, *gān cǎo's* actions are concurrently yīn and yáng; therefore, the *Shén Nóng Běn Cǎo Jīng* says: [*Gān cǎo*] governs the five viscera and the six bowels. The action of *rén shēn* specifically supplements the yīn [and], therefore, the *Shén Nóng Běn Cǎo Jīng* says: [*Rén shēn*] governs the five viscera. To eliminate the disease of

9. *Tàn* 炭 literally means "charcoal," but here it is used in combination with ice and denotes the contrast, so "fire" sounds more familiar to the Western reader.

10. *Tuó yuè* 橐籥: A bellows is a tool with a bag of air, which upon pressing two handles together, emits a stream of air, and is used to make the fire of a forge hotter. This is a metaphor for the lungs presiding over the qì, controlling the breathing and regulating the function of the qì mechanism.

cough, which also is because of physical cold and damage due to cold drinks, [Zhāng] Zhòngjǐng did not [find] this class of yīn cold medicinal appropriate.

Huáng Qí 黃耆
Root of Astragalus membranaceus

氣味甘、微溫，無毒。主癰疽，久敗瘡，排膿止痛，大風癩疾，五痔鼠瘻，補虛，小兒百病。

The qì and flavor are sweet, slightly warm, and non-toxic. [*Huáng qí*] governs welling and flat-abscesses, and enduring decaying sores. It expels pus, stops pain, [and treats] great wind leprosy,[11] the five kinds of hemorrhoids, and mouse fistulae.[12] [*Huáng qí*] supplements vacuity and [governs] the one hundred diseases of children.

生用、鹽水炒、酒炒、醋炒、蜜炙、白水炒。

It can be used fresh, stir-fried with brine, stir-fried with wine, stir-fried with vinegar, mix-fried with honey, or stir-fried in plain boiled water.

陳修園曰：黃耆氣微溫，稟少陽之氣，入膽與三焦。味甘無毒，稟太陰之味，入肺與脾。其主癰疽者，甘能解毒也。久敗之瘡，肌肉皮毛潰爛，必膿多而痛甚，黃耆入脾而主肌肉，入肺而主皮毛也。大風者，殺人之邪風也。黃耆入膽而助中正之氣，俾神明不為風所亂。入三焦而助決瀆之用，俾竅道不為風所壅。入脾而救受剋之傷。入肺而制風木之動，所以主之。

Chén Xiūyuán said: The qì of *huáng qí* is slightly warm, inherits the qì of shàoyáng, [and] enters the gallbladder and sānjiāo. [*Huáng qí's*] flavor is sweet, non-toxic, [and] inherits the flavor of tàiyīn [which] enters the lungs and the spleen. It governs welling and flat-abscesses; this is because the sweet is able to resolve toxin. [When there are] enduring decaying sores, where the flesh, skin and hair ulcerate, [then there] will be copious pus and severe pain. *Huáng qí* enters the spleen and

---

11. *Dà fēng lài jí* 大風癩疾 (great wind leprosy) is a transmissible disease that is characterized by localized numbing and red patches that swell and rupture. This can cause loss of the eyes, nose, and skin areas on the feet attributed to leprosy toxin stagnating in skin and muscles. See in Wiseman, 1998, under the topic: pestilential wind p. 431.

12. *Wǔ zhì* 五痔 (The five kinds of hemorrhoids) are male hemorrhoids, female hemorrhoids, vessel hemorrhoids, hemorrhoids of the intestines, and hemorrhoids of the blood. *Shǔ lòu* 鼠瘻 (mouse fistulae) refers to scrofula.

governs the flesh; it [also] enters the lungs and governs the skin and body hair. Great wind[13] refers to evil wind that kills people. *Huáng qí* enters the gallbladder and assists the right qì of the center enabling the *shén míng* (spirit) not to be confused by the wind.[14] [*Huáng qí*] enters the sānjiāo and it is used to assist in clearing the sluices,[15] [therefore] enabling the orifices not to be congested by wind. [*Huáng qí*] enters the spleen and rescues it from the damage by restraint. [Lastly, *huáng qí*] enters the lungs and controls the stirring of wind and wood. Therefore, [it] governs [all] of this.

癩疾，又名大麻風，即風毒之甚也。五痔者，五種之痔瘡，乃少陽與太陰之火陷於下，而此能舉其陷。鼠瘻者，瘰癧之別名，乃膽經與三焦之火鬱於上，而此能散其鬱也。其曰補虛者，是總結上文諸證，久而致虛，此能補之。非泛言補益之品也。

Another name for leprosy is "great numbing wind;" hence, this is a very severe wind toxin. The five hemorrhoids are the five kinds of hemorrhoid sores, so [this is] the fire of shàoyáng and tàiyīn sinking into the lower [body], and this [medicinal] is able to lift [what has] sunken. Mouse fistulae is another name for scrofula,[16] so [this] is the fire of the gallbladder channel and the sānjiāo that is depressed in the upper [body], and this [medicinal] is able to scatter the depression. When [the passage above] says supplementing vacuity, this summarizes all of the patterns mentioned above. [This is because] enduring [disease] causes vacuity, [and this medicinal] is able to supplement this, [but] it is not generally [considered] a supplementing medicinal.

葉天士云：小兒稚陽也。稚陽為少陽，少陽生氣條達則不病，所以概主小兒百疾也。余細味經文，俱主表證而言，如六黃湯之寒以除熱，熱除則汗止。耆附湯之溫以回陽，陽回則汗止。玉屏風散之散以驅風，風平則汗止。諸方皆借黃耆走表之力，領諸藥而速達於表而止汗，非黃耆自能止汗也。諸家固表及生用發汗、炒用止汗等說，貽誤千古，茲特正之。

Yè Tiānshì said: Children [have] immature yáng, [and] immature yáng is shàoyáng. When shàoyáng generates the qì and outthrusts, then there is no disease; therefore, [*huáng qí*] generally governs the hundred diseases of children. I [have] carefully pondered the writing of the classics, and [they] say that [*huáng qí*] always governs external patterns, for example [using] the cold [nature] of *Liù Huáng Tāng*[17] in order to eliminate heat, and by eliminating heat, then sweating will stop. [Use] the warmth of *Qí Fù Tāng* in order to return the yáng, and when the yáng returns, then the sweating will stop. [Use] the dispersing [nature] of *Yù Píng Fēng Sǎn* in order to expel wind, and when wind is calm, then sweating will stop. All these formulas make use of *huáng qí's* power of pen-

---

13. This is also pestilential wind leprosy. See the same citation as the Wiseman citation above.

14. When the *shén míng* 神明 is confused by wind, then there is epilepsy.

15. *Jué dú* 決瀆 (clear the sluices) means to dredge the waterways, which is one of the main responsibilities of the sānjiāo.

16. Scrofula means lymphadenitis.

17. This is an abbreviation for *Dāng Guī Liù Huáng Tāng* 當歸六黃湯 (Tangkuei Six Yellows Decoction).

etrating the exterior. It leads all the medicinals, quickly outthrusts [them] to the exterior, and stops sweating, [but] *huáng qí* by itself is not able to stop sweating. Various schools of thought say that it secures the exterior and promotes sweating when used fresh, or stops sweating when used stir-fried and so on. This theory has been misleading through the ages; therefore, [these mistakes have been] specially corrected.

Bái Zhú 白朮
Rhizome of Atractylodes macrocephala

氣味甘、溫，無毒。主風寒濕痹，死肌、痙、疸，止汗，除熱，消食。作煎餌，久服輕身，延年，不飢。

The qì and flavor are sweet, warm, and non-toxic. [*Bái zhú*] governs wind-cold-damp-impediment,[18] insensible flesh,[19] tetany, and jaundice. [It] stops sweating, eliminates heat, and disperses food. [One can] pan-fry [it into] cakes and when taken over a long period of time, it lightens the body,[20] prolongs life, and prevents hunger.

仲景有赤朮，即蒼朮也。功用略同，偏長於消導。汗多者大忌之。

Zhòng Jǐng [writes] *chì zhú* [which is] namely *cāng zhú*. The actions are about the same, and [he] tended to increase [this] for eliminating and guiding out.[21] For profuse sweating, it is greatly contraindicated.

陳修園曰：此為脾之正藥。其曰：風寒濕痹者，以風寒濕三氣合而為痹也。三氣雜至，以濕氣為主。死肌者，濕浸肌肉也。痙者，濕流關節也。疸者，濕鬱而為熱，熱則發黃也。濕與熱交蒸，則自汗而發熱也。脾受濕則失其健運之常，斯食不能消也。白朮功在除濕，所以主之。「作煎餌」三字另提。先聖大費苦心，以白朮之功用在燥，而所以妙處，在於多脂。

Chén Xiūyuán said: This is the correct medicinal for the spleen. This says: wind-cold-damp impediment, because the three qì of wind, cold, and damp combine and become impediment. Of

---

18. *Bì* 痹 (impediment) is a syndrome caused by a combination of the lingering pathogens wind, damp and cold. It is also translated as rheumatism. See: Nigel Wiseman, Feng Ye: *A Practical Dictionary of Chinese Medicine*. Brookline 1998, p. 295

19. *Sǐ jī* 死肌 (numb or insensible flesh) can also be necrosis, as literally, this term means "dead flesh."

20. In the following text, whenever "lightens the body" is spoken of, this does not mean a reduction of weight, but a sensation of lightness.

21. Wiseman: "abduction and dispersion."

the three qì, damp qì is the governor. Insensible flesh is [due to] damp soaking the flesh. Tetany is [caused by] damp flowing in the joints. Jaundice is depressed damp that becomes heat, [where] the heat results in yellowing. When damp and heat interact, steam [is formed], resulting in spontaneous sweating and fever. When the spleen contracts dampness, then it loses the regularity of its healthy transport [function]; thus food cannot be digested. *Bái zhú's* [primary] action is to eliminate damp; therefore, this is why it governs this. The three characters "to pan-fry [it into] cakes" are additions. The sages of former times expended a lot of effort to take the action of *bái zhú* as drying, but the reason it is marvelous lies in its greasiness.

張隱庵云：土有濕氣，始能灌溉四旁，如地得雨露，始能發生萬物。

Zhāng Yǐn'ān said: [Only when] the earth has damp qì, is it able to irrigate the four sides [of the body]. For example, when the earth receives the rain and dew, then it is able to create the ten thousand things.

今以生朮削去皮，急火炙令熟，則味甘溫而質滋潤，久服有延年不飢之效。可見今人炒燥、炒黑、土蒸、水漂等製，大失經旨。

Nowadays, raw [*bái*] *zhú* is scraped to remove the peel and thoroughly cooked with a fierce fire [for only a brief moment]. This results in a flavor [that] is sweet, warm and moist in nature. When taken over a long period of time, its effect is to prolong life and to prevent hunger. It can be seen that the people of today greatly fail the aim of the classics by dry-frying, or stir-frying until black, or earth-steaming, or long rinsing and [similar kinds of] processing.

Gān Cǎo 甘草
Root of Glycyrrhiza uralensis

氣味甘平，無毒。主五臟六腑寒熱邪氣，堅筋骨，長肌肉，倍氣力，金瘡[22]解毒。久服輕身延年。

The qì and flavor are sweet, neutral, and non-toxic. It governs the five viscera and six bowels, cold and heat, and evil qì; hardens the tendons and bones, grows the flesh, doubles the qì and strength, governs incised wounds with swelling, and resolves toxins. When taken over a long period of time, it lightens the body and prolongs life.

---

22. *Zhōng* 尰, is another word for swollen.

24

生用清火，炙用補中。

[When] used raw, it clears fire, [and when] used honey-fried, it supplements the center.

陳修園曰：物之味甘者，至甘草為極。甘主脾，脾為後天之本，五臟六腑皆
受氣焉。臟腑之本氣，則為正氣。外來寒熱之氣，則為邪氣。正氣旺則邪氣
自退也。筋者，肝所主也。骨者，腎所主也。肌肉者，脾所主也。氣者，肺
所主也。力者，心所主也。但使脾氣一盛，則五臟皆循環受益，而皆得其堅
之、長之、倍之之效矣。金瘡者，為刀斧所傷而成瘡，瘡甚而腫。脾得補而
肉自滿也。能解毒者，如毒物入土，則毒化也。土為萬物之母，土健則輕身
延年也。

Chén Xiūyuán said: Of [the] substances with a sweet flavor, arriving at *gān cǎo* is the ultimate. Sweet governs the spleen, the spleen is the root of later heaven,[23] and the five viscera and six bowels all receive [this] qì! The original qì of the viscera and bowels is the right qì. The qì of cold and heat that comes from the outside is evil qì, [and] when the right qì is exuberant, then the evil qì spontaneously abates. For the sinews, the liver is that which governs. For the bones, the kidneys are that which governs. For the muscles, the spleen is that which governs. For the qì, the lungs are that which governs. For strength, the heart is that which governs. However, [when] the spleen qì flourishes, then the five viscera [are able to] circulate and receive benefit, and all [the viscera] are able to receive [the spleen's] fortifying, promoting and multiplying effects! Incised wounds are caused by damage from knives and hatchets, becoming sores that are severe and swollen. When the spleen receives supplementation, the flesh naturally is filled. The ability to resolve toxins is like [when] a toxic substance enters the earth and the toxin is transformed. The earth is the mother of the myriad things, [and when] the earth is healthy, then this lightens the body and prolongs life.

Shǔ Yù 薯蕷
Root of Dioscorea opposita

氣味甘、平，無毒。主傷中，補虛羸，除寒熱邪氣，補中，益氣力，長肌
肉，強陰。久服耳目聰明，輕身，不飢，延年。

The qì and flavor are sweet, neutral, and non-toxic. [*Shǔ yù*] governs damage to the center, supplements vacuity emaciation, and eliminates the evil qì of cold and heat. It supplements the center, boosts the qì and strength, grows the flesh, and strengthens the yīn. When one takes [*shǔ yù*] over a

---

23. Later heaven means nutrition which is acquired after birth. The human constitution is composed of what is called pre- and post-heaven qì. Pre-heaven qì is what we would call genetic predisposition and is stored in the kidneys. Once it is used up, life ends. Later or post-heaven qì can be refilled with daily intake of food.

long period of time, it sharpens the hearing and brightens the vision. It lightens the body, prevents hunger, and prolongs life.

陳修園曰：此藥因唐代宗名蕷，避諱改為山藥。山藥氣平入肺，味甘無毒入脾。脾為中州而統血，血者陰也，中之守也。唯能益血，故主傷中。傷中愈，則肌肉豐，故補虛羸。肺主氣，氣虛則寒邪生。脾統血，血虛則熱邪生。血氣充而寒熱邪氣除矣。脾主四肢，脾血足則四肢健。肺主氣，肺氣充則氣力倍也。且此物生搗，最多津液而稠黏，又能補腎而填精，精足則陰強。目明、耳聰、不飢，是脾血之旺。輕身是肺氣之充。延年是夸其補益之效也。

Chén Xiūyuán said: Because the *Táng* emperor was named Yù, this medicinal's [name] was taboo and changed to *shān yào*. The qì of *shān yào* is neutral and enters the lungs, [while] the flavor is sweet, non-toxic, and enters the spleen. The spleen is in the region of the middle and gathers the blood; the blood is yīn, and the defender of the center. Only because [*shān yào*] is able to benefit the blood [does] it govern damage to the center. When damage to the center heals, the flesh is bountiful, and therefore [*shān yào*] supplements vacuity emaciation. The lungs govern the qì, [and if] the qì is vacuous, then cold evil is engendered. The spleen controls the blood, and if the blood is vacuous, then heat evil is engendered. When [both] blood and qì are full, then the cold and heat evil qì is eliminated! The spleen governs the four limbs, [and when] the spleen and blood are sufficient, then the four limbs are strong. The lungs govern the qì, [and when] the lungs and qì are full, then the qì and strength are doubled. Moreover, when this medicinal is freshly pounded, the fluids are the most copious, thick, and sticky. This is able to supplement the kidneys and replenish the essence. [When] the essence is sufficient, then the yīn is strong. That [*shān yào*] clears the sight, sharpens the hearing, and prevents hunger, is due to the exuberance of spleen blood. The effect of lightening the body is due to fullness of the lung qì. The prolonging of life is due to [*shān yào's*] great supplementing and boosting effects.

凡上品，俱是尋常服食之物，非治病之藥，故神農別提出久服二字。可見今人每服上品之藥，如此物及人參、熟地、葳蕤、阿膠、菟絲子、沙苑蒺藜之類，合為一方，以治大病，誤人無算。蓋病不速去，元氣日傷，傷及則死。凡上品之藥，法宜久服，多則終身，少則數年，與五穀之養人相佐，以臻壽考。若大病而需用此藥，如五穀為養脾第一品。脾虛之人，強令食穀，即可畢補脾之能事，有是理乎？然操此技者，未有不得盛名。薛立齋、張景岳、馮楚瞻輩，倡之於前。而近日之東延西請、日診百人者，無非是朮，誠可慨也！

In general, all the substances of the highest grade are common foods and not medicinals for treating disease. Therefore, Shén Nóng separately mentions the two characters "when taken over a long period of time." It can clearly be seen that [when] modern people take medicinals of the highest grade, like this substance, or *rén shēn, shú dì* [*huáng*], *wēi ruí, ē jiāo, tù sī zǐ* or *shā yuàn jí lí*, [and] then combine them into a formula in order to treat severe disease, the harm [they do] to people is incalculable. Now, when a disease is not quickly removed, then the original qì is damaged daily, [and when] the damage is at its utmost, this results in death. Generally, for medicinals of the highest grade, the appropriate method is to take them over a long period of time. Taking a lot means [over one's] entire life, taking a little means for several years, and with the nurturing assistance of the five grains,[24] one can reach longevity.[25] In case of a serious disease, when one needs this medicinal,[26] it resembles using the five grains which are the best for nurturing the spleen. [When] people with spleen vacuity are forced to eat grains, this [has the] capability of completely supplementing the spleen; is this logical? So, of those who grasp the skill [of handling this medicinal], there are none that have not obtained a famous reputation. The generation of Xuē Lìzhāi, Zhāng Jǐngyuè, and Féng Chǔdǎn[27] introduced this before, but recently of those who treat from the east reaching to the west, who examine one hundred people per day, [there are none that] do not use this technique. One [could] sincerely sigh!

Ròu Cōng Róng 肉蓯蓉
Fleshy stalk of Cistanche salsa

氣味甘、微溫，無毒。主五勞七傷，補中，除莖中寒熱痛，養五臟，強陰，益精氣，多子，婦人癥瘕。久服輕身。

The qì and flavor are sweet, slightly warm, and non-toxic. [*Ròu cōng róng*] governs the five taxations and the seven damages,[28] supplements the center, and eliminates cold and heat pain within the

24. The five grains are rice, millet, glutinous millet, wheat, and soybeans, but this term can also simply mean all kinds of grains.

25. *Shòu kǎo* 壽考 (longevity) means a natural life span. *Kǎo*, means old, or aged.

26. *Shān yào* 山藥.

27. For Xuē Lìzhāi 薛立齋 and Zhāng Jǐngyuè 張景岳 see Footnote 7 above, and Footnote 22 of the preface. Féng Chǔdǎn 馮楚瞻 (seventeenth century) was a specialist for pediatrics from Zhèjiāng. See: *Zhōng Guó Yī Rén Wù Cí Diǎn Zhǔ Biān Lǐ Jīng Wěi*, Shànghǎi Cí Shū Chū Bǎn Shè.《中國醫人物詞典》主編李經緯上海辭書出版社 Lǐ Jīng Wěi (Ed.) (Chinese Medical People Dictionary) Shanghai Dictionary Publishing House 1985, p. 198.

28. *Wǔ láo* 五勞 (the five taxations) have two possible variations. The first is: prolonged vision damages the blood, prolonged lying damages the qì, prolonged sitting damages the flesh, prolonged standing damages the bones, and prolonged walking damages the sinews. The second variation is: visceral taxation damage is defined as: lung taxation, liver taxation, heart taxation, spleen taxation, and kidney taxation. See: Nigel Wiseman, Feng Ye: *A Practical Dictionary of Chinese Medicine*. Brookline 1998, p. 207. *Qī shāng* 七傷 (The seven damages) also has two variations. The first is: damage due to food, damage due to anxiety, damage due to alcohol, damage due to sexual intemperance, damage due to hunger, damage due to taxation, or damage due to the channel network and construction-defense. The other variation is: great overeating damages the spleen; great anger and qì counterflow damage the liver; exertion or lifting heavy weights and long sitting on wet ground damage the kidneys; cold in the body and cold drinks damage the lungs; anxiety, worry, thought, and contemplation damage the heart; wind, rain, cold, and summer heat damage the body; great fear damages the mind. See: ibid, p. 526.

penis. It nourishes the five viscera, strengthens yīn, boosts the essence and qì, increases fertility, and [governs] women's abdominal masses.[29] When taken for a long period of time, it lightens the body.

陳修園曰：肉蓯蓉是馬精落地所生，取治精虛者，同氣相求之義也。凡五勞七傷，久而不愈，未有不傷其陰者。蓯蓉補五臟之精，精足則陰足矣。莖中者，精之道路，精虛則寒熱而痛，精足則痛已矣。又滑以去著。精生於五臟，而藏之於腎，精足則陽舉，精堅令人多子矣。婦人癥瘕，皆由血淤，精足則氣充，氣充則淤行也。

Chén Xiūyuán said: *Ròu cōng róng* grows where a horse's essence falls to the ground, and is taken to treat essence vacuity. This is similar to the meaning that [things with the same kind of] qì have an affinity to one another. In general, when the five taxations and the seven damages last for a long period of time without [being] cured, there is none that does not damage the yīn. [*Ròu*] *cōng róng* supplements the essence of the five viscera. If the essence is sufficient, then the yīn is [also] sufficient! Within the penis means the pathway of essence. If the essence is vacuous, then there is cold or heat and pain. If the essence is sufficient, then the pain will stop! *In addition, slippery [medicinals] are taken in order to remove the fixed [sediment].* Essence is generated in the five viscera and stored in the kidneys: if the essence is sufficient, then yáng is lifted; if the essence is fortified [it] causes increased fertility! Women's abdominal masses all derive from blood stasis. If essence is sufficient, then the qì is full, [and] if qì is full, then the stasis moves.

葉天士注：癥瘕之治，謂其鹹以軟堅，滑以去著，溫以散結，猶淺之乎測蓯蓉也。

Yè Tiānshì commented: The treatment of abdominal masses refers to [using] the salty [flavor] in order to soften hardness, [using] slippery in order to remove the fixed [sediment, and using] warmth to dissipate binds; [this is] a shallow measure of [*ròu*] *cōng róng*.

張隱庵曰：馬為火畜，精屬水陰。蓯蓉感馬精而生，其形似肉，氣味甘溫，蓋稟少陰水火之氣，而歸於太陰坤土之藥也。土性柔和，故有「從容」之名。

Zhāng Yǐn'ān said: The horse is a firery domestic animal, [but] the essence belongs to water and yīn. [*Ròu*] *cōng róng* contracts the horse's essence and life, and in appearance [the *cōng róng*] resembles flesh. The qì and flavor are sweet and warm; thus it inherits the qì of shàoyīn water and fire, but it is [also] affiliated with medicinals of tàiyīn *kūn*[30] earth. The nature of earth is soft and gentle; therefore it is called: *cōng róng* (calm and leisurely).

29. Concretions and conglomerations. See Wiseman, 1998. p. 92.

30. This is one of the eight trigrams and corresponds to yīn earth. See Volume 9 of *Zhēn Jiǔ Dà Chéng*, Footnote 93, p 85. (Wilcox, The Chinese Medicine Database, 2011).

Dì Huáng 地黄
Root of Rehmannia glutinosa

氣味甘、寒，無毒。主折跌絕筋，傷中，逐血痹，填骨髓，長肌肉。作湯除寒熱積聚，除痹。生者尤良。久服輕身不老。

The qì and flavor are sweet, cold, and non-toxic. It governs broken bones, severed sinews, and damage to the center. [It] expels blood impediment, replenishes bone marrow, and grows flesh. When made into a decoction, it eliminates cold and heat, accumulations and gatherings, and syndromes of impediment. Fresh [roots] are especially good. When taken over a long period of time, it lightens the body and prevents aging.

參葉天士：地黃氣寒，入足少陰腎經。味甘無毒，入足太陰脾經。氣味重濁，陰也。陰者，中之守也。傷中者，守中真陰傷也。地黃甘寒，補中焦之精汁，所以主之。血痹者，血虛閉而不運也。地黃味甘以滋脾血，氣寒以益腎氣，氣血行而閉者開矣。腎主骨，益腎則水足而骨髓充。脾主肌肉，潤脾則土滋而肌肉豐也。作湯除寒熱積聚者，湯者蕩也，或寒或熱之積聚，湯能蕩之也。蓋味甘可以緩急，性滑可以去著也。又曰：除痹者，言不但逐血痹，更除皮肌筋骨之痹也。除皮肉筋骨之痹，則折跌絕筋亦可療矣。久服輕身不老，以先後二天交換，元氣與穀氣俱納也。生者尤良，謂其本性俱在也。

A comparison by Yè Tiānshì: Dì huáng's qì is cold and enters the foot shàoyīn kidney channel. The flavor is sweet, non-toxic, and enters the foot tàiyīn spleen channel. The qì and flavor are heavy and turbid, which is yīn. The yīn is the guardian of the center. Damage to the center, is damage to the true yīn, [which] guards the center. *Dì huáng* is sweet, cold, and it supplements the essence fluid[31] of the middle *jiāo*, and thus [*dì huáng*] governs this. Blood impediment is blood which is vacuous, blocked, and unable to move. The sweet flavor of *dì huáng* is used to enrich the spleen blood. The cold qì is used to boost the qì of the kidneys. [Therefore, when the] qì and blood move, the blocked is unblocked! The kidneys govern the bones. [When *dì huáng*] boosts the kidneys, then the water is sufficient and the bone marrow is full. The spleen governs the flesh. [When *dì huáng*] moistens the spleen, then the earth is enriched and the flesh becomes abundant. Make as a decoction to eliminate cold or heat or accumulations and gatherings; this is [because] decoctions [act to] flush away. For accumulations and gatherings of cold [or] heat, a decoction is able to flush this [away]. Now, the sweet flavor can be used to relax tension, and the slippery nature can remove adhesions. Moreover, it is said to eliminate impediment. This means it not only expels blood impediment, but further eliminates impediment of the skin, muscle, sinew, or bone. Because it can eliminate impediment of the skin, muscle, sinew, and bone, then bone fractures and severed sinews can also

---

31. "Essence fluid" could refer to either blood or gall, but in this instance blood makes more sense.

be cured [with *dì huáng*]! When taken over a long period of time, it lightens the body and prevents aging by the interaction and exchange of pre- and post-heaven, [whereby] both the original qì and grain qì are absorbed. The fresh [medicinal] is especially good, which means its original nature still exists.

陳修園曰：地黃，《 本經 》名地髓，《 爾雅 》名芐，又名芑 。唐以後九蒸九曬為熟地黃，苦味盡除，入於溫補腎經丸劑，頗為相宜 。

Chén Xiūyuán said: *Dì huáng*, called *dì suǐ*[32] in the [*Shén Nóng*] *Běn* [*Cǎo*] *Jīng* 《 本經 》 and in the *Ěr Yǎ* 《 爾雅 》 (Approaching the Refined)[33] it is called *hù* 芐,[34] another name is *qǐ* 芑.[35] After the *Táng* dynasty, the [*dì huáng*] was steamed nine times and sun-dried[36] nine times [and this] made *shú dì huáng*. [Using this process], the bitter flavor is completely eliminated, so ingesting this as a preparation of *Wēn Bǔ Shèn Jīng Wán* is considered quite appropriate.

若入湯劑及養血涼血等方，甚屬不合 。蓋地黃專取其性涼而滑利流通，熟則膩滯不涼，全失其本性矣 。徐靈胎辨之甚詳，無如若輩竟執迷不悟也 。

If ingested as a decoction or with a prescription that nourishes or cools the blood and similar formulas, it is quite inappropriate. Now, *dì huáng* specifically applies the cool and slippery nature to promote circulation. Thoroughly cooking results in a cloying and stagnant [substance] which is not cool, so it completely loses its original nature! Xú Lingtāi[37] distinguished [between the raw and cooked] very explicitly, however, [later] generations after all [this], persist in their confusion without comprehending.

又曰：百病之極，窮必及腎 。及腎，危證也 。有大承氣湯之急下法，有桃花湯之溫固法，有四逆湯 、白通湯之回陽法，有豬苓湯 、黃連雞子黃湯之救陰法，有真武湯之行水法，有附子湯之溫補法，皆所以救其危也 。張景岳自創邪說，以百病之生，俱從腎治 。誤以《 神農本經 》上品服食之地黃，認為治病之藥 。

---

32. Literally: "earth-marrow."

33. This book is the oldest extant Chinese dictionary and it was compiled in the *Qín* dynasty or earlier. See: Weldon Coblin: *Ěr Yǎ* in Michael Loewe (ed.): *Early Chinese Texts: A Bibliographical Guide.* Berkeley 1993, pp 94–99.

34. This character means: *dì huáng* 地黃 (rehmannia).

35. Actually: "white millet," but here it also means *dì huáng* 地黃.

36. In fact, this processing technique does not necessarily stipulate that it has to be steamed and sun dried for nine times, but can simply mean several times.

37. This is the scholar physician Xú Lingtāi 徐靈胎 (1693–1771 in Jiāng Sū), whose commentary on the *Shén Nóng Běn Cǎo Jīng* was first published in 1736.

[Chén] further said: When the hundred diseases [are at their most] extreme, exhaustion will reach the kidneys. [That which] reaches the kidneys is a critical pattern. All of the [following] methods are used to rescue critical patterns: the method of urgently purging with *Dà Chéng Qì Tāng*, the method of warming and securing with *Táo Huā Tāng*, the method of restoring yang with *Sì Nì Tāng* and *Bái Tōng Tāng*, the method of rescuing yīn with *Zhū Líng Tāng*, and *Huáng Lián Ē Jiāo Jī Zǐ Tāng*, the method of moving water with *Zhēn Wǔ Tāng*, and the method of warmly supplementing with *Fù Zǐ Tāng*. Zhāng Jǐngyuè himself introduced the heresy, that generation of the one hundred diseases can all be treated beginning with the kidneys. [However], it is a mistake to think that *dì huáng*, which belongs to the highest class of herbs taken as food in the *Shén Nóng Běn [Cǎo] Jīng*, is a medicine for treating diseases.

《內經》云：五穀為養，五果為助，五菜為充，毒藥攻邪。神農所列上品，多服食之品，即五穀、五果、五菜之類也，玩「久服」二字可見。聖人藥到病瘳，何以云「久服」？凡攻邪以去病，多取毒藥。

In the Nèi Jīng it said: "The five grains act to nourish, the five fruits[38] act to assist, the five vegetables[39] act to fulfill, and the toxic medicinals attack evils. What Shén Nóng arranged under the highest class, are mostly foods, then of the categories of the five grains, the five fruits, and the five vegetables. This can be seen from the repeated usage of the two words "taken over a long period of time." If the sage had been speaking of medicines for healing diseases, why would he have said "taken over a long period of time?" In general, [when one] attacks evil in order to eliminate disease, [one] often [will] take toxic medicinals."[40]

滋潤膠黏，反引邪氣斂存於少陰而無出路，以後雖服薑、附不熱，服芩、連不寒，服參、朮不補，服硝、黃不下，其故何哉？蓋以熟地黃之膠黏善著。

The moist, glue-like and sticky [nature] of [*shú dì huáng*], contrary [to expectation], leads evil qì to be constrained and retained in shàoyīn. [The evil qì is] without a path from which to issue forth, and [therefore,] later on when [the patient] takes [*gān*] *jiāng* or *fù* [*zǐ*], they are not hot, or if they take [*huáng*] *qín* or [*huáng*] *lián*, they are not cold, or if they take [*rén*] *shēn* or [*bái/ cāng*] *zhú*, they are not supplemented, or if they take [*pò*] *xiāo* or [*dà*] *huáng* they are not purged. What is the reason for this? This is because the glue-like and sticky [nature] of of *shú dì huáng* tends to be adhesive.

---

38. The five fruits are: peach, plum, apricot/almond, chestnut, and date/jujube.

39. The five vegetables are: sunflower, leek, bean, scallion, and green onion.

40. See: *Huáng Dì Nèi Jīng Sù Wèn* 《黃帝內經素問》 (Inner Canon of the Yellow Emperor, Plain Questions), Chapter 7.

女人有孕服四物湯為主，隨證加入攻破之藥而不傷，以四物湯中之熟地黃能護胎也。知其護胎之功，便可悟其護邪之害。膠黏之性最善著物，如油入面，一著遂不能去也。凡遇有邪而誤用此藥者，百藥不效。病家不咎其用熟地黃之害，反以為曾用熟地黃而猶不效者，定為敗症，豈非景岳之造其孽哉？

[When] a woman is pregnant, it is important to take *Sì Wù Tāng*, [then] follow the signs [by] adding in medicinals [which] attack and break, but [do] not damage. Because *shú dì huáng* is within *Sì Wù Tāng*, it is able to safeguard the fetus. When [one] knows [*shú dì huáng's*] function of safeguarding the fetus, [one] easily can comprehend the harm of safeguarding evil, as the nature [of *shú dì huáng*] is extremely glue-like and sticky, and it tends to adhere to things. This is like oil added to flour: once it successfully adheres, [the oil] cannot be removed. Generally, [in an] encounter where there is evil and [one] misuses this medicinal, a hundred medicinals will not be effective. The patient and their family will not blame the harm on the use of *shú dì huáng*, [but] on the contrary they will believe that on a previous use of *shú dì huáng*, [it] also was not effective, and this is determined because the pattern is defeated, [but] was it not [Zhāng] Jǐngyuè who committed the evil [with his heresy]?

Tiān Mén Dōng 天門冬
Tuber of Asparagus cochinchinensis

氣味苦、平，無毒。主諸暴風濕偏痹，強骨髓，殺三蟲，去伏尸。久服輕身、益氣、延年、不飢。

The qì and flavor are bitter, neutral, and non-toxic. It governs all sudden wind-damp and hemi-lateral impediment, strengthens the bone marrow, kills the three parasites,[41] and removes hidden corpse.[42] When taken over a long period of time it lightens the body, boosts the qì, prolongs life, and prevents hunger.

【參】天門冬稟寒水之氣，而上通於天，故有天冬之名。主治諸暴風濕偏痹者，言風濕之邪暴中於人身，而成半身不遂之偏痹。天冬稟水天之氣，環轉營運，故可治也。強骨髓者，得寒水之精也。三蟲伏尸皆濕熱所化，天冬味苦可以祛濕，氣平可以清熱，濕熱下逐，三尸伏蟲皆去也。太陽為諸陽主氣，故久服輕身，益氣。天氣通貫於地中，故延年不飢。

---

41. *Sān chóng* 三蟲: The three worms: the three most frequently seen kinds of intestinal parasites in children, namely *cháng chóng* 長蟲 longworm (tapeworm), *chì chóng* 赤蟲 redworm (roundworm), and *náo chóng* 蟯蟲 pinworm. See: *Cháo Shì Zhū Bìng Yuán Hòu Zǒng Lùn* 《巢氏諸病源候總論》(Treatise on the Origins and Symptoms of Disease by Master Cháo, *Suí* dynasty), Chapter 18.

42. *Fú shī* 伏尸 (hidden corpse) is an old disease name. The corpse diseases are illnesses caused by incurring the displeasure of the dead body qì. Hidden corpse or consumption is a relatively latent and long lasting type of [disease]. See: Ibid., Chapter 23.

Comparison: *Tiān mén dōng* inherits the qì of cold and water, and ascends to connect with heaven; therefore, it is named *tiān dōng* (heaven winter). By governing the treatment of all sudden wind-damp and hemilateral impediment, this means that the evils of wind and damp suddenly strike the human body, and form the one-sided impediment of hemiplegia. [When] *tiān dōng* inherits the qì of water and heaven, it circulates and transports the nourishment, and therefore this can treat the [impediment]. By strengthening the bone marrow, this obtains the essence of cold water. The three parasites and hidden corpse in all cases [are] damp-heat which has transformed. *Tiān dōng's* bitter flavor can be used to dispel dampness, while the neutral qì can be used to clear heat. [When] the damp and heat are purged and expelled, the three parasites and the hidden corpse in all cases are eliminated. Tàiyáng acts to govern the qì of all the yáng;[43] therefore, when taken over a long period of time, [*tiān dōng*] lightens the body and boosts the qì. Heavenly qì connects and pierces to the center of the earth; therefore, it prolongs the life and prevents hunger.

張隱庵曰：天、麥門冬，皆稟少陰水精之氣。麥門冬，稟水精而上通於陽明。天門冬，稟水精而上通於太陽。夫冬主閉藏，門主開轉，鹹名門冬者，鹹能開轉閉藏而上達也。後人有天門冬補中有瀉，麥門冬瀉中有補之說，不知何處引來，良可嘆也。

Zhāng Yǐn'ān said: *Tiān [mén dōng]* and *mài mén dōng* both inherit the qì of shàoyīn water essence. *Mài mén dōng* inherits the water essence, and ascends to connect with yángmíng. *Tiān mén dōng* inherits the water essence, and ascends to connect with tàiyáng. *Dōng* 冬 (winter) governs closure and storage; *mén* 門 (gate) governs opening and revolving. All[44] things with the name *mén dōng* 門冬 (door of winter) are able to open, revolve, close, store, and outthrust upward. The people of later generations have a saying that *tiān mén dōng* supplements the center [while] draining, [and that] *mài mén dōng* drains the center [while] supplementing, [but it is] not known where this comes from. [I can only] greatly sigh [about this].

---

43. This refers to the three yáng: tàiyáng (the small intestine and bladder channels), yángmíng (the large intestine and stomach channels), and shàoyáng (the sānjiāo and gallbladder channels). The three yīn are: tàiyīn (the lung and spleen channels), shàoyīn (the pericardium and liver channels), and juéyīn (the heart and kidney channels).

44. *Xián* 鹹 here means "all, or whole."

Mài Mén Dōng 麥門冬
Tuber of Ophiopogon japonicus

氣味甘、平，無毒。主心腹結氣，傷中傷飢，胃脈絕，羸瘦短氣。久服輕身不老，不飢。

The qì and flavor are sweet, neutral, and non-toxic. It governs bound qì in the heart and abdomen, damage to the center, damage due to hunger, expiration of the stomach vessel, marked emaciation, and shortness of breath. When taken over a long period of time, it lightens the body, prevents aging, and prevents hunger.

張隱庵曰：麥冬，本橫生，根顆連絡。有十二枚者，有十四枚者，有十五、六枚者，蓋合於人身十二絡。加任之屏翳，督之長強，為十四絡。又加脾之大絡名大包，共十五絡。又加胃之大絡名虛裏，共十六絡。

Zhāng Yǐn'ān said: The roots of mài mén dōng grow horizontally, and the tubers are connected with the roots. There are [plants] with twelve tubers, with fourteen tubers, and those with fifteen or sixteen tubers; thus the tubers are congruent with the twelve collaterals in the human body. In addition to the [acupuncture points] Píng Yì 屏翳 (CV 1) on the conception vessel and Cháng Qiáng 長強 (GV 1) on the governing vessel, there are fourteen collaterals. Moreover if [one] adds the great collateral point of the spleen channel called Dà Bāo 大包 (SP 21), together there are fifteen collaterals. If [one] further adds the great collateral of the stomach called Xū Lǐ 虛裏 (apical pulse),[45] together there are sixteen collaterals.

唯聖人能體察之，用之以通脈絡，並無「去心」二字。後人不詳經義，不窮物理，相沿「去心」久矣，今特表正之。《經》云：主心腹結氣，傷中傷飢，胃絡脈絕者，以麥冬根顆連絡不斷，能通達上下四旁，令結者解，傷者復，絕者續，皆借中心之貫通也。

Only the sages [were] able to observe this and used [mài mén dōng] in order to free the vessels and collaterals, and further [the text is] without the two words "remove the hearts," [as instructions for processing the medicinals]. The people of later generations did not understand the meaning of the details of the classics, and did not thoroughly [comprehend] the logic, so the custom of "removing the hearts" has been handed down year after year for a long time! Now, [I would] especially [like to] correct this. The Classic[46] said: [Mài mén dōng] governs bound qì in the heart and abdomen, dam-

---

45. This region is located below the left nipple, where the pulsation of the heart can be felt. See: Wiseman 1998, p. 653.

46. Shén Nóng Běn Cǎo Jīng.

34

age to the center, damage due to hunger, [as well as] expiration of the stomach collateral vessel; this is because the tubers of *mài* [*mén*] *dōng* are continuously connected, and are able to reach upwards and downwards to the four sides [of the body. *Mài mén dōng*] causes the binds to resolve, the damage to recover, and the expiry to replenish. This all depends on the link to the heart center.

又主羸瘦短氣者，補胃自能生肌，補腎自能納氣也 。久服輕身不老 、不飢者，先天與後天俱足，斯體健而耐飢矣 。

Furthermore, [*mài mén dōng*] governs marked emaciation and shortness of breath; this is because supplementing the stomach naturally engenders the flesh, [while] supplementing the kidney naturally [promotes] absorption of [the lung] qì. When taken over a long period of time, it lightens the body, prevents aging, and prevents hunger; this is because [when] both pre-heaven and post-heaven are sufficient, the whole body is strengthened and [is able to] withstand hunger!

《崇原》曰：麥冬氣味甘平， 質性柔潤， 凌冬青翠， 蓋稟少陰冬水之精， 與陽明胃土相合。

In the [*Běn Cǎo*] *Chóng Yuán*[47] 《 崇原 》 [Zhāng Yǐn'ān] said: "The flavor of *mài* [*mén*] *dōng* is sweet and neutral, its nature is soft and moist, and it survives the cold of winter fresh and green; thus, it inherits the shàoyīn essence of winter and water, and unites together with yángmíng stomach earth.

又曰：凡物之涼者， 其心必熱， 熱者陰中之陽也 。人但知去熱， 而不知用陽， 得其陽而後能通陰中之氣 。

[Zhāng] further said: Generally, the coolness of a substance is because the heart will have heat, and this heat is the yáng within yīn. People only know to eliminate heat, but do not know to use yáng. [If one first] obtains the yáng, then after, [one] is able to free the qì within yīn.

---

47. *Běn Cǎo Chóng Yuán* 《 本草崇原 》 (Honored Originals of the Materia Medica) was written by Zhāng Yǐn'ān 張隱庵 in 1674.

Xì Xīn 細辛
Complete plant including root of Asarum heteropoides

氣味辛、溫，無毒。主咳逆上氣，頭痛腦動，百節拘攣，風濕痹痛，死肌。久服明目，利九竅，輕身長年。

The qì and flavor are acrid, warm, and non-toxic. It governs counterflow cough qì ascent, headache and brain stirring,[48] hypertonicity of the hundred joints, wind-damp impediment pain, and numbness.[49] When taken over a long period of time, it brightens the eyes, disinhibits the nine orifices, lightens the body, and prolongs life.

張隱庵曰：細辛氣味辛溫，一莖直上，其色赤黑，稟少陰泉下之水陰，而上交於太陽之藥也。少陰為水臟，太陽為水腑，水氣相通行於皮毛，內合於肺。若循行失職，則病咳逆上氣，而細辛能治之。太陽之脈，起於目內眥，從巔絡腦。若循行失職，則病頭痛腦動，而細辛亦能治之。太陽之氣主皮毛，少陰之氣主骨髓，少陰之氣不合太陽，則風濕相侵。痹於筋骨，則為百節拘攣。痹於腠理，則為死肌，而細辛皆能治之。其所以能治之者，以氣勝之也。

Zhāng Yǐn'ān said: *Xì xīn's* qì and flavor are acrid and warm, the stalk grows straight upwards, and the color is reddish black. It inherits the shàoyīn yīn-water of the lower spring,[50] and is a medicinal that ascends and interacts in tàiyáng. Shàoyīn is the water viscus, and tàiyáng is the water bowel. The water and qì communicate and circulate in the skin and body hair, and inside [the water and qì] unite with the lungs. If the circulation is impaired, then there is disease of counterflow cough with qì ascent, and *xì xīn* is able to treat this. The vessel of tàiyáng begins in the inner canthus of the eye and follows [along] the vertex of the head to wrap the brain. If the circulation is impaired, then there is disease of headache and brain stirring, and *xì xīn* is also able to treat this. The qì of tàiyáng governs the skin and body hair, [while] the qì of shàoyīn governs the bone marrow. If the qì of shàoyīn does not unite with tàiyáng, then wind and damp will mutually invade. When there is impediment in the sinews and bones, then there is hypertonicity of the hundred joints. When there is impediment in the interstices, then there is numbness, and *xì xīn* is able to treat all of this. It therefore is able to treat [these diseases], because [*xì xīn*] uses [its] qì to dominate this.

---

48. *Nǎo dòng* 腦動 (brain stirring) is likely epilepsy or vein deformity, a migraine, or anything having to with stirring of the brain.

49. The term *sǐ jī* 死肌 can also mean necrosis.

50. Namely, the kidneys.

神農本草經讀 · 卷一

久服明目利九竅者，水精之氣濡於空竅也。九竅利，則輕身而延年矣。

When taken over a long period of time, it brightens the eyes and disinhibits the nine orifices; [this is] because the qì of the water and essence moisten the orifices. When the nine orifices are disinhibited, then this lightens the body and prolongs life!

又曰：宋元佑·陳承謂細辛單用末，不可過一錢，多則氣閉不通而死。近醫多以此語忌用，而不知辛香之藥豈能閉氣？上品無毒之藥何不可多用？方書之言，類此者不少。學人不詳察而遵信之，伊芳黃之門，終身不能入矣！

[Zhāng] further said: Chén Chéng[51] of the *Sòng Yuán Yòu* period[52] states that *xì xīn* should be used separately as a powder not to exceed one *qián*;[53] if one uses more, then the qì will be blocked or obstructed, and [the patient] will die. In recent years, doctors often used these words to avoid using [*xì xīn*], but how could they not know that acrid and fragrant medicinals are able to block the qì? The medicinals of the highest category are non-toxic; why should more be used? The entries of a formula book are similar to this and numerous. The scholar who does not carefully investigate and observe the signs will not be able to get an official post for the rest of his life!

Chái Hú 柴胡
Root of Bupleurum chinense

氣味苦、平，無毒。主心腹腸胃中結氣，飲食積聚，寒熱邪氣，推陳致新。久服輕身、明目、益精。

The qì and flavor are bitter, neutral, and non-toxic. It governs bound qì within the heart, abdomen, intestines and stomach, food and drink accumulation and gatherings, and cold and heat evil qì. It pushes out the old to bring forth the new. When taken over a long period of time it lightens the body, brightens the eyes, and boosts the essence.

---

51. Chén Chéng 陳承 (12th century) is a physician from Sìchuān, whose expertise was in using cooling herbs. See: Lǐ, 1985, p. 311.

52. *Sòng Yuán Yòu* 宋元佑 is a reign device of Emperor Zhé Zōng 哲宗 (1086-1094).

53. This unit equals to 3.7 grams in the *Qīng* dynasty, but in the *Sòng*, it was around 4 grams.

按：經文不言發汗，仲聖用至八兩之多，可知性純，不妨多服，功緩必須重用也。

Commentary: The writing of the classic does not mention promotion of sweating; [however] the sage [Zhāng] Zhòng[jǐng] used up to eight *liàng* or more.[54] Clearly, [if] the nature is pure, there is no harm in taking more [of the medicinal]. Its function is mild, so one must make heavy use of it.

葉天士曰：柴胡氣平，稟天中正之氣。味苦無毒，得地炎上之火味。「膽者，中正之官，」相火之腑。所以獨入足少陽膽經。氣味輕升，陰中之陽，乃少陽也。其主心腹腸胃中結氣者，心腹腸胃，五臟六腑也。臟腑共十二經，凡十一臟，皆取決於膽。

Yè Tiānshì said: *Chái hú's* qì is neutral, and it inherits the qì of heavenly justice. [*Chái hú's*] flavor is bitter, non-toxic, [and] obtains the fire flavor of earth [which] flames upward.[55] The gallbladder is the office of justice,[56] and the bowel of ministerial fire; therefore, [*chái hú*] alone enters the foot shàoyáng gallbladder channel. Its qì and flavor are light, upbearing, and the yáng is within the yīn; therefore this is shàoyáng. [*Chái hú*] governs bound qì within the heart, abdomen, intestines, and stomach; this is because the heart, abdomen, intestines, and stomach are the five viscera and the six bowels. The viscera and bowels together have twelve channels, [and] altogether the eleven viscera depend on the gallbladder.

柴胡輕清，升達膽氣，膽氣條達，則十一臟從之宣化，故心腹腸胃中凡有結氣皆能散之也。其主飲食積聚者，蓋飲食入胃散精於肝，肝之疏散又借少陽膽為生發之主也。柴胡升達膽氣，則肝能散精，而飲食積聚自下矣。

Chái hú is light and clear, it upbears and thrusts out the gallbladder qì, and if the gallbladder qì is thrust out, then the eleven viscera follow, diffusing and transforming. Therefore, if the heart, abdomen, intestines, and stomach all have bound qì, then in all cases [*chái hú*] is able to disperse this. It governs food and drink accumulations and gatherings; this is because food and drink enter the stomach, [and the stomach] dissipates the essence to the liver. The coursing and dissipation of the liver moreover depends on the shàoyáng gallbladder as the governor of development. [When] *chái hú* upbears and thrusts out the gallbladder qì, then the liver is able to dissipate the essence, and the food and drink accumulations and gatherings naturally are purged!

---

54. One *liàng* 兩 was 37.7 grams in the *Qīng*, but during the Eastern *Hàn* dynasty, it was only about 14.4 grams. It is not clear whether Chén 陳 was aware of this difference.

55. The qì is of heaven, and the flavor is of earth.

56. This sentence is a quotation from the *Huáng Dì Nèi Jīng Sù Wèn*《黃帝內經素問》(Inner Canon of the Yellow Emperor Plain Questions), Chapter 8.

少陽經行半表半裏，少陽受邪，邪並於陰則寒。邪並於陽則熱。柴胡和解少陽，故主寒熱之邪氣也。春氣一至，萬物俱新。柴胡得天地春升之性，入少陽以生氣血，故主推陳致新也。久服清氣上行，則陽氣日強，所以輕身。五臟六腑之精華上奉，所以明目。清氣上行，則陰氣下降，所以益精。精者，陰氣之英華也。

The shàoyáng channel circulates half in the exterior and half in the interior, [and when] shàoyáng contracts evil, the evil is simultaneously in the yīn, and then [there is] cold. If the evil is simultaneously in the yáng, then [there is] heat. *Chái hú* harmonizes and resolves shàoyáng; therefore, it governs the evil qì of cold or heat. When the spring qì first arrives, the ten thousand things all are new. *Chái hú* obtains the nature of heaven, earth, spring, and upbearing, which enters the shàoyáng in order to engender qì and blood; therefore, it governs pushing out the old to bring forth the new. When taken over a long period of time, the clear qì ascends and circulates, and then the yáng qì strengthens by the day; therefore, this lightens the body. The essence of the five viscera and six bowels is received in the upper body, therefore brightening the eyes. If the clear qì ascends and cirulates, then the yīn qì descends and downbears, and therefore this boosts the essence. The essence is the quintessence of yīn qì.

Huáng Lián 黃連
Rhizome of Coptis chinensis

氣味苦、寒，無毒。主熱氣目痛、眥傷淚出，明目，腸澼，腹痛，下痢，婦人陰中腫痛。久服令人不忘。

The qì and flavor are bitter, cold, and non-toxic. [*Huáng lián*] governs heat qì and pain in the eyes, damage and tearing at the canthus of the eye; it brightens the eyes, [and governs] intestinal afflux,[57] abdominal pain, diarrhea, and female vaginal swelling and pain. When taken over a long period of time, it prevents forgetfulness.

陳修園曰：黃連氣寒，稟天冬寒水之氣，入足少陰腎。味苦無毒，得地南方之火味，入手少陰心。氣水而味火，一物同具，故能除水火相亂而為濕熱之病。其云：主熱氣者，除一切氣分之熱也。目痛、眥傷、淚出、不明，皆濕熱在上之病。腸澼，腹痛，下痢，皆濕熱在中之病。婦人陰中腫痛，為濕熱在下之病。黃連除濕熱，所以主之。

Chén Xiūyuán said: *Huáng lián's* qì is cold, it inherits the qì of heaven, winter, cold, and water, and enters the foot shàoyīn kidney channel. [*Huáng lián's*] flavor is bitter, non-toxic, obtains the fire

---

57. *Cháng pì* 腸澼 (intestinal afflux) is dysentery or bloody spurting of stool due to intestinal stasis. See: Wiseman 1998, p.317.

flavor of the earth and the southern direction, [and] enters the hand shàoyīn heart channel. [*Huáng lián's*] qì is that of water, but its flavor is that of fire. It is one substance with similar qualities; therefore, it is able to eliminate water and fire's confusion with each other [which] becomes a disease of damp-heat. [Shén Nóng] said that [*huáng lián*] governs heat qì, and therefore eliminates all [types of] heat from the qì aspect. Eye pain, canthus damage, tearing, and unclear vision, are all diseases of damp-heat located in the upper body. Intestinal afflux, abdominal pain, and diarrhea are all diseases of damp-heat located in the center. Female vaginal swelling and pain is a disease of damp-heat located in the lower body. *Huáng lián* eliminates damp-heat, and therefore, it governs [this].

久服令人不忘者，苦入心即能補心也。然苦為火之本味，以其味之苦而補之。而寒能勝火，即以其氣之寒而瀉之。千古唯仲景得《本經》之秘。《金匱》治心氣不足而吐血者，取之以補心。《傷寒》寒熱互結心下而痞滿者，取之以瀉心。厥陰之熱氣撞心者，合以烏梅。下利後重者，合以白頭翁等法。真信而好古之聖人也。

When it is taken over a long period of time, it prevents forgetfulness. This is because bitter enters the heart, and hence it is able to supplement the heart. So, bitter is the root flavor of fire; [therefore,] the bitter flavor [is used to] supplement [the heart]. Yet cold is able to dominate fire; [therefore,] the cold qì is used to drain [the fire]. Through the ages, only [Zhāng] Zhòngjǐng obtained the secrets of the *Shén Nóng Běn Cǎo Jīng*. [In his] *Jīn Gùi Yào Lüè* (Essential Prescriptions of the Golden Cabinet),[58] [Zhòngjǐng] treated heart qì insufficiency and spitting of blood by applying [*huáng lián*] in order to supplement the heart. The *Shāng Hán Lùn* (Discussion on Cold Damage), [said that when] cold and heat mutually bind below the heart and [there is] glomus and fullness, apply [*huáng lián*] in order to drain the heart. If the heat qì of juéyīn strikes the heart, [then] use [*huáng lián*] combined with *wū méi*. If [there is] diarrhea and after heaviness, [then] use [*huáng lián*] combined with *bái tóu wēng* and other similar methods.[59] The sage [Zhāng Zhòngjǐng] truly believed in and loved the ancient [traditions]!

---

58. See: *Jīn Gùi Yào Lüè* 《金匱要略》(Essential Prescriptions of the Golden Cabinet), Chapter 16.

59. See: Craig Mitchell et al: *Shāng Hán Lùn* 《傷寒論》(On Cold Damage), Paradigm Publications, Brookline 1999, p. 228 - 241, 526, 557.

Fáng Fēng 防風
Root of Ledebouriella divaricata

氣味甘、溫，無毒。主大風，頭眩痛，惡風，風邪目盲無所見，風行周身，骨節疼痛、身重。久服輕身。

The qì and flavor are sweet, warm, and non-toxic. It governs great wind,[60] dizziness and headache, aversion to wind, wind evil, and blindness without [the ability] to see, wind moving in the whole body, bone and joint pain, and generalized heaviness. When taken over a long period of time, it lightens the body.

陳修園曰：防風氣溫，稟天春木之氣而入肝。味甘無毒，得地中土之味而入脾。「主大風」三字提綱，詳於巴戟天注，不贅。風傷陽位，則頭痛而眩。風傷皮毛，則為惡風之風。邪風害空竅，則目盲無所見。風行周身者，經絡之風也。骨節疼痛者，關節之風也。身重者，病風而不能矯捷也。防風之甘溫發散，可以統主之。

Chén Xiūyuán said: *Fáng fēng's* qì is warm; inherits the qì of heaven, spring, and wood; and enters the liver. The flavor is sweet and non-toxic, obtains the flavor of earth and center-earth, and enters the spleen. This outlines the three characters of "governs great wind" and is comprehensively explained in *bā jǐ tiān's* commentary, so [I will] not repeat [it here]. If wind damages yáng's location, then [there is] headache and dizziness. If wind damages the skin and body hair, then the wind causes aversion to wind.[61] If evil wind harms the orifices, then [there is] blindness without [the ability] to see. Wind moving in the whole body is [due to] wind in the channels and collaterals. The bone and joint pain is [due to] wind in the joints. The generalized heaviness is a wind disease [where the patient] is unable to [be] vigorous or nimble. The sweet, warm, and dispersing [nature] of *fáng fēng* is able to control and govern this.

然溫屬春和之氣，入肝而治風。尤妙在甘以入脾，培土以和木氣，其用獨神。此理證之易象，於剝復二卦而可悟焉。兩土同崩則剝，故大病必顧脾胃。土木無忤則復，故病轉必和肝脾。防風驅風之中，大有回生之力。李東垣竟目為卒伍卑賤之品，真門外漢也。

So, the warm [nature] belongs to the qì of spring and harmony, enters the liver, and treats wind. Particularly wonderful is the sweet [nature] in order to enter the spleen, bank up the earth in order

---

60. The term *dà fēng* 大風 means pestilential wind, as well as leprosy, but this also could simply be a bad cold.

61. Because wind in general can cause shivering, this sentence could also be translated as: "If wind damages the skin and body hair, one has shivering as of aversion to wind."

to harmonize the wood qì, and this use alone is divine. The *Yì Jīng* 《易經》 shape[62] of this logical pattern can be comprehended by [looking at] the two hexagrams *bō* and *fù*![63] When the two earths[64] collapse together it is *bō* (decline); therefore, in major diseases [one] must look after the spleen and stomach. When earth and wood are without hostility, then [this is] *fù* (prosperity). Therefore, when disease shifts, [one] must harmonize the liver and spleen. *Fáng fēng's* expulsion of wind strike has great power to return life. Surprisingly, Lǐ Dōngyuán actually cataloged it as a lowly and worthless medicinal for soldiers. [He] truly was a layman!

Xù Duàn 續斷
Root of Dipsacus asper

氣味苦、微溫，無毒。主傷寒，補不足，金瘡，癰瘍，折跌，續筋骨，婦人乳難。久服益氣力。

The qì and flavor are bitter, slightly warm, and non-toxic. It governs cold damage, supplements insufficiency, [governs] incised wounds, welling abscesses, broken [bones] and falls, joins [severed] sinews and bones, and [governs] women's difficult lactation. When taken over a long period of time, it boosts the qì and power.

參：此以形為治。續斷有肉有筋，如人筋在肉中之象，而色帶紫、帶黑，為肝腎之象。氣味苦溫，為少陰、陽明火土之氣化。故寒傷於經絡而能散之，癰瘍結於經絡而能療之，折跌筋骨有傷，而能補不足、續其斷絕。以及婦人乳難，而能通其滯而為乳。久服益氣力者，亦能強筋骨之功也。

Comparison: This [medicinal] uses the form to act as the treatment.[65] *Xù duàn* has flesh as well as sinews, which are similar to the appearance of a person's sinews located within the flesh, and appear to have bands of purple and black, while [the leaves] are the shape of the liver and kidneys. The qì and flavor are bitter and warm, [which] cause qì transformation of shàoyīn and yángmíng fire and earth.[66] Therefore, [*xù duàn*] is able to disperse cold damage from the channels and collaterals,

---

62. *Yì xiàng* 易象 (shape of changes) means the outward appearance of a certain issue as depicted in the eight trigrams from the *Book of Changes*.

63. These two hexagrams from the *Yì Jīng* 《易經》 can be literally translated as "fall" and "return." Together they are used as "prosperity and decline." The hexagram for *bō* 剝 is ䷖ and the hexagram for *fù* 復 is ䷗.

64. The two earths are stomach and spleen.

65. Similar to the doctrine of signatures, this medicinal is believed to cure because of its shape.

66. This means, that because of the bitter flavor, *xù duàn* assists the shàoyīn fire (heart), and because of its warmth, *xù duàn* assists the yángmíng earth (stomach). Chén corresponds each flavor or qì-quality with the symptoms listed under the main indications.

[and] is able to cure welling abscesses, and binds in the channels and collaterals. If there are broken [bones] and falls, or damage to [severed] sinew and bone, it is able to supplement insufficiency, and replenish that which has been interrupted and cut off. When it comes to women's difficult lactation, [*xù duàn*] is able to free the stagnation and produce milk. When taken over a long period of time, it boosts the qì and power, and is also able to strengthen the function of the sinews and bones.

Niú Xī 牛膝
Root of Achyranthes bidentata

氣味苦，酸，平，無毒。主寒濕痿痺，四肢拘攣，膝痛不可屈伸，逐血氣，傷熱火爛，墮胎。久服輕身耐老。

The qì and flavor are bitter, sour, neutral, and non-toxic. It governs cold-damp wilting impediment, hypertonicity of the four limbs, and knee pain with inability to bend and stretch. [*Niú xī*] expels blood, qì, damage from heat, fire erosion, and induces abortion. When taken over a long period of time, it lightens the body and makes [one] resistant to old age.

陳修園曰：牛膝氣平，稟金氣而入肺。味苦，得火味而入心包。味酸，得木味而入肝。唯其入肺，則能通調水道而寒濕行，胃⁶⁷熱清而痿愈矣。唯其入肝，肝藏血而養筋，則拘攣可愈，膝亦不痛而能屈伸矣。唯其入心包，苦能泄實，則血因氣凝之病可逐也。苦能瀉火，則熱湯之傷與火傷之爛可完也。苦味本伐生生之氣，而又合以酸味，而遂大申其涌泄之權，則胎無不墮矣。久服輕身耐老者，又統言其流通血脈之功也。

Chén Xiūyuán said: *Niú xī's* qì is neutral; [it] inherits the metal qì, and enters the lungs. The bitter flavor is the fire flavor, and enters the pericardium. The sour flavor is the wood flavor, and enters the liver. Only by [the neutral qì] entering the lungs, is [*niú xī*] then able to regulate the waterways and move the cold and damp, clear the stomach heat, and cure the wilting! Only by [the sour flavor] entering the liver, [is] the liver [able to] store the blood and nourish the sinews; then the hypertonicity can be cured. The knee also is not painful and can bend and stretch! Only by [the bitter flavor] entering the pericardium, is the bitter able to discharge repletion; then the blood disease [which] causes the qì to congeal can be expelled. Bitter is able to drain fire. As a result, the damage from hot decoctions and erosion due to fire damage can be overcome. The bitter flavor essentially quells the multiplication of qì, and moreover [when the bitter flavor] is united with the sour flavor, and consequently greatly extends the powers of ejection and discharge, then the fetus always is aborted! When taken over a long period of time, it lightens the body and makes [one] resistant to old age. This also [can be] gathered into one saying: that [*niú xī's*] function is to free flow the blood and vessels.

---

67. *Wèi* 胃 (stomach), this character is suspected to be a typographical mistake for *fèi* 肺 (lungs).

Bā Jǐ Tiān 巴戟天
Root of Morinda officinalis

氣味甘、微溫，無毒。主大風邪氣，陰痿不起，強筋骨，安五臟，補中增志益氣。酒焙。

The qì and flavor are sweet, slightly warm, and non-toxic. It governs great wind, evil qì, impotence, and failure [of the penis] to rise. [*Bā jǐ tiān*] strengthens the sinews and bones, quiets the five viscera, supplements the center, increases the will, and boosts the qì. *Stone-bake [or soak in] alcohol.*

陳修園曰：巴戟天氣微溫，稟天春升之木氣而入足厥陰肝。味辛甘無毒，得地金土二味入足陽明燥金胃。雖氣味有木土之分，而其用則統歸於溫肝之內。佛經以風輪主持大地，即是此義。

Chén Xiūyuán said: *Bā jǐ tiān's* qì is slightly warm, inherits the wood qì of heaven, spring, upbearing, and enters the foot juéyīn liver [channel]. The flavor is acrid,[68] sweet and non-toxic; by obtaining earth and metal, [these are] the two flavors of earth [which] enter the foot yángmíng dry metal[69] stomach. While the qì and flavor have aspects of wood and earth, their principal use is to gather and return the warmth inwardly to the liver. According to Buddhist scripture: the "wind wheel" governs and controls the planet earth, then this is the meaning.[70]

---

68. The original text of the *Shén Nóng Běn Cǎo Jīng* does not mention an acrid flavor.

69. Hand and foot yángmíng are thought to have a dry and metallic nature. This is also part of the *Wǔ Yùn Liù Qì Xué Shuō* 五運六氣學説 (Theory on the Five Transformations and Six Qì). See Footnote 55 in the Preface. The seasonal changes of the six stages are also described in the: *Huáng Dì Nèi Jīng Sù Wèn* 《 黃帝 内經素問 》 (Inner Canon of the Yellow Emperor Plain Questions), Chapter 21:
風化厥陰，熱化少陰，溼化太陰，火化少陽，燥化陽明，寒化太陽。

Wind transforms juéyīn, heat transforms shàoyīn, damp transforms tàiyīn, fire transforms shàoyáng, dry transforms yángmíng, and cold transforms tàiyáng.

70. According to Buddhist belief, the "wind wheel" (*fēng lún* 風輪) is one of the *sì lún* 四輪 (four wheels): these are the *jīn lún* 金輪 (metal wheel), *shuǐ lún* 水輪 (water wheel), *fēng lún* 風輪 (wind wheel), and *kòng lún* 空輪 (emptiness wheel). The metal wheel is our planet earth, which in this system is believed to flow on water, the water dwells on wind, and below the wind is emptiness. (See: *The Chinese Buddhist Order of Sangha in Thailand: A Dictionary of Buddhism,* Bangkok 1976, p.19) However, this does not really make so much sense here. It is more likely, that Chén is talking about the medical *fēng lún* 風輪 (wind wheel), which in medical texts usually denotes that the cornea and iris are related to the liver, and earth would be the "flesh ring," that is the eyelids. This is called the *Wǔ Lún Xué Shuō* 五輪學説 (Theory of the Five Wheels), namely the five regions of the eyes correlating with the five viscera. The liver belongs to wood, and wood controls earth. See: Ed. Raymund Pothmann: *33 Fallbeispiele zur Akupunktur aus der VR China. (Thirty-three acupuncture cases from the People´s Republic of China).* Stuttgart, 1996, p. 44.

《本經》以「主大風」三字提綱兩見：一見於巴戟天，一見於防風。陰陽造化之機，一言逗出。《金匱》云：風能生萬物，亦能害萬物。防風主除風之害，巴戟天主得風之益，不得滑口讀去。蓋人居大塊之中，乘氣以行，鼻息呼吸，不能頃刻去風。風即是氣，風氣通於肝，和風生人，疾風殺人。其主大風者，謂其能化疾風為和風也。邪氣者，五行正氣不得風而失其和。木無風則無以遂其條達之情，火無風則無以遂其炎上之性，金無風則無以成其堅勁之體，水無風則潮不上，土無風則植不蕃。一得巴戟天之用，則到處皆春而邪氣去矣。邪氣去而五臟安，自不待言也。況肝之為言敢也，肝陽之氣，行於宗筋而陰痿起。行於腎臟，腎藏志而志增，腎主骨而骨強。行於脾臟，則震坤合德，土木不害而中可補。「益氣」二字，又總結通章之義。氣即風也，逐而散之。風散即為氣散，生而亦死。益而和之，氣和即為風和，死可回生。非明於生殺消長之道者，不可以語此也。

The *Shén Nóng Běn Cǎo Jīng* uses the three words "govern great wind," as a key point [that] has two appearances: one appears in *bā jǐ tiān*; the other appears in *fáng fēng*. [I want to] speak on the mechanism of creation and transformation of yīn and yáng for a while. The *Jīn Gùi [Yào Lüè]* said: "The wind is able to generate the ten thousand things, and is also able to harm the ten thousand things."[71] *Fáng fēng* governs the elimination of harmful wind, [while] *bā jǐ tiān* governs the increased contraction of wind; it would not be plausible to leave the study here. People [who] live within nature, take advantage of qì in order to move, breathe the breath, and cannot for a short moment eliminate wind. Wind then is qì, and the wind qì communicates in the liver; a breeze [gives] life to people [while] a storm kills people. [*Bā jǐ tiān's* ability to] govern great wind refers to the ability to transform a storm into a breeze. Evil qì is when the five phases and the right qì can not receive wind and lose their harmony. If the wood is without wind, then the absence subsequently affects [the wood's ability to] outthrust. If fire is without wind, then the absence subsequently affects [the fire's ability to] upwardly flame. If metal is without wind, then the absence [affects] the formation of the body's fortification and strength. If water is without wind, then the tides can not rise. If earth is without wind, then plants can not flourish. As soon as one obtains the use of *bā jǐ tiān*, everywhere will be spring and the evil qì will be eliminated! When the evil qì is eliminated and the five viscera are quiet, there is nothing left to be said. Moreover, [I] venture to speak of the liver: the qì of liver yáng moves in the ancestral sinew[72] and the yīn wilt [will] rise. [When the qì of liver yáng] moves in the kidney viscus, the kidney stores the *zhì* (will), and so the will increases, the kidney governs the bones, and the bones strengthen. [When the qì of liver yáng] moves in the spleen viscus, then *zhèn* (thunder) and *kūn* (earth) will unite in virtue,[73] earth and wood are not harmed, and the center can be supplemented. The two words "boost the qì" additionally generally summarize the meaning of

---

71. The original text is: 風氣雖能生萬物，亦能害萬物。 The wind qì, although able to give birth to ten thousand things, also is able to harm the ten thousand things." See: *Jīn Gùi Yào Lüè* 《金匱要略》 (Essential Prescriptions of the Golden Cabinet), Chapter 1.

72. Here, ancestral sinew means penis.

73. The trigrams for these characters are: *zhèn* 震 ☳ (thunder) and *kūn* 坤 ☷ (earth). They can be combined either as the above-mentioned hexagram *fù* 復 ䷗ (prosperity), or as *yù* 豫 ䷏ (comfort). *Zhèn* 震 (thunder) belongs to the wood element, so wind and liver are associated. If wood and earth are combined in virtue, there will be prosperity or comfort.

this chapter. Qì, then, is wind; it [can be] expelled and dispersed [by *fáng fēng*. If] wind is dispersed, then [this] causes the qì to disperse: it can mean life, but also death. [By using *bā jǐ tiān* to] boost and harmonize this, [if] the qì is harmonized, then [this] causes the wind [to be] harmonized, and death can be returned to life. Those who are not clear about the Dào of life and death, [or] decline and growth, can not speak about this.

葉天士云：淫羊藿治陰虛陰痿，巴戟天治陽虛陰痿 。

Yè Tiānshì said: *Yín yáng huò* treats yīn vacuity yīn wilt (impotence), while *bā jǐ tiān* treats yáng vacuity yīn wilt (impotence).

Shí Hú 石斛
Whole plant of Dendrobium nobile

氣味甘、平，無毒 。主傷中，除痺，下氣，補五臟虛勞羸瘦，強陰益精 。久服厚腸胃 。

The qì and flavor are sweet, neutral, and non-toxic. [*Shí hú*] governs damage to the center, eliminates impediment, descends the qì, and supplements vacuity taxation of the five viscera with marked emaciation. It strengthens the yīn and boosts the essence. When taken over a long period of time, it thickens the intestines and stomach.

葉天士曰：石斛氣平入肺，味甘無毒入脾 。甘平為金土之氣味，入足陽明胃、手陽明大腸 。陰者，中之守也 。陰虛則傷中，甘平益陰，故主傷中 。痺者，脾病也 。風、寒、濕三氣而脾先受之，石斛甘能補脾，故能除痺 。上氣，肺病也 。火氣上逆則為氣喘，石斛平能清肺，故能下氣 。五臟皆屬於陰，而脾名至陰，為五臟之主 。石斛補脾而蔭及五臟，則五臟之虛勞自復，而肌肉之消瘦自生矣 。陰者宗筋也 。精足則陰自強 。精者，陰氣之精華也 。納穀多而精自儲 。腸者，手陽明大腸也 。胃者，足陽明胃也 。陽明屬燥金，久服甘平清潤，則陽明不燥，而腸胃厚矣 。《新訂》 。

Yè Tiānshì said: The qì of *shí hú* is neutral and enters the lungs; the flavor is sweet, non-toxic, and enters the spleen. Sweet and neutral are the qì and flavor of metal and earth, [and] enter the foot yángmíng stomach and the hand yángmíng large intestine. The yīn guards the center. If the yīn is vacuous, then [there is] damage to the center. The sweet and neutral [flavors] boost the yīn; therefore, [these] govern damage to the center. Impediment is a disease of the spleen, and the spleen is the first to contract the three qì of wind, cold, and damp. *Shí hú's* sweetness [is] able to supplement the spleen; therefore, [it is] able to eliminate impediment. Ascending qì is a disease of the lungs.

46

神農本草經讀・卷一

When fire qì ascends counterflow, it results in wheezing. *Shí hú's* neutral [flavor is] able to clear the lungs, therefore it is able to descend the qì. The five viscera all belong to yīn, and the spleen is called the consummate yīn, because [it is] the governor of the five viscera. *Shí hú* supplements the spleen and protects[74] the five viscera, so that the vacuity taxation of the five viscera spontaneously recovers, and the emaciation of the flesh generates spontaneously! The yīn, is the ancestral sinew. When the essence is sufficient, then the yīn will naturally be strong. The essence is the essence and bloom of the yīn qì. When [the patients] add more grains [to their diet], the essence is naturally saved. The intestines are hand yángmíng large intestine, [and] the stomach is foot yángmíng stomach. The yángmíng belongs to the dry metal; [therefore, if one] takes sweet, neutral, clear, and moist [medicinals] over a long period of time, then the yángmíng will not be dry and the intestines and stomach will thicken! *Newly revised.*

張隱庵曰：石斛生於石上，得水長生，是稟水石之專精而補腎。味甘色黃，不假土力，是奪中土之氣化而補脾。斛乃量名，主出主入，能運行中土之氣而愈諸病也。

Zhāng Yǐn'ān said: *Shí hú* grows on top of stones; by obtaining water [one] promotes life.[75] [*Shí hú*] inherits the concentrated essence of water and stone, and supplements the kidneys. The sweet flavor and yellow color [of *shí hú*] are truly the strength of earth; this completes the qì transformation of center-earth and supplements the spleen.[76] *Hú* 斛 is a name [for] measuring;[77] it governs issuing forth and entering, and is able to move the qì of center-earth and cure all diseases.

Zé Xiè 澤瀉
Rhizome of Alisma plantago-aquatica

氣味甘、寒，無毒。主風寒濕痹，乳難，養五臟，益氣力，肥健，消水。久服耳目聰明，不飢，延年，輕身，面生光，能行水上。

The qì and flavor are sweet, cold, and non-toxic. It governs wind-cold-damp impediment[78] and difficult lactation, nourishes the five viscera, boosts the qì and strength, fattens and strengthens, and disperses water [swelling]. When taken over a long period of time, it sharpens the hearing and brightens the vision, prevents hunger, prolongs life, and lightens the body. [*Zé xiè*] generates luster of the face and is able to move water upwards.

---

74. *Yīn* 蔭 means to shade, to shelter, to protect.
75. This passage could also be translated as: …receives the growth and generation of water.
76. This means, *shí hú* receives strong earth qualities though not growing in earth but on top of stones.
77. *Hú* 斛 is an ancient measure for grain and is equal to fifty liters.
78. Note that here, this is a cold medicinal used for cold impediment.

陳修園曰：澤瀉氣寒，水之氣也。味甘無毒，土之味也。生於水而上升，能
啟水陰之氣上滋中土也。其主風、寒、濕痹者，三氣以濕為主，此能啟水氣
上行而復下，其痹即從水氣而化矣。其主乳難者，能滋水精於中土而為汁
也。其主「養五臟，益氣力，肥健」等句，以五臟主藏陰，而脾為五臟之
原，一得水精之氣則能灌溉四旁，俾五臟循環而受益，不特肥健消水不飢，
見本臟之功。而肺得水精之氣而氣益，心得水精之氣而力益，肝得水精之氣
而目明，腎得水精之氣而耳聰，且形得水精之氣而全體輕，色得水精之氣而
面生光輝，一生得水精之氣而延年，所以然者，久服之功。能行在下之水而
使之上也。此物形圓，一莖直上，無下行之性，故其功效如此。今人以鹽水
拌炒，則反掣其肘矣。

Chén Xiūyuán said: The cold qì of *zé xiè* is the qì of water. The sweet and non-toxic flavor is the
flavor of earth. It grows in the water, and rises upwards. [It] is able to open the qì of water yīn,
[and] raise and enrich the center-earth. [*Zé xiè*] governs wind-cold-damp-impediment, because of
[these] three qì, damp is [that which] governs. This [medicinal] is able to open the water qì to move
upwards and return it downward, so the impediment then, follows the water qì and transforms! [*Zé
xiè*] governs difficult lactation: this is [because it] is able to enrich the water essence in the center-
earth and make the milk. It governs "nourishing the five viscera, boosts the qì and strength, fattens
and strengthens" and so on. [These] sentences [are mentioned] because the five viscera govern the
storage of yīn, and the spleen is the source of the five viscera. [The spleen, which is] first to receive
the qì of water and essence, then is able to irrigate the four sides, and enable the five viscera to
circulate and receive benefit. Not only [does it] fatten and strengthen, disperse water [swelling] and
prevent hunger, but it appears to [improve the] function of the original viscus. [When] the lungs
receive the qì of water and essence, this boosts the qì. [When] the heart receives the qì of water and
essence, this boosts the strength. [When] the liver receives the qì of water and essence, the eyes
are brightened. [When] the kidneys receive the qì of water and essence, the hearing is sharpened.
Furthermore, [when] the form receives the qì of water and essence, the entire body is lightened.
[When] the complexion receives the qì of water and essence, [then] the face [becomes] radiant.
[When one] receives the qì of water and essence throughout one's life, [then this] prolongs life. The
reason for this, is that as a result of taking [*zé xiè*] over a long period of time, [one] is able to move
water located in the lower [body] and cause it to ascend. The shape of this plant is round, its stalk is
straight upright, and it does not have any downward-moving characteristics; therefore, its action is
like this. Nowadays, people use salt water to stir-fry it, [and this] results in adverse hindrance![79]

---

79. *Chè zhǒu* 掣肘 literally means: "to hold somebody by the elbow."

神農本草經讀・卷一

Wǔ Wèi Zǐ 五味子
Fruit of Schisandra chinensis

氣味酸，溫，無毒。主益氣，咳逆上氣，勞傷羸瘦，補不足，強陰，益男子精。

The qì and flavor are sour, warm, and non-toxic. [*Wǔ wèi zǐ*] governs boosting the qì, counterflow cough qì ascent, [and] taxation damage with marked emaciation. [It] supplements insufficiency, strengthens the yīn, and boosts the male essence.

陳修園曰：五味子氣溫味酸，得東方生長之氣而主風。人在風中而不見風，猶魚在水中而不見水。人之鼻息出入，頃刻離風則死，可知人之所以生者，風也。風氣通於肝，即人身之木氣。莊子云：「野馬也，塵埃也，生物之息以相吹也。」「息」字有二義：一曰「生息」，二曰「休息」。五味子溫以遂木氣之發榮，酸以斂木氣之歸根。生息，休息，皆所以益其生生不窮之氣。倘其氣不治，治，安也。咳逆上氣者，風木挾火氣而乘金也。為勞傷、為羸瘦、為陰痿、為精虛者，則《金匱》所謂「虛勞諸不足，風氣百疾」是也。風氣通於肝，先聖提出虛勞大眼目，惜後人不能申明其義。五味子益氣中，大具開闔升降之妙，所以概主之也。唐、宋以下，諸家有謂其具五味而兼治五臟者。有謂其酸以斂肺，色黑入腎，核似腎而補腎者。想當然之說，究非定論也。然肝治五臟，得其生氣而安，為《本經》言外之正旨。仲景佐以乾薑，助其溫氣，俾氣與味相得而益彰，是補天手段。

Chén Xiūyuán said: The qì of *wǔ wèi zǐ* is warm and the flavor is sour. It receives the qì of east, generates growth, and governs wind. Humans are within wind,[80] but cannot see the wind, like a fish is within water, but cannot see the water. The breath of man exits and enters;[81] [if one is] deprived of wind for a short moment, it results in death. It is clear that in order for man to live [there must be] wind. The wind qì communicates in the liver, [which] is namely the wood qì of the human body. Zhuāng Zǐ said: [In regards to the wind caused by the wings of the mythological bird the roc]: "It is a wild horse [never standing still], it is dust [quivering in a sunbeam], it is the breath of living creatures [constantly] blown against each other."[82] The character "breath" has two different meanings: one is "to live" and the other one is "to rest."[83] *Wǔ wèi zǐ's* warmth is used to bring about the flourishing of wood qì; *wǔ wèi zǐ's* sourness is used to collect and return the wood qì to the

---

80. This means that humans are surrounded by wind.

81. This passage can also be translated as: "the human breath is exhaled and inhaled."

82. Zhuāng Zǐ 莊子, actually named Zhuāng Zhōu 莊周, (369-286 B.C.) is the most influential philosopher in daoism. His work has been fully translated by James Legge. This quotation is part of the inner chapters of the book *Zhuāng Zǐ* 《莊子》 (Zhuāng zǐ), Xiāo Yáoyóu 《逍遙遊》 (Enjoyment in Untroubled Ease), 1.

83. Another way to read these two sets of characters is "life" and "death."

roots.[84] Living and resting both, therefore, boost the qì's endless multiplication. Supposing the qì is not managed (*[in this case] managed means rested*), [and] there is counterflow cough qì ascent, this is [because] the wind and wood are coerced by the qì of fire and take advantage of metal. [This] causes taxation damage, marked emaciation, yīn wilt (impotence), and essence vacuity. This is then what is referred to in the *Jīn Gùi [Yào Lüè* where it] says: "Vacuity taxation and all insufficiency [are due to] wind qì and the hundred diseases."[85] When the wind qì communicates in the liver, the sages of former generations proposed [that if one has] vacuity taxation, [then one will have] big eyes,[86] [but] regretfully, later generations were unable to clearly explain the true meaning [of this phrase]. *Wǔ wèi zǐ* boosts the qì and center and is a great and miraculous tool for opening and closing, upbearing and downbearing; therefore, it generally governs [the above-mentioned diseases]. After the *Táng* and *Sòng* [dynasties], all physicians were of the opinion that [*wǔ wèi zǐ*] possesses five flavors and simultaneously treats the five viscera, and they were of the opinion that the sour flavor of [*wǔ wèi zǐ* was] used to constrain the lungs: the black color enters the kidneys, and the kernels resemble the kidneys, and thus supplement them. In theory [it is easy] to believe, [however,] when studied carefully, these are not accepted arguments. It is correct that the liver manages the five viscera, and upon receiving [*wǔ wèi zǐ's*] vital qì, [the liver] is quiet. This is the real implied aim of the text in the *Shén Nóng Běn Cǎo Jīng*. Zhòngjǐng assists [*wǔ wèi zǐ* with] *gān jiāng* to reinforce the warm qì and enables the qì and flavor to both receive [while] distinctly [being] boosted. This supplements the method of heaven.[87]

Yì Yǐ Rén 薏苡仁
Seed kernel of Coix lachryma-jobi

氣味甘、微寒，無毒。主筋急拘攣，不可屈伸，久風濕痹，下氣。久服輕身益氣。

The qì and flavor are sweet, slightly cold, and non-toxic. [*Yì yǐ rén*] governs tension and hypertonicity of the sinews, inability to bend or stretch [the limbs], chronic wind-damp-impediment, and lower [body] qì. When taken over a long period of time, [*yì yǐ rén*] lightens the body and boosts the qì.

---

84. This sentence describes the growth of a tree that, no matter how tall it is, returns its own nutrient matter to the roots by shedding its leaves.

85. See: *Jīn Gùi Yào Lüè* 《金匱要略》 (Essential Prescriptions of the Golden Cabinet), Chapter 6, Line 16.

86. It is not quite clear which source Chén is referring to here.

87. *Bǔ tiān* 補天 is a Daoist method to preserve health.

陳修園曰：薏苡仁夏長秋成，味甘色白，稟陽明金土之精。金能制風，土能勝濕，故治以上諸證。久服輕身益氣者，以濕行則脾健而身輕，金清則肺治而氣益也。

Chén Xiūyuán said: *Yì yǐ rén* grows in the summer and ripens in the autumn. The flavor is sweet, the color is white, [and *yì yǐ rén*] inherits the essence of yángmíng metal and earth. The metal is able to control wind, and the earth is able to dominate dampness, therefore it treats all the above-mentioned patterns. When taken over a long period of time, [*yì yǐ rén*] lightens the body and boosts the qì; this is [because when] dampness moves, then the spleen is fortified and the body is lightened. Clearing metal, then treats the lungs and boosts the qì.

神農本草經讀 · 卷一

卷之二

Chapter Two

閩吳航陳念祖修園甫著
男 元豹道彪古愚元犀道照靈石同挍字

Written by Chén Niànzǔ Xiūyuán from Mǐn Wúháng.
Revised by Yuánbào Dàobiāo Gǔyú and Yuánxī Dàozhào Língshí.

上品

Medicinals of the Highest Grade

Tù Sī Zǐ 菟絲子
Seed of Cuscuta chinensis

氣味辛、平，無毒。主續絕傷，補不足，益氣力，肥健人，汁去面䵣。久服明目，輕身，延年。

The qì and flavor are acrid, neutral, and non-toxic. [*Tù sī zǐ*] governs continuing damage due to expiration, supplements insufficiency, boosts the qì and strength, fattens and strengthens people, and the juice removes soot-black patches[88] from the face. When taken over a long period of time, [*tù sī zǐ*] brightens the eyes, lightens the body, and prolongs life.

陳修園曰：菟絲氣平稟金氣，味辛得金味，肺藥也。然其用在腎而不在肺。子中脂膏最足，絕類人精，金生水也。主續絕傷者，子中脂膏如絲不斷，善於補續也。補不足者，取其最足之脂膏，以填補其不足之精血也。精血足，則氣力自長，肥健自增矣。汁去面䵣者，言不獨內服得其填補之功，即外用亦得其滑澤之效也。久服，腎水足則目明，腎氣壯則身輕。華元化云：腎者，性命之根也。腎得補則延年。

Chén Xiūyuán said: The qì of *tù sī zǐ* is neutral, and inherits the metal qì. The flavor is acrid, obtains the metal flavor, [and] is a lung medicinal. However, this [medicinal] is used for the kidneys and not for the lungs. The fat inside the seeds is the most complete [with an] exceptional resemblance to human essence, [thus] metal generates water. [*Tù sī zǐ*] governs and replenishes expiry damage; this is [because] the fat inside the seeds is uninterrupted like silk, and [is] good at supplementing and replenishing. To supplement insufficiency, take [*tù sī zǐ's*] most complete fat in order to replenish and supplement the essence and blood insufficiency. If essence and blood are sufficient, then the qì and strength naturally grow, and the fat and strength naturally increase! The juice [of *tù sī zǐ*] removes soot-black patches in the face; this means [that the] action of replenishing and supplementing is not only obtained from taking this internally, but even when used externally [one] also obtains its glossy and moistening effects. [When this is] take over a long period of time, [then] the kidney water [becomes] sufficient, the eyes are brightened, and when the kidney qì is strong, then

---

88. *Miàn gān* 面䵣 are soot-black patches or face moles.

53

the body [becomes] light. Huà Yuánhuà said: The kidneys are the root of life.[89] When the kidneys are supplemented, then the life is prolonged.

Wēi Ruí 葳蕤
Rhizome of Polygonatum odoratum

氣味甘、平，無毒。主中風暴熱，不能動搖，跌筋結肉，諸不足。久服去面黑皯，好顏色，潤澤，輕身不老。

The qì and flavor are sweet, neutral, and non-toxic. It governs wind strike with fulminant heat [effusion], inability to stir and shake, falling sinews and bound flesh; [these] are all insufficiencies. When taken over a long period of time, it eliminates soot-black patches from the face, [fosters] a complexion [that is] good, moisturizes, lightens the body, and prevents aging.

張隱庵曰：葳蕤氣味甘平，質多津液，稟太陰濕土之精以資中焦之汁。主中風暴熱不能搖動者，以津液為邪熱所灼也。跌筋者，筋不柔和也。結肉者，肉無膏澤也。諸不足者，申明以上諸證皆屬津液不足也。久服則津液充滿，故去面上之黑皯，好顏色而肌膚潤澤，且輕身不老也。

Zhāng Yǐn'ān said: The qì and flavor of *wēi ruí* is sweet and neutral, its nature increases fluids, [and] it inherits the essence of tàiyīn damp earth in order to support the juices of the middle *jiāo*. [*Wēi ruí*] governs wind strike with fulminant heat [effusion] and inability to shake and stir; this is because the fluids are scorched by evil heat. Falling sinews [occur when] the sinews are not soft and flexible. Bound flesh [occurs when] the flesh is without fat and moisture. All kinds of insufficiencies, [this] explains that the various signs above all belong to insufficiency of fluids. When taken over a long period of time, then the fluids are filled. Therefore, [*wēi ruí*] eliminates soot-black patches from the face, [fosters] a complexion [that is] good, and moisturizes the flesh and skin; moreover [it] lightens the body, and prevents aging.

又曰：陰柔之藥，豈堪重用？古人除治風熱以外，絕不敢用。自李時珍有不寒不燥，用代參，耆之說，時醫信為補劑，虛證仗此，百無一生，咎其誰職耶？

[Zhāng Yǐn'ān] further said: How can a yīn medicinal [which] softens be an important [medicinal] to use? The people of antiquity did not dare to use it, except in the treatment of wind heat. From Lǐ

---

89. Namely Huà Tuó 華佗; see Footnote 61 of the preface for Huà Yuánhuà 華元化. Unfortunately, Huà's writings have not been preserved, so Chén Xiūyuán seems to mention his name here in order to enhance the authority of what he says.

Shízhēn onward, [*wēi ruí*] was listed as not cold, not dry, and [was] said to be used as a substitute for [*rén*] *shēn* and [*huáng*] *qí*. Present-day physicians believe it to be a supplementing formula, [but if one] relies on this [herb] with vacuity patterns, not even one out of one hundred [patients] will survive. Who is to be blamed for this, eh?

Shā Shēn 沙參
Root of Adenophora tetraphylla

氣味苦、微寒，無毒。主血結，驚氣，除寒熱，補中，益肺氣。

The qì and flavor are bitter, slightly cold, and non-toxic. [*Shā shēn*] governs blood bind, fright qì, eliminates cold and heat, supplements the center, and boosts the lung qì.

參葉天士：沙參氣微寒，稟水氣而入腎。味苦無毒，得火味而入心。謂其得水氣，以瀉心火之有餘也。心火亢，則所主之血不行而為結，而味之苦可以攻之。心火亢，則所藏之神不寧而生驚，而氣之寒可以平之。心火稟炎上之性，火鬱則寒，火發則熱，而苦寒能清心火，故能除寒熱也。陰者，所以守中者也，苦寒益陰，所以補中。補中則金得土生，又無火剋，所以益肺氣也。

A comparison by Yè Tiānshì: The qì of *shā shēn* is slightly cold, inherits the qì of water, and enters the kidneys. [*Shā shēn's*] flavor is bitter, non-toxic, [and] obtains the fire flavor [which] enters the heart. [This] says that [*shā shēn*] obtains the water qì in order to drain the surplus heart fire. [When the] heart fire is hyperactive, [then] the blood, which it governs, cannot move and is bound, and [thus] the bitterness of [*shā shēn's*] flavor can be used to attack this. [When the] heart fire is hyperactive, [then] the *shén* which [is] stored, is not tranquil and generates fright, and [thus] the coldness of [*shā shēn's*] qì can be used to calm [the fright]. The heart fire inherits the nature of flaming upwards. [When the] fire is depressed, then [there is] cold; [when] the fire emerges, then [there is] heat; but bitter and cold are able to clear heart fire. Therefore, [*shā shēn*] is able to eliminate cold and heat. Yīn, therefore protects the center. Bitter and cold boost the yīn, therefore supplementing the center. If the center is supplemented, then [when] metal is obtained earth is generated, [and] moreover is without the restraint of fire; therefore, [*shā shēn*] boosts the lung qì.

Yuǎn Zhì 遠志
Root of Polygala tenuifolia

氣味苦、溫，無毒。主逆咳傷中，補不足，除邪氣，利九竅，益智慧，耳目聰明，不忘，強志，倍力。久服輕身不老。

The qì and flavor are bitter, warm, and non-toxic. [*Yuǎn zhì*] governs counterflow cough due to center damage, supplements insufficiency, eliminates evil qì, disinhibits the nine orifices, sharpens the wits, sharpens the hearing, brightens the vision, prevents forgetfulness, strengthens the will, and multiplies the power. When taken over a long period of time, it lightens the body and prevents aging.

按：遠志氣溫，稟厥陰風木之氣，入手厥陰心包。味苦，得少陰君火之味，入手少陰心。然心包為相火，而主之者，心也。火不刑金，則咳逆之病愈。火歸土中，則傷中之病愈。主明則下安，安則不外興利除弊兩大事，即「補不足，除邪氣」之說也。心為一身之主宰，凡九竅耳目之類，無一不待其使令，今得遠志以補之，則九竅利，智慧益，耳聰目明，善記不忘，志強力壯，所謂「天君泰，百體從令」者此也。

Commentary: The qì of *yuǎn zhì* is warm, inherits the qì of juèyīn wind and wood, and enters the hand juèyīn pericardium [channel]. The flavor is bitter, obtains the flavor of the sovereign fire shàoyīn, [and] enters the hand shàoyīn heart [channel]. Now, the pericardium is the ministerial fire, and is what governs the heart. If fire does not punish metal, then the disease of counterflow cough is cured. If fire returns to center-earth, then the disease of center damage is cured. If the governor is clear, then the subjects will be at peace. [If the subjects are at] peace, then there is nothing more [important than these] two major issues: promotion [of that which is useful] and elimination [of that which does] harm. This is namely the doctrine of "supplementing [what is] insufficient and eliminating the evil qì." The heart is the ruler of the whole body. Among each of the nine orifices, such as ears and eyes, there is none that does not await [the heart's] orders. Now, when *yuǎn zhì* is used to supplement this, then the nine orifices are disinhibited, the wits are sharpened, hearing is sharpened, and the vision is brightened; [one] is good at remembering, and does not forget, the will is strengthened, and power is fortified. This is what is called "if the heavenly monarch[90] is peaceful, the one hundred body [parts] follow [the monarch's] commands."[91]

---

90. This refers to the heart viscus.

91. This passage is quoted from: Zhū Xī 朱熹 (1130-1200): *Sì Shū Zhāng Jù Jí Zhù, Gào Zǐ Zhāng Jù Shàng* 《四書章句集注·孟子集注》告子章句上 (Collection of Commentaries to Writings from The Four Books, Collection of Comments to Mèngzǐ, first chapter of Gàozǐ's writings), Chapter 4, first chapter on *Gàozǐ*, Line 15. Originally, the idea of the heart as ruler stems from the ancient classic of *Xúnzǐ*: "心居中虛，以治五官，夫是之謂天君。 The heart dwells in the thoracic cavity and governs the five organs, so it is called heavenly ruler." See: *Xún Zǐ, Tiān Lùn* 《荀子》天論 (Xúnzǐ, Discussion on Heaven), Chapter 17, Line 4.

又云：「久服輕身不老者」，即《內經》所謂：「主明則下安，以此養生則壽」之說也。夫曰養生，曰久服，言其為服食之品，不可以之治病，故經方中絕無此味。今人喜用藥丸為補養，久則增氣而成病。唯以補心之藥為主，又以四臟之藥為佐，如四方諸侯，皆出所有以貢天子，即乾綱剛振，天下皆寧之道也。諸藥皆偏，唯專於補心，則不偏。

Shén Nóng further said: "When taken over a long period of time, it lightens the body and prevents aging." This is namely what the *Nèi Jīng* calls: "If the governor is clear, then the subjects [will be at] peace. [If one] uses this [herb] to nurture life, then longevity [can be obtained]."[92] What is spoken of as "nurturing life" and "taking over a long period of time," cannot be used to treat disease; therefore, this is not mentioned in the classical formulas. The people of today are fond of taking medicinal pills to supplement and nurture, [and when this is done over] a long period of time, then there is an increase of qì and formation of disease. Only by using medicinals [that] act to govern and supplement the heart, and by using medicinals [that] act as assistants to the four viscera, [this is] like the feudal princes of the four directions, who pay what they possess as tribute to the Son of Heaven. This means to consolidate the monarchial power,[93] and is always the "way" of peace in the land under heaven. All medicinals always [have] tendencies, [however] only [when a medicinal] specializes in supplementing the heart, then [the medicinal does] not have tendencies.

抱朴子謂：「陵陽子仲，服遠志二十七年，有子三十七人。」開書所視，記而不忘，著其久服之效也。若以之治病，則大失經旨矣。

Bào Pùzǐ[94] said: "Língyáng Zǐzhòng ingested *yuǎn zhì* for twenty-seven years [and] had thirty-seven sons,"[95] [and] what he read in books, he could memorize without forgetting. This proves the efficacy of his taking [*yuǎn zhì*] over a long period of time.[96] If one used [*yuǎn zhì*] to treat diseases, then [this would be] greatly missing the purpose of the classics!

---

92. This passage is quoted from: *Huáng Dì Nèi Jīng Sù Wèn · Líng Lán Mì Diǎn Lùn* 《黃帝內經素問·靈蘭秘典論》 (Inner Canon of the Yellow Emperor, Plain Questions · Discussion on the Profound Canons of the Yellow Emperor's Library) Chapter 8, Line 2.

93. *Qiān gāng kè zhèn* 乾綱剋振 (to arouse the capability of monarchical power), this means to sufficiently consolidate the monarchical power.

94. Bào Pùzǐ 抱朴子 is the nickname of Gě Hóng 葛洪 (284-363 or 283-343), the famous physician, Daoist, alchemist, natural scientist, and chemist from Jiāngsū. *Bào Pùzǐ* 《抱朴子》 is also the title of one of his works. It is divided into inner and outer parts. The former deals with miscellaneous episodes of Gě Hóng's Daoist life; the latter contains Gě Hóng's opinions on Daoist practices. See: Lǐ, 與遠志自上以行於下者有別 1985, p. 596.

95. Daughters were usually not counted, so it is likely, he had around twice as many children.

96. See: *Bào Pùzǐ, Nèi Piān, Xiān Yào* 《抱朴子·內篇，仙藥》 (Bào the name of an immortal. Zǐzhòng 子仲 seems to be a variant for Zǐ Míng 子明, who was an immortal in Chinese folklore.)

Chāng Pú 菖蒲
Rhizome of Acorus gramineus

氣味辛、溫，無毒。主風寒濕痹，咳逆上氣，開心竅，補五臟，通九竅，明耳目，出聲音。主耳聾，癰瘡，溫腸胃，止小便利。久服輕身，不忘，不迷惑，延年，益心智，高志不老。

The qì and flavor are acrid, warm, and non-toxic. [*Chāng pú*] governs wind-cold-damp-impediment and counterflow cough qì ascent, opens the orifice of the heart,[97] supplements the five viscera, frees the nine orifices, clears the ears and eyes, and frees the voice. [*Chāng pú*] governs deafness, welling-abscess sores, warms the intestines and stomach, and stops disinhibited urination. When taken over a long period of time it lightens the body, prevents forgetfulness, prevents confusion, prolongs life, boosts wisdom, heightens the will, and prevents aging.

陳修園曰：菖蒲性用略同遠志，但彼苦而此辛，且生於水石之中，受太陽寒水之氣。其味辛，合於肺金而主表。其氣溫，合於心包絡之經，通於君火而主神。

Chén Xiūyuán said: The nature and use of *chāng pú* is approximately the same as *yuǎn zhì*, but that [medicinal] is bitter and this one is acrid. [*Chāng pú*] grows amongst the water and stones [in creeks, ponds, or marshes], and receives the qì of tàiyáng cold water. The flavor is acrid, unites with lung metal, and governs the exterior. The qì is warm, unites with the channel of the pericardium, communicates with the sovereign fire,[98] and governs the *shén*.

其主風寒濕痹、咳逆上氣者，從肺驅邪以解表也。「開心竅」至末句，皆言補心之效，其功同於遠志。聲音不出，此能入心而轉舌，入肺以開竅也。癰瘡為心火，而此能寧之。心火下濟而光明，故能溫腸胃而止小便利也。但菖蒲稟水精之氣，外通九竅，內濡五臟，其性自下以行於上，與遠志自上以行於下者有別。

[*Chāng pú*] governs wind-cold-damp-impediment and counterflow cough qì ascent. [This] expels evils from the lungs by resolving the exterior. [When this says] "opens the orifice of the heart" at the end of the sentence, all [of this] speaks to the effectivenss of [*chāng pú* in] supplementing the heart. [*Chāng pú's*] action is similar to that of *yuǎn zhì*. If the voice does not issue forth, [*chāng pú*] is able to enter the heart and rotate the tongue, [and it] enters the lungs in order to open the orifices. Welling-

---

97. This means consciousness, spirit mind as well as tongue. See: Wiseman, *Bào Pùzǐ · Inner Part, Medicinals of Immortality*) Chapter 11, Line 20. Língyáng Zǐzhòng 陵陽子仲 1998, p. 421.

98. Heart.

abscess sores are heart fire, and this [medicinal] is able to pacify them. [*Chāng pú*] aids in the descent of heart fire and shines. Therefore, [*chāng pú*] is able to warm the intestines and stomach, and stops disinhibited urination. However, *chāng pú* inherits the qì of water and essence. On the outside, it frees the nine orifices, [and] on the inside, it moistens the five viscera. Compared to [*yuǎn zhì*], the nature [of *chāng pú*] spontaneously descends [heart fire] in order to circulate in the upper body, and *yuǎn zhì* spontaneously ascends [clear qì] in order to circulate in the lower body.

Chì Jiàn 赤箭
Rhizome of Gastrodia elata

氣味辛、溫，無毒。主殺鬼精物，蠱毒惡風。久服益氣力，長陰，肥健。

The qì and flavor are acrid, warm, and non-toxic. [*Chì jiàn*] governs killing demons, *gǔ* 蠱 venom,[99] and malign wind. When taken over a long period of time, [*chì jiàn*] boosts qì and strength, grows the yīn, fattens, and fortifies.

張隱庵曰：赤箭氣味辛溫，其根名天麻者，氣味甘平。蓋赤箭辛溫屬金，金能制風，而有弧矢之威，故主殺鬼精物。天麻甘平屬土，土能勝濕，而居五運之中，故能治蠱毒惡風。天麻形如芋魁，有游子十二枚周環之，以仿十二辰。十二子在外，應六氣之司天。天麻如皇極之居中，得氣運之全，故功同五芝，力倍五參，為仙家服食上品，是以久服益氣力，長陰，肥健。

Zhāng Yǐn'ān said: The qì and flavor of *chì jiàn* is acrid and warm; its root is called *tiān má* (literally: Heavenly Hemp),[100] of which the qì and flavor are sweet and neutral. Now, the acridity and warmth of *chì jiàn* belong to metal, as metal is able to control wind, and has the influence of a bow and arrow,[101] thus it governs killing demonic creatures. The sweetness and neutrality of *tiān má* belongs to earth; earth is able to overcome damp, and it resides in the center of the five movements.[102] Therefore, [*tiān má*] is able to treat *gǔ* venom and malign wind. *Tiān má's* shape resembles

---

99. *Gǔ* 蠱 is a term for a legendary venomous worm. Generally, this refers to the toxin of poisonous insects that damage the liver and spleen with drum distension. According to Wiseman, it denotes various severe conditions, e.g. scrub typhus, severe hepatitis, or amoebic dysentery. See: Wiseman, 1998, p. 250.

100. Today, there is no differenciation between *chì jiàn* 赤箭 and *tiān má* 天麻. Both are gastrodia rhizome. See: Dan Bensky et al.: *Chinese Herbal Medicine. Materia Medica*, 3rd Edition, Eastland Press, Seattle, 2004, p. 972.

101. This connotes a very powerful bow and arrow for shooting the demons, because *chì jiàn* 赤箭 literally means "crimson arrow." Bows and arrows have traditionally been regarded as extremely powerful. For example, there is the myth of Yì the archer, who shot nine suns in order to save the Chinese world from getting scorched.

102. The *wǔ yùn* 五運, the five movements are fire, earth, metal, water and wood. Also see Footnote 55 in the preface.

a large taro [root with] twelve irregular sprouts [which] encircle [the root, and] imitate the twelve earthly branches. The twelve branches [which are] located outside, correspond to the management of the six qì of heaven. *Tiān má* resembles the emperor, who dwells in the center and receives all of the movements of qì. Therefore, [*tiān má's*] function is similar to the five kinds of mushrooms;[103] its power is twice as strong as the five kinds of ginseng,[104] [and] is a medicinal for immortals of the highest grade. Therefore, [if this is] taken over a long period of time, it boosts the qì and strength, fosters the yīn, and fattens and fortifies.

李時珍曰：補益上藥，天麻第一，世人止用之治風，良可惜也！

Lǐ Shízhēn said: Among the supplementing and boosting medicinals of the highest grade, *tiān má* is the best. That the common people stopped using it for treating wind is really a pity!

Chē Qián Zǐ 車前子
Seed of Plantago asiatica

氣味甘、寒，無毒。主氣癃止痛，利水道，通小便，除濕痹。久服輕身耐老。

The qì and flavor are sweet, cold, and non-toxic. [*Chē qián zǐ*] governs qì dribbling block and stops pain, disinhibits the waterways, frees the urine, and eliminates damp impediment. When taken over a long period of time, it lightens the body and makes [one] resistant to old age.

張隱庵曰：車前草，《本經》名當道，《毛詩》名芣苢。

Zhāng Yǐn'ān said: The herb *chē qián* in the *Shén Nóng Běn Cǎo Jīng* is called *dāng dào* 當道 (to be in power) and is called *fóu yǐ* 芣苢 (plantago major) in the *Máo Shī* 《毛詩》 (Book of Odes by the Two Máo).[105]

---

103. According to *Bào Pùzǐ*, *wǔ zhī* 五芝 are the five kinds of mushrooms: *shí zhī* 石芝 (stone ganoderma), *mù zhī* 木芝 (wood ganoderma), *cǎo zhī* 草芝 (grass ganoderma), *ròu zhī* 肉芝 (flesh ganoderma), *jūn zhī* 菌芝 (fungus ganoderma). See: *Bào Pù Zǐ, Nèi Piān, Xiān Yào* 《抱朴子内篇・仙藥》 (Bàopùzǐ Inner Section・Medicinals of Immortality) Chapter 11, Line 2. However, in more recent texts, they are listed as variants in color (greenish-blue, purple, scarlet, yellow, white, and black) of ganoderma lucudum and Ganoderma sinense.

104. The *wǔ shēn* 五參 five kinds of ginseng are: *rén shēn* 人參 (ginseng), *xuán shēn* 玄參 (scrophularia), *dān shēn* 丹參 (salvia), *shā shēn* 沙參 (adenophora), and *kǔ shēn* 苦參 (sophora).

105. This book is listed in the Dynastic History of the *Hàn* as being compiled by father Máo Hēng 毛亨 and son Máo Cháng 毛萇 around the beginning of the Western *Hàn* dynasty (206-23 B.C.). They are regarded as being in the direct lineage of Kǒngzǐ's disciples.

乾坤有動靜，夫坤其靜也翕，其動也辟。車前好生道旁，雖牛馬踐踏不死，蓋得土氣之用，動而不靜者也。氣癃，膀胱之氣閉也。閉則痛，痛則水道不利。車前得土氣之用，土氣行則水道亦行而不癃，不癃則不痛，而小便長矣。土氣行則濕邪散，濕邪散則濕痹自除矣。久服土氣升而水氣布，故能輕身耐老。

Qiān and *kūn*[106] are movement and stillness. *Kūn* is stillness [and] also to gather together, [while *qiān* is] movement [and] also to ward off. *Chē qián* likes to grow beside the road, and although oxen and horses trample on it, [*chē qián*] does not perish. This is because it is able to use the earth qì; [*chē qián*] moves and is not still. Qì dribbling block is blocked qì of the urinary bladder. [When there is] blockage, then [there is] pain. [When there is] pain, then the waterways are inhibited. *Chē qián* is able to use the earth qì, and if the earth qì moves, then the waterways also move, and there is no dribbling block. If there is no dribbling block, then there is no more pain, and urination is fostered! If the earth qì moves, then damp evils are dispersed. If damp evils are dispersed, then the damp impediment is spontaneously eliminated! When taken over a long period of time, the earth qì upbears and water qì spreads throughout. Therefore, [*chē qián*] is able to lighten the body and makes [one] resistant to old age.

《神仙服食經》云：「車前，雷之精也。震為雷為長男。」《詩》言：「采采芣苢」，亦欲妊娠而生男也。

The *Shén Xiān Fú Shí Jīng* 《神仙服食經》 (Dietary Classic of the Immortals)[107] says: "*Chē qián* has the essence of thunder. [The trigram] *zhèn* is thunder and stands for the eldest son."[108] In the *Shī [Jīng]* 《詩[經]》 (Book of Odes) there is a saying that goes: "We gather plantago major…."[109] [The women] also desire to get pregnant and give birth to a son!

---

106. *Qiān* 乾 (heaven) ☰ and *kūn* 坤 (earth) ☷ are trigrams from the *Yì Jīng* 《易經》 (Book of Changes). In combination, they stand for the two polarities heaven and earth, yáng and yin, male and female and so on.

107. This book is first mentioned in the *Suí* dynasty history under the heading of a religious text of medical kind and was probably written by Wèi Huàcún 魏華存 of the *Jìn* dynasty (265-420). See: *Suí Shū, Jīng Jí Zhì, Yī Fāng Lèi Zù Lù* 《隋書》《經籍志》《醫方類著录》 [Dynastic History] of the *Suí* Dynasty, Register of Texts, Recorded Books of Medical Category).

108. The trigram of *zhèn* 震 (to shake or vibrate as with the clap of thunder) ☳ has the nature of *léi* 雷 (thunder) and the family position of eldest son. There is also a hexagram called *zhén wèi léi* 震為雷 (shock) ䷲. It is said to be very auspicious and blesses people with strong children.

109. This is a poem on collecting plantago that was sung by women while picking this herb. See: *Shī Jīng, Guŏ Fēng, Zhōu Nán, Fú Yĭ* 《詩經》《國風》《周南》《芣苢》 (Book of Odes, Lessons from the States, Odes of Zhōu and the South, Plantago). James Legge has translated this complete poem; please see the bibliography for links.

Qiāng Huó 羌活
Root of Notopterygii

氣味苦、甘、辛，無毒。主風寒所擊，金瘡止痛，奔豚，癇痓，女子疝瘕。
久服輕身耐老。一名獨活。

The qì and flavor are bitter, sweet, acrid, and non-toxic. [*Qiāng huó*] governs wind and cold attacks, stops pain in incised wounds, running piglet,[110] epilepsy and tetany, and women's mounting conglomeration.[111] When taken over a long period of time, it lightens the body and makes [one] resistant to old age. *Another name is dú huó.*[112]

陳修園曰：羌活氣平，稟金氣而入肺。味苦甘無毒，得火味而入心，得土味
而入脾。其主風寒所擊者，入肺以御皮毛之風寒，入脾以御肌肉之風寒，入
心助太陽之氣以御營衛之風寒也。其主金瘡止痛者，亦和營衛，長肌肉，完
皮毛之功也。奔豚乃水氣上凌心火，此能入肺以降其逆，補土以制其水，入
心以扶心火之衰，所以主之。

Chén Xiūyuán said: The qì of *qiāng huó* is neutral, inherits the qì of metal, and enters the lungs. The flavor is bitter, sweet, non-toxic, [and] obtains the fire flavor [which] enters the heart, [as well as] the earth flavor [which] enters the spleen. In regards to its governing of wind and cold attack, [*qiāng huó*] enters the lung thereby warding off wind and cold in the skin and hair. It enters the spleen there by warding off wind and cold in the flesh. It enters the heart and assists the qì of tàiyáng to ward off wind and cold in the construction and defense. Concerning its governing of stopping pain in incised wounds, [*qiāng huó*] also harmonizes the construction and defense, grows the flesh, and completes the work of the skin and hair. Running piglet, then, is water qì ascending and intimidating the heart fire, and this [medicinal] is able to enter the lungs thereby downbearing the counterflow. [*Qiāng huó*] supplements the earth, thereby controlling the water, and it enters the heart thereby supporting the debilitated heart fire. Therefore, [*qiāng huó*] governs these [diseases].

癇痓者，木動則生風，風動則挾木勢而害土，土病則聚液而成痰，痰迸於心
則為痓為癇。此物稟金氣以制風，得土味而補脾，得火味以寧心，所以主
之。女子疝瘕，多經行後血假風濕而成，此能入肝以平風，入脾以勝濕，入
心而主宰血脈之流行，所以主之。久服輕身耐老者，著其扶陽之效也。

---

110. This pattern includes kidney accumulation by yīn cold of kidney or liver qì fire. See: Wiseman 1998, p. 510.

111. Mounting conglomeration is a conglomeration of wind, heat, and damp in the small intestine and urinary bladder. See: Wiseman 1998, p. 400.

112. *Dú huó* 獨活 today is pubescent angelica root, so now *qiāng huó* 羌活 and *dú huó* 獨活 are considered to be two different species of medicinal. See: Bensky 2004, p. 323.

Epilepsy and tetany are [caused by] stirring wood [which] results in the generation of wind. Stirring wind then complicates wood's dynamic and harms the earth. When the earth is diseased, then fluids collect and form phlegm. The phlegm spurts into the heart, then causes tetany and epilepsy. This plant inherits the qì of metal in order to control the wind, obtains the flavor of earth, and supplements the spleen. It obtains the flavor of fire thereby quieting the heart. Therefore, [*qiāng huó*] governs these [diseases]. Women's mounting conglomeration is [caused by] false wind and damp forming in the blood after heavy menstruation.[113] This [medicinal] is able to enter the liver, thereby calming the wind; enters the spleen, thereby dominating the damp; and enters the heart, which then governs the circulation of the blood and vessels. Therefore, [*qiāng huó*] governs these [diseases]. When taken over a long period of time, it lightens the body and makes [one] resistant to old age; this is due to [*qiāng huó's*] effect of supporting yáng.

張隱庵曰：此物生苗，一莖直上，有風不動，無風自動，故名獨活。後人以獨活而出於西羌者，名羌活。出於中國，處處有者，名獨活。今觀肆中所市，竟是二種。有云羌活主上，獨活主下，是不可解也。

Zhāng Yǐn'ān said: This plant produces sprouts and its stalk grows straight upward. When it is windy, [*qiāng huó*] does not stir, [but when] the wind is absent, [*qiāng huó*] spontaneously stirs; therefore this is called *dú huó*.[114] The people of later times used the *dú huó* [which is] grown in the western Qiáng area,[115] and called this *qiāng huó*. The [medicinal which] grows everywhere in China, [the ancient people] called this *dú huó*. Currently, [the medicinals that] one sees on display in the markets, are actually two [different] species. Some people say that *qiāng huó* governs the upper [part of the body], while *dú huó* governs the lower; this can not be explained.

Shēng Má 升麻
Rhizome of Cimifuga foetida

氣味甘、平、苦、微寒，無毒。主解百毒，殺百精老物殃鬼，辟瘟疫瘴氣邪氣，蠱毒入口皆吐出，中惡腹痛，時氣毒癘，頭痛寒熱，風腫諸毒，喉痛口瘡。久服不夭，輕身延年。

The qì and flavor are sweet, neutral, bitter, slightly cold, and non-toxic. [*Shēng má*] governs resolving the hundred toxins; kills the one hundred kinds of spirits, old creatures[116] and damage [from]

---

113. The heavy menstruation is due to vacuity in the blood vessels, which causes the internal wind to rise.

114. This is a literal translation, as in moveable by itself, or self-moving.

115. *Xī Qiáng* 西羌 is a term for a tribe that lived in the western part of China. Today it is an ethnic minority in Sìchuān.

116. This means spirits of the dead, ghosts, and wandering souls.

ghosts; repels the evil qì of epidemic disorders and miasmic qì; [repels] *gǔ* toxins that enter the mouth [and] in all cases cause vomiting, as well as nausea and abdominal pain. [*Shēng má*] repels seasonal qì and toxic pestilence with headache, chills and fever, and all toxins [that cause] wind swelling, throat pain, and sores of the mouth. When taken over a long period of time, it prevents premature death, lightens the body, and prolongs life.

張隱庵曰：升麻氣味甘、苦、平，甘者土也，苦者火也，主從中土而達太陽之氣，太陽標陽本寒，故微寒。蓋太陽稟寒水之氣而行於膚表，如天氣之下連於水也。太陽在上，則天日當空，光明清湛。清湛故主解百毒，光明故殺百精老物殃鬼。太陽之氣行於膚表，故辟瘟疫瘴氣邪氣。

Zhāng Yǐn'ān said: The qì and flavor of *shēng má* are sweet, bitter, and neutral. Sweetness belongs to earth; bitterness belongs to fire. [*Shēng má*] governs the qì from within earth and outthrusts the tàiyáng. Tàiyáng is the outward manifestation[117] of yáng, but the root is cold; therefore [*shēng má*] is slightly cold. In this case, tàiyáng inherits the qì of cold water and moves in the skin and exterior. This resembles the descent of heavenly qì which combines with water.[118] When tàiyáng is in the upper [part of the body], then the sun in the heavens is located high above, shining bright and clear. This clarity therefore governs the resolution of the one hundred toxins, and the shining brightness therefore kills the one hundred kinds of spirits, old creatures, and damage [from] ghosts. The qì of tàiyáng circulates in the skin and exterior, therefore, [*shēng má*] repels the evil qì of epidemic disorders and miasmic qì.

太陽之氣行於地中，故蠱毒入口皆吐出。治蠱毒，則中惡腹痛自除。辟瘟疫瘴氣邪氣，則時氣毒癘、頭痛寒熱自散。寒水之氣滋於外而濟於上，故治風腫諸毒、喉痛口瘡。久服，則陰精上滋，故不夭。陽氣盛，故輕身。陰陽充足，則長年矣。

The qì of tàiyáng [also] circulates in center earth. Therefore, [*shēng má* repels] *gǔ* toxins which enter the mouth and in all cases cause vomiting. When [*shēng má*] treats the *gǔ* toxins, then the nausea and abdominal pain are spontaneously eliminated. By repelling the evil qì of epidemic disorders and miasmic qì, then the seasonal qì and toxic pestilence with headache, chills, and fever spontaneously disperse. The qì of cold water enriches the exterior and aids the upper [body]. Therefore, [*shēng má* is able to] treat all toxins with wind swelling, throat pain, and mouth sores. When taken over a long period of time, then the yīn and essence are enriched in the upper [body], and therefore [*shēng má*] prevents premature death. [When] yáng qì is abundant, [it] causes lightness of the body. When yīn and yáng are sufficient, then life is prolonged!

---

117. Also translated as "tip," as in the root and tip or root and branch.

118. Zhāng Yǐn´ān here describes the condensation process that supplies the skin with clear steam from the kidneys and spleen. This forms the defense qì and is compared to the formation of the weather.

嘗考：凡物紋如車輻者，皆有升轉循環之用。防風、秦艽、烏藥、防己、木通、升麻，皆紋如車輻，而升麻更覺空通，所以升轉甚捷也。

Test: All plants with linear markings like spokes of a carriage wheel, are all used to upbear, shift, and circulate. *Fáng fēng, qín jiāo, wū yào*, [*guǎng*] *fáng jǐ, mù tōng*, and *shēng má* all have linear markings like spokes of a carriage wheel, but *shēng má* further feels [that it is] hollow and continuous; therefore [because of this, *shēng má*] upbears and shifts very quickly.

Yīn Chén [Hāo] 茵陳[蒿]
Shoots and leaves of Artemisia capillaris

氣味苦、平、微寒，無毒。主風濕寒熱邪氣，熱結黃疸。久服輕身，益氣，耐老，面白悅，長年。白兔食成仙。

The qì and flavor are bitter, neutral, slightly cold, and non-toxic. [*Yīn chén hāo*] governs the evil qì of wind, damp, cold, and heat, [as well as] heat bind and jaundice. When taken over a long period of time, it lightens the body, boosts the qì, makes [one] resistant to old age, [creates] a luster[119] in the face, and prolongs life. When [this was] eaten by the white rabbit, it became immortal.[120]

張隱庵曰：《經》云：「春三月，此謂發陳。」茵陳因舊苗而春生，蓋因冬令水寒之氣，而具陽春生發之機。主治風濕寒熱邪氣，得生陽之氣，則外邪自散也。結熱黃疸，得水寒之氣，則內熱自除也。久服則生陽上升，故輕身益氣耐老。因陳而生新，故面白悅、長年。兔乃純陰之物，喜食陽春之氣，故白兔食之成仙。

Zhāng Yǐn'ān said: The classic said: "The three months of spring, this speaks of emerging from the old."[121] [For this] reason the old sprouts of *yīn chén* [*hāo*] grow in spring. [This is] because winter's qì is water-cold, and [this] provides the mechanisms of yáng, spring, growth, and emergence. [*Yīn chén hāo*] governs the treatment of the evil qì of wind, damp, cold, and heat, and when the generation of yáng qì is obtained, then the external evils are spontaneously dispersed. In heat bind and jaundice, [when *yīn chén hāo*] obtains the qì of water-cold, then inner heat is spontaneously eliminated. When taken over a long period of time, [*yīn chén hāo*] generates the ascending and upbearing of

---

119. *Bái yuè* literally means white and pleasant.

120. According to Chinese mythology, a white rabbit and a toad live on the moon and produce the elixir of immortality.

121. This is a quotation from the *Huáng Dì Nèi Jīng Sù Wèn* 《黄帝內經素問》 (Inner Canon of the Yellow Emperor Plain Questions), Chapter 1. The beginning of spring in Chinese lunar calendar is between the end of January and the middle of February. *Fā chén* 發陳 "Creating from the old" means: when the vitality of spring blossoms, old things are pushed aside in order to generate new ones.

yáng, therefore it lightens the body, boosts the qì, and makes [one] resistant to old age. Because the old [sprout] generates the new [plant], there is a luster in the face and [one's] life is prolonged. Moreover, rabbits are animals [that] belong to pure yīn. They are fond of eating the qì of yáng and spring. Therefore, the white rabbit became immortal upon eating [*yīn chén hāo*].

[Gān] Jú Huā [甘]菊花
Flower of Chrysanthemum morafolii

氣味苦、平，無毒。主諸風頭眩腫痛，目欲脫淚出，皮膚死肌，惡風，濕痺。久服利血氣，輕身耐老延年。

The qì and flavor are bitter, neutral, and non-toxic. It governs all cases of wind with swollen, painful head and dizzy vision, where the eyes desire to shed tears, [there is] numbness of the skin and muscles, aversion to wind, and damp impediment. When taken over a long period of time, [*gān jú huā*] benefits the blood and qì, lightens the body, makes [one] resistant to old age, and prolongs life.

徐靈胎曰：凡芳香之物皆能治頭目肌表之疾。但香則無不辛燥者，惟菊得天地秋金清肅之氣而不甚燥烈，故於頭目風火之疾尤宜焉。

Xú Língtāi said: In general, all aromatic plants have the ability to treat diseases of the head, eyes, and fleshy exterior. However, there are no aromatic [medicinals] without an acrid and drying [effect]; only [*gān*] jú huā obtains the clearing and clarifying qì of autumn and metal qì from heaven and earth, while [it also is] not severely drying and harsh. Therefore, [*gān jú huā*] is especially suitable for [treating] wind and fire diseases in the head and eyes!

Lóng Dǎn 龍膽
Root and rhizome of Gentiana scabra

氣味苦、澀、大寒，無毒。主骨間寒熱，驚癇邪氣，續絕傷，定五臟，殺蟲毒。

The qì and flavor are bitter, astringent, greatly cold, and non-toxic. [*Lóng dǎn*] governs heat and cold in-between the bones, fright epilepsy, and evil qì. [It] replenishes damage [from] expiry, stabilizes the five viscera, and kills *gǔ* toxins.

張隱庵曰：龍乃東方之神，膽主少陽甲木，苦走骨，故主骨間寒熱。澀類酸，故除驚癇邪氣。膽主骨，肝主筋，故續絕傷。五臟六腑皆取決於膽，故定五臟。山下有風曰蠱，風氣升而蠱毒殺矣。

Zhāng Yǐn'ān said: Dragons are the deities of the East; bile[122] governs *jiǎ* wood.[123] The bitter [flavor] penetrates the bones. Therefore, [*lóng dǎn*] governs cold and heat in-between the bones. Astringent belongs to the category of sour. Therefore, [*lóng dǎn*] eliminates fright epilepsy and evil qì. The gallbladder governs the bones, and the liver governs the tendons; therefore, [*lóng dǎn*] replenishes damage [from] expiry. The five viscera and the six bowels all depend on the gallbladder. Therefore, [*lóng dǎn*] stabilizes the five viscera. On the foot of mountains there is a wind called *gǔ*.[124] Wind and qì upbear and [when one takes *lóng dǎn*] the *gǔ* is killed!

Zǐ Sū 紫蘇
Foliage of Perilla frutescens

氣味辛、微溫，無毒。主下氣，殺穀除飲食，辟口臭，去邪毒，辟惡氣。久服通神明，輕身耐老。

The qì and flavor are acrid, slightly warm, and non-toxic. [*Zǐ sū*] governs the descent of qì, kills the grains,[125] eliminates food and drink [amassment], repels bad breath, removes evil toxins, and repels malign qì. When taken over a long period of time, [*zǐ sū*] improves the mental abilities,[126] lightens the body, and makes [one] resistant to old age.

述：紫蘇氣微溫，稟天之春氣而入肝。味辛，得地之金味而入肺。主下氣者，肺行其治節之令也。殺穀除飲食者，氣溫達肝，肝疏暢而脾亦健運也。辟口臭、去邪毒、辟惡氣者，辛中帶香，香為天地之正氣，香能勝臭，即能解毒，又能勝邪也。久服則氣爽神清，故通神明，輕身耐老。其子下氣尤速。其梗下氣寬脹，治噎膈反胃，止心痛。旁小枝通十二經關竅脈絡。

Narration: The qì of *zǐ sū* is slightly warm, inherits the qì of spring from heaven, and enters the liver. The flavor is acrid, obtains the metal flavor of earth, and enters the lung. [*Zǐ sū*] governs the descent

---

122. Zhāng Yǐn'ān speaks of dragons and bile, because the literal translation of *lóng dǎn* 龍膽 is: dragon bile.

123. S1 wood *jiǎ mù* 甲木 is the first of the ten heavenly stems and stands for the foot shàoyáng gallbladder meridian.

124. *Shān xià yóu fēng, gǔ.* 山下有風，蠱。 (When there is wind below the mountains, it is *gǔ*.) This is a citation from a commentary to the *Zhōu Yì, Gǔ Gǔ* 《周易》《䷑蠱》 (Book of Changes, Hexagram *Gǔ* 蠱䷑), Chapter 18, line 1. This hexagram stands for compensation.

125. "Kills the grains" is a metaphor which means "to cause swift digestion."

126. This sentence can also be translated as: facilitates the enlightenment of the spirit.

of qì; this is [because] lung's movement causes this [to be] managed and regulated.[127] [Zǐ sū] kills the grains, eliminates food and drink [amassment]; this is [because] the warm qì outthrusts the liver. [When one] facilitates the coursing of the liver, then the spleen's transportation [function] is also strengthened. [Zǐ sū] repels bad breath, removes evil toxins, and repels malign qì; this is [because] of the acrid fragrance within [zǐ sū], and the fragrance is the right qì of heaven and earth. [What is] fragrant is able to dominate [that which] smells; accordingly [zǐ sū] is able to resolve toxins, and it is further able to dominate evil [qì]. When taken over a long period of time, the qì is invigorated and the spirit clears. Therefore, [zǐ sū] improves the mental abilities, lightens the body, and makes [one] resistant to old age. [Zǐ sū's] seeds (fruits) are particularly quick at descending the qì. Its stalks descend the qì and loosen distention. [Zǐ sū] cures dysphagia-occlusion[128] and stomach reflux, and stops heart pain. The small twigs on the sides [of zǐ sū] open the twelve channels [which] pass [through] the orifices, vessels, and collaterals.

Ǒu Shí, Jīng 藕實，莖
Node of Nelumbo nucifera

氣味甘、平。主補中養神，益氣力，除百疾。久服輕身耐老，不飢延年。

The qì and flavor are sweet and neutral. [Ǒu shí, jīng] governs the supplementation of the center, nourishes the spirit, boosts the qì and strength, and eliminates the hundred diseases. When taken over a long period of time, it lightens the body, makes [one] resistant to old age, prevents hunger, and prolongs life.

---

127. In *Huáng Dì Nèi Jīng Sù Wèn* 《黃帝內經素問》 (Inner Canon of the Yellow Emperor, Plain Questions), Chapter 8, it says: "肺者，相傅之官，治節出焉。 The lung is the organ of the assistant, and [it] manages the regulation and issuing forth." Then in the *Lèi Jīng* 《類經》 (Categorized Classic) in Chapter 3, Section 1, Zhāng Jǐngyuè 張景岳 commented: 肺與心皆居膈上，位高近君，猶之宰輔，故稱相傅之官。肺主氣，氣調則營衛臟腑無所不治，故曰治節出焉。節，制也。 Lung and heart both reside above the diaphragm; [their] position is high near the sovereign, and this is similar to governing and supporting. Therefore it is the organ of assistance and balance. The lung governs the qì. [When] the qì is regulated, then [as to] the *yíng* and *wèi*, and viscera and bowels, there is nothing that cannot be treated. Therefore this says: [This] manages the regulation and issuing forth. Regulation is to control. (JS)

128. Dysphagia-occlusion is difficulty in swallowing and vomiting of food [which has] just been eaten. Wiseman 1998, p. 163.

Jī Tóu Shí 雞頭實
Seeds of Euryale ferox

氣味甘、平。主濕痹，腰脊膝痛，補中，除暴疾，益精氣，強志，令耳目聰明。久服輕身不飢，耐老，神仙。

The qì and flavor are sweet and neutral. [*Jī tóu shí*] governs damp impediment, lower-back and knee pain, supplements the center, eliminates fulminant diseases, boosts the essence and qì, strengthens the will, and causes the hearing to sharpen and the vision to brighten. When taken over a long period of time, [*jī tóu shí*] lightens the body, prevents hunger, makes [one] resistant to old age, and [when ingested, bestows] immortality.

Hēi Zhī Má 黑芝麻
Black seeds of Sesamum indicum

氣味甘、平，無毒。主傷中虛羸，補五內，益氣力，生長肌肉，填髓腦。久服輕身不老。色黑者良。

The qì and flavor are sweet, neutral, and non-toxic. [*Hēi zhī má*] governs damage to the center with vacuity emaciation. It supplements the five internal organs, boosts the qì and strength, generates and grows the flesh, and replenishes the marrow and brain. When taken over a long period of time, [*hēi zhī má*] lightens the body, and prevents aging. *Black [hēi zhī má] are excellent.*

Yì Mǔ Cǎo Zǐ 益母草子
Seeds of Leonurus artemisia

氣味辛，甘、微溫，無毒。主明目益精，除水氣。久服輕身延年。

The qì and flavor are acrid, sweet, slightly warm, and non-toxic. [*Yì mǔ cǎo zǐ*] governs brightening the eyes, boosting the essence, and eliminating water qì. When taken over a long period of time, [*yì mǔ cǎo zǐ*] lightens the body, and prolongs life.

今人奉為女科專藥，往往誤事，且其獨具之長反掩。

People of today esteem [yì mǔ cǎo zǐ] as a special medicinal for gynecology, [but] frequently this is a mistake. Moreover, [yì mǔ cǎo zǐ's] unique talents and strong points are on the contrary hidden from view.[129]

Qiàn Cǎo [Gēn] 茜草[根]
Root of Rubia cordifolia

氣味苦、寒，無毒。主寒濕風痹，黃疸，補中。

The qì and flavor are bitter, cold, and non-toxic. [*Qiàn cǎo gēn*] governs cold-damp-wind-impediment, jaundice, and supplements the center.

陳修園曰：氣味苦寒者，得少陰之氣化也。風寒濕三氣合而為痹，而此能入手足少陰，俾上下交通而旋轉，則痹自愈矣。上下交通則中土自和，斯有補中之效矣。中土和則濕熱之氣自化，而黃疸愈矣。

Chén Xiūyuán said: The qì and flavor are bitter and cold; this is [because *qiàn cǎo*] obtains the qì transformation of shàoyīn. The three qì of wind, cold, and damp combine and become impediment. This [medicinal] is able to enter the hand and foot shàoyīn, [which] enables communication [between] the upper and lower body and reverses the condition; then the impediment is spontaneously cured! When there is communication between the upper and lower body, then the center earth naturally harmonizes, so this [medicinal] is effective at supplementing the center! When the center earth is harmonized, then the qì of damp and heat naturally transform, and [thus] jaundice is cured!

又《素問》以蘆茹一兩，烏鰂魚骨四兩，丸以雀卵，飲以鮑魚汁，治氣竭肝傷、脫血、血枯，婦人血枯經閉，丈夫陰痿精傷，名曰四烏鰂骨一蘆茹丸。

Furthermore, in the *Sù Wèn* [there is the following passage]: take one *liàng*[130] of *lú rú*,[131] four *liàng* of *wū zéi yú gǔ* and make them into pills as big as a sparrow's egg. Then [swallow the pills by] drink-

---

129. Thank you to Eran Even and Lorraine Wilcox for giving second and third renderings of this line. The gist of this line according to Wilcox is: "The author is saying that even though people today use it for women's issues, that isn't correct; however, what it is especially good for... we don't know."

130. In modern times, one *liàng* equals to approximately 15.6 grams (when assumed that the *Sù Wèn* was compiled between the first and second century B.C.). During the first and second century B.C., a *liǎng* during the era of the *Shén Nóng Běn Cǎo Jīng*, equaled about 14.4 grams; so in this case, four *liàng* is about 60 grams.

131. The character combination *lú rú* 蘆茹 is today reversed into *rú lú* 茹蘆.

ing with abalone juice. This treats qì exhaustion, liver damage, blood desertion, blood desiccation, women's blood desiccation and menstrual block, as well as men's impotence, and seminal damage. The name [for this famous prescription] is: *Sì Wū Zéi Gǔ Yī Lú Rú Wán* 四烏鰂骨一蘆茹丸.[132]

lú rú	蘆茹	一兩	15 grams
wū zéi yú gǔ	烏鰂魚骨	四兩	60 grams

蘆茹即茜草也，亦取其入少陰以生血，補中宮以統血 。汁可染絳，似血而能行血歟 。

Lú rú is namely *qiàn cǎo*. [One can] also apply [the medicinal to] enter the shàoyīn channel in order to engender blood, [and] supplement the central palace in order to control the blood. The juice of [*qiàn cǎo gēn*] can dye [things] a crimson [color, which] resembles blood and [this juice] is able to move blood!

後人以此三味入烏骨白絲毛雞腹內， 以陳酒、 童便煮爛， 烘乾為丸。以百勞水下五七十丸， 治婦人倒經血溢於上、 男子咳嗽吐血、 左手關脈弦， 背上畏寒， 有瘀血者。

The people of later generations use these three ingredients,[133] inside the abdomen of a wū gǔ bái sī máo jī,[134] and decoct with chén jiǔ and tóng biàn until soft, oven-dry, and make into pills. Swallow five, seven, or ten pills with bǎi láo shuǐ.[135] This treats women's inverted menstruation with blood spilling over in the upper body, men's coughing and spitting of blood, a wiry left guān pulse, fear of cold on the upper back, and blood stasis.

132. *Four of Cuttlefish Bone One of Rubia Root Pill*. This passage is not a literal quotation. See: *Huáng Dì Nèi Jīng, Sù Wèn·Fù Zhōng Lùn* 《黃帝內經素問·腹中論》 (Inner Canon of the Yellow Emperor Plain Questions·Discussion on the Inner Abdomen), Chapter 40, Line 2.

133. Rubia root, cuttlefish bone, and abalone juice.

134. *Wū gǔ bái sī máo jī* 烏骨白絲毛雞 (black-boned silky fowl) is Gallus gallus domesticus Brisson, a chicken with silky white feathers and black skin, meat and bones. Another name is *yào jī* 藥雞 (medicinal chicken). See: Bensky 2004, p. 504.

135. *Bǎi láo shuǐ* 百勞水 (medically prepared water) refers to flowing water that has been stirred intensely with a spoon for "one thousand" times to produce bubbles, and subsequently is used for decocting the medicine. The method was invented by Zhāng Zhòngjǐng and is called *gān lán shuǐ fǎ* 甘瀾水法 (the method of worked water). The idea is to turn water, which is salty and heavy, into a sweet and light substance. See: *Zhōng Guo Yī Xuě Dà Cí Diǎn* 《中國醫學大辭典》 (Great Dictionary of Chinese Medicine), 1988, Volume 1, p. 817.

Fú Líng 茯苓
Dried fungus of Poria cocos

氣味甘、平，無毒。主胸脅逆氣，憂恚驚邪恐悸，心下結痛，寒熱煩滿咳逆，口焦舌乾，利小便。久服安魂養神，不飢延年。

The qì and flavor are sweet, neutral, and non-toxic. [*Fú líng*] governs counterflow qì of the chest and rib-sides, anxiety, anger, fright evil, fear palpitations, painful binds below the heart, chills and fever with vexation and fullness, counterflow cough [qì ascent], parched mouth, and dry tongue, and it disinhibits urination. When taken over a long period of time, [*fú líng*] pacifies the *hún*, nourishes the *shén*, prevents hunger, and prolongs life.

陳修園曰：茯苓氣平入肺，味甘入脾。肺能通調，脾能轉輸，其功皆在於「利小便」一語。胸為肺之部位，脅為肝之部位，其氣上逆則憂恚驚邪恐悸，七情之用因而弗調。心下為太陽之部位，水邪停留則結痛。水氣不化則煩滿。凌於太陰則咳逆。客於營衛則發熱惡寒。內有宿飲則津液不升，為口焦舌乾，唯得小便一利，則水行而氣化，諸疾俱愈矣。久服安魂養神、不飢延年者，以肺金為天，脾土為地，位一身之天地，而明其上下交和之效也。

Chén Xiūyuán said: The neutral qì of *fú líng* enters the lungs, and the sweet flavor enters the spleen. The lung is able to clear and harmonize, the spleen is able to shift and transport. In one word, [*fú líng's*] function consists entirely of "disinhibiting urination." The chest is the place of the lungs and the rib-sides are the place of the liver. If the [patient's] qì ascends counterflow, then [there is] anxiety, anger, fright evil, and fear palpitations; therefore the application of the seven emotions is not regulated. [The region] below the heart is the place of the tàiyáng, [and when] water evil collects and lodges here, then [there are] painful binds. [When] the water qì is not transformed, there is vexation and fullness. [When the water] intimidates tàiyīn, then [there is] counterflow cough [qì ascent. If the water evil] "visits" the *yíng* and *wèi*, then [there is] fever and aversion to cold. If there is abiding rheum in the inner body, then the fluids cannot upbear, and this causes the mouth to be parched and tongue to be dry. Only when the urination is completely disinhibited, then the water moves and the qì transforms, and the various diseases are all cured! When taken over a long period of time, [*fú líng*] pacifies the *hún* and nourishes the *shén*. It prevents hunger and prolongs life, because lung metal acts as heaven, [and] spleen earth acts as earth. [In this case], heaven and earth [act] as the whole body, and [for this reason *fú líng*] is clearly effective in harmonizing the communication of above and below.

Zhū Líng 豬苓
Polyporus umbellatus

氣味甘、平，無毒。主痎瘧，解毒，蠱疰不祥，利水道。久服輕身耐老。

The qì and flavor are sweet, neutral, and non-toxic. [*Zhū líng*] governs malaria, resolves toxins, [governs] inauspicious summer influx,[136] and disinhibits the waterways. When taken over a long period of time, it lightens the body and makes [one] resistant to old age.

陳修園曰：豬苓氣平，稟金氣而入肺。味甘無毒，得土味而入脾。肺主治節，脾主轉輸，所以能利水道。又考此物，出土時帶甘，久則淡然無味，無味則歸於膀胱。膀胱為太陽，其說有二：一曰經絡之太陽，一曰六氣之太陽。

Chén Xiūyuán said: The qì of *zhū líng* is neutral, inherits the qì of metal, and enters the lungs. The flavor is sweet and non-toxic, obtains the earth flavor [and] enters the spleen. The lungs govern management and regulation and the spleen governs shifting and transport; therefore, [*zhū líng*] is able to disinhibit the waterways. Further investigation into this medicinal [shows that] at the time it is dug from the earth [*zhū líng*] is sweet. [After] a long period of time, then [it] becomes bland and flavorless, and what is flavorless belongs to the urinary bladder. [In regards to] the urinary bladder being tàiyáng, there are two theories: the first says [that] tàiyáng [is] the channel and collateral, and the second says [that] tàiyáng [is one of] the six qì.

何謂經絡之太陽？其腑在下而主水，得上焦肺氣之化，中焦脾氣之運，則下焦愈治。所謂上焦如霧，中焦如漚，下焦如瀆。俾決瀆之用行於州都，則州都中自有雲行雨施之景象，利水如神，有由來也，且不獨利水道也。

What is the tàiyáng channel and collateral? The bowel is located below and governs water. [When] it obtains the transformation of the lung qì from the upper *jiāo*, and the transportation of spleen qì from the middle *jiāo*, then the lower *jiāo* recovers. What is called the upper *jiāo* is like fog, the middle *jiāo* is like foam, and the lower *jiāo* is like a sluice. If the movement of the urinary bladder is used to keep the sluices clear, then within the urinary bladder naturally [this] has the appearance of moving the clouds and distributing rain. [*Zhū líng's* ability to] disinhibit water is as if divine [and this] is [where this] comes from. Moreover, [*zhū líng*] does not only disinhibit the waterways.

---

136. *Gǔ zhù* 蠱疰 (summer influx or infixation) is one kind of damp obstruction caused by summer-heat. See: Wiseman 1998, p. 592.

六氣之太陽名曰巨陽，應天道居高而衛外，乃君心之藩籬也。凡風寒初感，無非先入太陽之界，治不得法，則留於膜原而為瘧，久則為痎「即傷寒雜病似瘧非瘧者，皆在此例」。但得豬苓之通利水道，水行氣化，水精四布，濈濈汗出，則營衛和而諸邪俱解。仲景五苓散、桂枝去桂加茯苓白朮湯非於此得其悟機乎？

Tàiyáng of the six qì is called the great yáng. [Great yáng] corresponds to the Dào of heaven, dwells high above, and guards the outside [of the body, and] therefore is the barrier of the sovereign heart. Ordinarily [when] wind-cold is initially contracted, [the wind-cold] only first enters the boundary of tàiyáng, and as a rule if this is not treated, then [the wind-cold] will lodge in the membrane source and cause malaria. [If the malaria is] chronic, then [it will] become malaria. ([This is] then [why] the *Shāng Hán Zá Bìng Lùn* 《傷寒雜病論》 (Treatise on Cold Damage and the Various Diseases) [said]: "This resembles malaria, but is not malaria,"[137] [and] this is always the case.) Nevertheless, [because] *zhū líng* is able to unblock and disinhibit the waterways, the water moves, the qì transforms, [and] the water essence spreads throughout the four [limbs. When the] sweat issues forth in streams, then the *yíng* and *wèi* are harmonized and the various evils all resolve. Is it not on the basis of *Wǔ Líng Sǎn* and *Guì Zhī Qù Guì Jiā Fú Líng Bái Zhú Tāng* that Zhòngjǐng obtained his insight?

若陽明之渴欲飲水，小便不利，少陰之咳嘔而渴，心煩不眠，熱瘧多兼此症。總於利水道中，布達太陽之氣，使天水循環，滋其枯燥，即仲景豬苓湯之義也。且太陽為天，光明清湛，清湛則諸毒可解，光明則蠱疰不祥自除。

For example, [with] the thirst of yángmíng [patterns, there is] desire to drink water, [with] inhibited urination. In shàoyīn [patterns, there is] cough, retching, and thirst, as well as vexation of the heart with inability to sleep. In heat malaria, these symptoms often exist concurrently. In general, [the ability of *zhū líng* is] to disinhibit the waterways, spread throughout, and thrust out the qì of tàiyáng, causing heavenly water to circulate [and] enrich [that which is] dessicated and dry. [This] then is the significance of Zhòngjǐng's *Zhū Líng Tāng*. Moreover, tàiyáng is heaven; [it] shines bright and clear. The clear then can resolve all toxins. The shining and brightness, then naturally eliminate the inauspicious summer influx.

又云：久服輕身耐老者，溺得陽氣之化而始長，溺出不能遠射，陽氣衰於下也。溺出及溺已時頭搖者，頭為諸陽之會，從下以驗其上之衰也。此皆老態，得豬苓助太陽之氣而可耐之。然此特聖人開太陽之治法，非謂豬苓平淡之可賴也。

[Shén Nóng] further said: "When taken over a long period of time, [*zhū líng*] lightens the body and makes [one] resistant to old age." [This is because] the urine obtains the transformation of yáng qì

---

137. See: Mitchell et al., 1999, p. 125.

and begins to grow. [However], when the urine issues forth, [but] is unable to shoot far, [this is because the] yáng qì is debilitated in the lower [body. If the patient] has shaking of the head from the time the urine issues forth until urination ceases, this is because the head is the confluence of all the yáng channels. Observe the lower [body] in order to check the debilitation of the upper [body]. These are all conditions of the elderly, [and because] *zhū líng* is able to assist the qì of tàiyáng, the [elderly] can resist these [conditions]. So, [in] this distinguished sage's treatment method of opening tàiyáng, [Zhòngjǐng] does not say [that one] can rely on *zhū líng's* neutral and bland [flavors].

Mǔ Guì 牡桂
Bark of Cinnamonum cassia[138]

氣味辛、溫，無毒。主上氣咳逆，結氣喉痹，吐吸，利關節，補中益氣。久服通神，輕身不老。

The qì and flavor is acrid, warm, and non-toxic. [*Mǔ guì*] governs qì ascent, counterflow cough, bound qì, throat impediment,[139] [and difficulties with the rhythm of] exhalation and inhalation.[140] [It also] disinhibits the joints, supplements the center, and boosts qì. When taken over a long period of time, [*mǔ guì*] frees the *shén*, lightens the body, and prevents aging.

牡，陽也。牡桂者，即今之桂枝、桂皮也、菌根也。菌桂即今之肉桂、厚桂也。然生發之機在枝乾，故仲景方中所用俱是桂枝，即牡桂也。時醫以桂枝發表，禁不敢用，而所用肉桂，又必刻意求備，皆是為施治不愈，卸罪巧法。

Male[141] is yáng. *Mǔ guì*, then, is today's *guì zhī* (cinnamon twig), *guì pí* (cinnamon bark), and *jūn gēn* (the root of incense wood). *Jūn* [*gēn*], then, is today's *ròu guì* (cassia) and *hòu guì* (thick cinnamon). So the mechanism of [*mǔ guì*] emerges and grows in the twigs and stems, and therefore within Zhòngjǐng's formulas that which is used, without exception, is *guì zhī*, [which] is namely *mǔ guì*. Contemporary physicians do not dare to use *guì zhī* in order to effuse the exterior, but use *ròu guì* and [therefore] must be meticulous and demanding [in their] preparation. However, [the prepara-

---

138. *Mǔ guì* 牡桂 is male cinnamon. The soft branches of the camphor tree family of cinnamomum cassiae are *guì zhī* 桂枝 (cinnamon twig); the trunk bark and branch bark of cinnamomum cassiae are *ròu guì* 肉桂, and what is referred to in this passage as male cinnamon and the species of cassia are in reality one and the same thing. The so called *jūn guì* 菌桂 (incense wood) is the same as today's highest-quality cinnamon (official cinnamon).

139. *Hóu bì* 喉痹 (throat impediment) is a generic name for swelling and soreness of the throat and is usually caused by either externally contracted wind-heat or yīn vacuity. See: Wiseman, 1998, p. 611.

140. This pattern could be compared to what is now called chronic obstructive pulmonary disease (COPD).

141. The *mǔ* 牡 of *mǔ guì* 牡桂 means: male animal.

tion] is all a clever method for shifting the blame in case there is no recovery [after the] treatment [is] applied.

張隱庵曰：桂本凌冬不凋，氣味辛溫，其色紫赤，水中所生之木火也。肺腎不交，則為上氣咳逆之證。桂啟水中之生陽，上交於肺，則上氣平而咳逆除矣。結氣喉痹者，三焦之氣不行於肌腠，則結氣而為喉痹。桂稟少陽之木氣，通利三焦，則結氣通而喉痹可治矣。吐吸者，吸不歸根即吐出也。桂能引下氣與上氣相接，則吸入之氣直至丹田而後出，故治吐吸也。

Zhāng Yǐn'ān said: The root of *guì* does not wither in winter. Its qì and flavor are acrid and warm. The color is purplish-red; wood and fire are generated from within water. [When the] lungs and kidneys do not interact, then there are the signs of qì ascent and counterflow cough. [*Mǔ*] *guì* initiates the generation of yáng within water, which ascends to interact in the lungs, [and] results in calming the qì ascent and eliminating the counterflow cough! In regards to the bound qì and throat impediment, [when] the qì of the sānjiāo does not move in the interstices of the flesh, then the qì is bound and causes throat impediment. [When *mǔ*] *guì* inherits the wood qì of shàoyáng, and unblocks and disinhibits the sānjiāo, then the bound qì is freed and the throat impediment can be treated! The [difficulties with the rhythm of] exhalation and inhalation, [occur because] the inhalation does not return to its root[142] and then is released. [*Mǔ*] *guì* is able to guide the descending qì joining [this] together with the ascending qì. Then the breath of inhalation [is drawn in] until [it reaches] the *dān tián*[143] and afterwards is exhaled. Therefore, [*mǔ guì*] treats [difficulties with the rhythm of] exhalation and inhalation.

關節者，兩肘、兩腋、兩髀、兩膕皆機關之室，周身三百六十五節，皆神氣之周行。桂助君火之氣，使心主之神氣而出入於機關，游行於骨節，故利關節也。補中益氣者，補中焦而益上下之氣也。久服則陽氣盛而光明，故通神明。三焦通會元真於肌腠，故輕身不老。

The joints, [namely] both elbows, both armpits, both hips, and the two popliteal fossa, are all the internal workings of the mechanism [of movement]. The whole body has three hundred and sixty-five joints, and they all circulate the *shén* qì.[144] [*Mǔ*] *guì* assists the qì of sovereign fire. It enables the *shén* qì, [which is] governed by the heart, to exit and enter from the mechanism, and travel into the joints; therefore, [*mǔ guì* is able to] disinhibit the joints. [It] supplements the center and boosts the qì [because] it supplements the middle *jiāo* and boosts the qì of the upper and lower [body]. When taken over a long period of time, the yáng qì is abundant and shines. Therefore, [*mǔ guì*] frees the

---

142. This means: returning to the kidneys.

143. *Dān tián* 丹田 (cinnabar field) is the region three inches below the umbilicus. Wiseman, 1998, p. 62.

144. *Shén qì* 神氣 (spirit qì) refers to the spirit, the channel qì, the right qì, the blood, and the yáng qì of the viscera and bowels. See: Wiseman, 1998, p. 55.

shén míng. The sānjiāo connects and gathers the true origin[145] into the interstices of the flesh. There-fore, [*mǔ guì*] lightens body, and prevents aging.

徐忠可曰：近來腎氣丸、十全大補湯俱用肉桂，蓋雜溫暖於滋陰藥中，故無礙。至桂枝湯，因作傷寒首方，又因有春夏禁用桂枝之說，後人除有汗發熱惡寒一證，他證即不用，甚至春夏則更守禁藥不敢用矣。不知古人用桂枝，取其宣通血氣，為諸藥向導。即腎氣丸古亦用桂枝，其意不止於溫下也。

Xú Zhōngkě[146] said: Lately in both *Shèn Qì Wán* and *Shí Quán Dà Bǔ Tāng, ròu guì* is used. There-fore, [one can] mix warm [medicinals] into yīn-enriching medicinals, without hindering [the yīn-enriching medicinals. Thus one] arrives at *Guì Zhī Tāng*, because it is the chief formula for cold damage, and also because of the theory that the use of *guì zhī* is prohibited in spring and summer. People of later generations [only use *Guì Zhī Tāng*] for the single pattern of sweating with aversion to cold and fever; for other patterns, then [*Guì Zhī Tāng* is] not used. Even more, [upon] the arrival of spring and summer, then [one] further observes the prohibition and does not dare to use [this medicinal! Contemporary physicians] do not know that the people of antiquity used *guì zhī* to diffuse and free the blood and qì, [and that it] is a guide for all other medicinals. Hence, in antiq-uity *Shèn Qì Wán* also contained *guì zhī*, and the intention [of this formula] is not limited to warm precipitation.

他如《金匱》論虛損十方，而七方用桂枝。孕妊用桂枝湯安胎。又桂苓丸去癥。產後中風面赤，桂枝、附子、竹葉並用。產後乳子煩亂，嘔逆，用竹皮大丸。內加桂枝，治熱煩。又附方於建中加當歸為內補。然則，桂枝豈非通用之藥？若肉桂則性熱下達，非下焦虛寒者不可用，而人反以為通用，宜其用之而多誤矣。餘自究心《金匱》以後，其用桂枝取效，變幻出奇，不可方物，聊一拈出以破時人之惑。

This is like the ten prescriptions for vacuity detriment[147] discussed in the *Jīn Guì Yào Lüè*: [where] seven of these formulae use *guì zhī*. [When] used in pregnancy, *Guì Zhī Tāng* quiets the fetus. Fur-ther, *Guì Líng Wán* eliminates concretions. [In] postpartum wind strike with red face, *guì zhī, fù zǐ,* and *zhú yè* also are used. [In] postpartum vexation and confusion of a suckling child with counter-flow retching, use *Zhú Pí Dà Wán.* When *guì zhī* is added, [this] treats heat vexation. Moreover, the

---

145. *Yuán zhēn* 元真 or *zhēn yuán* 真元 (true origin) is original qì in its relationship to the kidneys. See: Wiseman, 1998, p. 629. Another possibility is: original qì (kidney qì) plus true qì (congenital qì and grain qì). The meaning is the same.

146. Xú Zhōngkě 徐忠可 is Xú Bīn 徐彬 (seventeenth century), a physician who wrote an important com-mentary to the *Jīn Guì Yào Lüè* 《金匱要略》 (Essential Prescriptions of the Golden Cabinet) with the title *Jīn Guì Yào Lüè Lùn Zhù* 《金匱要略論注》 (Treatise on the Essential Prescriptions of the Golden Cabinet) published 1671. See: Lǐ, 1985, p. 507.

147. *Xū sǔn* 虛損 (vacuity detriment) is any kind of severe chronic insufficiency of qì, yīn, yáng, or blood. See: Wiseman, 1998, p. 646.

attached formula [in the *Jīn Gùi Yào Lüè*] of *Jiàn Zhōng Jiā Dāng Guī* (Fortify the Center with Dāng Guī Added) acts to supplement the interior.[148] If this is the case, how can it be that *guì zhī* is not a commonly used medicinal? If *ròu guì's* nature is hot and outthrusts to the lower [body, then if there is] not vacuity cold of the lower *jiāo*, this cannot be used. Conversely when people regard it as commonly used, there are many mistakes made in [*ròu guì's*] proper usage! After I personally studied the *Jīn Gùi Yào Lüè* with concentration, I applied *guì zhī* effectively, [without] unusual fluctuations, [and for those who] cannot distinguish, I merely have to draw [upon] one of these [prescriptions] to break contemporary people's doubts.

陳修園曰：《 金匱 》謂氣短有微飲，宜從小便出之，桂苓甘朮湯主之，腎氣丸亦主之 。

Chén Xiūyuán said: The *Jīn Gùi Yào Lüè* says, if in shortness of breath there is mild fluid retention, it is appropriate to discharge through urine, [therefore both] *Guì Líng Gān Zhú Tāng*[149] and *Shèn Qì Wán* govern this.

喻嘉言注：呼氣短，宜用桂苓甘朮湯以化太陽之氣 。吸氣短，宜用腎氣丸以納少陰之氣 。二方俱借桂枝之力，市醫不曉也 。第桂枝為上品之藥，此時卻塞於遇，而善用桂枝之人，亦與之同病 。

Yù Jiāyán[150] comments: [If there is] shortness of breath on exhale, it is appropriate to use *Guì Líng Gān Zhú Tāng* in order to transform the qì of tàiyáng. [If there is] shortness of breath on inhale, it is appropriate to use *Shèn Qì Wán* in order to take in the qì of shàoyīn.[151] The two prescriptions both rely on the power of *guì zhī*, [but] marketplace doctors cannot comprehend this. *Guì zhī* is a medicinal of the highest grade. Nowadays, however, it is difficult to come across [*guì zhī*], and those who are good at applying it, also suffer the same destiny.[152]

癸亥歲，司馬某公之媳，孀居數載，性好靜，長日閉戶獨坐，得咳嗽病，服生地 、麥冬 、百合之類，一年餘不效 。延餘診之，脈細小而弦緊，純是陰霾四布，水氣滔天之象，斷為水飲咳嗽，此時若不急治，半月後水腫一作，盧扁莫何 ！

---

148. This is from Chapter 21 of the *Jīn Gùi Yào Lüè*《 金匱要略 》(Essential Prescriptions of the Golden Cabinet), and the full name of the formula is *Qiān Jīn Nèi Bǔ Dāng Guī Jiàn Zhōng Tāng*《 千金 》內補當歸建中湯.

149. Also known as *Líng Guì Zhú Gān Tāng* 苓桂朮甘湯 (Poria, Cinnamon Twig, Ovate Atractylodes, and Licorice Decoction).

150. Yù Jiāyán 喻嘉言 is the physician Yù Chāng 喻昌 (1585-1664) from Jiāngxī. See: Lǐ, 1985, p. 607.

151. This passage is paraphrasing *Yī Mén Fǎ Lǜ · Lùn Líng Guì Zhú Gān Tāng Shèn Qì Wán Èr Fāng*《 醫門法律· 論苓桂朮甘湯腎氣丸二方 》(Regulations of Medicine · Discussion on the Two Prescriptions Poria, Cinnamon Twig, Ovate Atractylodes, and Licorice Decoction and Kidney Qì Pill) by Yù Chāng 喻昌.

152. That is, that people who are good at applying *guì zhī* are equally rare.

In the year of *guǐ hài* 癸亥 (1803), a certain Sir Sīmǎ's daughter-in-law had been living as widow for a couple of years. Her nature was very quiet and for extended days she had kept her door closed and sat alone, [and when] she contracted a cough, [she] took medicinals like fresh *dì* [*huáng*], *mài* [*mén*] *dōng*, and *bǎi hé* for more than one year, [but] without effect. I was sent to examine her. The pulse was fine, small, stringlike, and tight. This simply was depression [which had] spread throughout the [entire person,[153] and is] comparable to the water qì [which] overflows [from] heaven.[154] [I] concluded [that this was] because of water-rheum cough, and that if [this was] not urgently treated now, after half a month [this would] become water swelling. [Then even] Lú Biǎn[155] would not know what to do!

言之未免過激，診一次後，即不復與商。嗣腫病大作，醫者用檳榔、牽牛、葶藶子、厚朴、大腹皮、蘿卜子為主，加焦白朮、熟地炭、肉桂、附子、茯苓、車前子、牛膝、當歸、芍藥、海金砂、澤瀉、木通、赤小豆、商陸、豬苓、枳殼之類，出入加減。計服二個月，其腫全消，人瘦如柴，下午氣陷腳腫，次早亦消，見食則嘔，冷汗時出，子午二時煩躁不寧，咳嗽輒暈。醫家以腫退為效，而病人時覺氣散不能自支。

[My] words were unavoidably drastic, and after examining her once, then she did not consult me again. Subsequently, she developed severe edema, and [another] physician used *bīng láng, qiān niú, tíng lí zǐ, hòu pò, dà fù pí,* and *luó bó zǐ* as the main [ingredients] and added [other medicinals] like *jiāo bái zhú, shú dì tàn, ròu guì, fù zǐ, fú líng, chē qián zǐ, niú xī, dāng guī, sháo yào, hǎi jīn shā, zé xiè, mù tōng, chì xiǎo dòu, shāng lù, zhū líng,* and *zhǐ ké* [in such a way that] the modifications were inconsistent. [I] reckon she took this for two months, and her edema completely dispersed, [but] she was emaciated like firewood. In the afternoons she had sinking qì and edema in the legs, [and by] the next morning this also dispersed. [However,] at the appearance of food, then [she would] retch, have frequent issuing forth of cold sweats, and [between] the two times of *zǐ* (11pm to 1am) and *wǔ* (11am to 1pm) she felt vexed, agitated, and restless, and while coughing, [she would] suddenly [become] dizzy. The physician took the reduction of swelling for success, but, the patient frequently felt her qì disperse and was unable to prop herself up.

又數日，大汗、嘔逆、氣喘欲絕。又延余診之，脈如吹毛，指甲黯，四肢厥冷。

After several days, she had great sweating, retching counterflow, [and] panting [as if the breath was] about to expire. I was called again to examine [the patient]. The pulse was like blown downy [hair], her fingernails were dark, and she had reversal cold of the four limbs.

---

153. Literally, *yīn mái sì bù* 陰霾四布 (a yīn dust-storm in all directions), this is figurative for deep depression.

154. Therefore, the water is in excess.

155. Lú Biǎn 盧扁 is a nickname of the famous ancient physician Biǎn Què 扁鵲 (407-310 B.C.), because he was from the city of Lú. He is said to have invented pulse diagnosis. See: Lǐ, 1985, p. 458.

余驚問其少君曰：「前此直言獲咎，以致今日病不可為，余實不能辭其責
也。但尊大人於庚申夏間將入都，沾恙一月，余進藥三劑全愈，迄今三載，
尚守服舊方，精神逾健，豈遂忘耶？茲兩次遵命而來，未准一見，此症已束
手無策，未知有何面諭？ 」

Appalled, I asked her son[156]: "I am to be blamed for my previous frank words, as a result, today the disease cannot be [accounted for, therefore] I truly am unable to dismiss my responsibility. However, when your honorific grandfather was about to enter the capital city in the summer of the year *gēng shēn* 庚申 (1800), he was infected by sickness for one month. [After taking] three doses of the medicine I recommended, [he] completely recovered. So far, it has been three years, and he still guards [himself] by taking the old prescription. His essence and spirit have become much stronger; how can this consequently be forgotten, eh? Both times, I have followed [his] command and arrived, but he did not allow [me to] see him once. [Now, with] this condition, my hands are already bound.[157] I do not know what his personal instructions are [now]?"

渠少君云：「但求氣喘略平。」所以然者，非人力也。余不得已，以《金
匱》苓桂朮甘湯小劑應之茯苓二錢、白朮、桂枝、炙甘草各一錢。次日
又延，余知術拙不能為力，固辭之，別延醫治。後一日歿。旋聞醫輩私議，
苓桂朮甘湯為發表之劑，於前證不宜。夫苓桂朮甘湯豈發表劑哉？祇緣湯中
之桂枝一味，由來被謗，余用桂枝，宜其招謗也。噫！桂枝之屈於不知己，
將何時得以大申其用哉？

The son replied: "But, I beseech you to slightly calm the panting." This being so, it is not up to human power. I had no choice but to use small dosages of *Líng Guì Zhú Gān Tāng*[158] from the *Jīn Gùi Yào Lüè* (*two qián of fú líng. Bái zhú, guì zhī, and zhì gān cǎo each one qián*). The next day, I was called again. I knew that the method was clumsy and not powerful, and [I would] undoubtedly be dismissed, [and a] different doctor [would be] called to treat. One day later [the patient] died. Not long after this, a well-known doctor personally criticized [me, saying] *Líng Guì Zhú Gān Tāng* is a formula for effusing the exterior, and was inappropriate from the previous signs. How come *Líng Guì Zhú Gān Tāng* is an exterior-effusing formula? Only because the decoction contains *guì zhī*, this single flavor that has been defamed up to now? When I use *guì zhī*, I should attract libel. Yeah! *Guì zhī's* inferior position lies in its being unfamiliar [to most physicians,] when will we get greater explanations on its use?

桂枝性用，自唐宋以後，罕有明其旨。叔父引張隱庵之注，字字精確。又引
徐忠可之論，透發無遺。附錄近日治案，幾於痛哭垂涕而道之。其活人無己
之心，溢於筆墨之外。吾知桂枝之功用，從此大彰矣！

---

156. *Shǎo jūn* 少君 means: young gentleman, or son.

157. Chén is unable to change the current situation.

158. Chapter 12.

神農本草經讀・卷二

The importance of *guì zhī*'s nature and usage was rarely clarified after the *Táng* and *Sòng* dynasties. My father's younger brother quotes Zhāng Yǐn'ān's commentary, which is accurate in each word. He also quotes from Xú Zhōngkě's discussions, which are thoroughly issued without omissions. He made an appendix recently with treatment of cases, several [of which he] spoke of with tears and hanging snivel. His mind is selfless [regarding the] saving of people, [and] overflows beyond the writing. I know that *guì zhī*'s actions will henceforth be greatly known!

又按：仲景書桂枝條下，有「去皮」二字。葉天士《醫林指南》方中，每用桂枝末，甚覺可笑。蓋仲景所用之桂枝，祇取梢尖嫩枝，內外如一，若有皮骨者去之，非去枝上之皮也。諸書多未言及，特補之。受業侄鳳騰、鳴岐注。

Additional commentary: In Zhòngjǐng's book following *guì zhī*'s [preparation instructions], there are the two characters "remove the bark." In Yè Tiānshì's *Yī Lín Zhǐ Nán*,[159] the formulas each use the tips of *guì* [*zhī*, which] is very ridiculous. This is because the *guì zhī* [which] Zhòngjǐng [makes] use of is only the very tips of the soft branches. They are the same inside and outside, and if there were bark and bones,[160] he would remove those. It is not that he removed the peel on top of the branches. Of all books, many have not yet said enough [about *guì zhī*], and this has to be especially amended. *The disciple and paternal nephew Fèng Téng cawed this divergent commentary.*[161]

Jūn Guì 菌桂
Bark of Cinnamonum cassia

氣味辛、溫、無毒。主百病，養精神，和顏色，為諸藥先通聘使。久服輕身不老，面生光華，媚好常如童子。

The qì and flavor are acrid, warm, and non-toxic. [*Jūn guì*] governs the hundred diseases, nourishes essence and spirit, harmonizes the facial complexion, and is an envoy for various medicinals. When taken over a long period of time, it lightens the body, prevents aging, generates a bright luster in the face, and makes [one's] beauty constant like [that of a] child.

---

159. The *Yī Lín Zhǐ Nán* 《醫林指南》 (Medical Guide Book) is most likely the same as *Lín Zhèng Zhǐ Nán Yī Àn* 《臨證指南醫案》 (Guide to Clinical Practice in Cases).

160. This means, when there was a piece of the branch, where the bark and inner stalk were separated, then because they were not soft enough, Zhòngjǐng did not use these parts.

161. Chén Xiūyuán's 陳修園 nephew Fèng Téng 鳳騰 (?-?). His speaking of himself as a cawing bird is probably a wordplay, because his name can literally be translated as "rising phoenix."

陳修園曰：性用同牡桂。養精神者，內能通達臟腑也。和顏色者，外能通利血脈也。為諸藥先通聘使者，辛香能分達於經絡，故主百病也。與牡桂有輕重之分，上下之別，凡陰邪盛與藥相拒者，非此不能入。

Chén Xiūyuán said: The nature and usage is the same as that of *mǔ guì*. [*Jūn guì*] nourishes the essence and spirit, because internally it is able to freely penetrate the viscera and bowels. It harmonizes the facial complexion, because externally it is able to free the blood vessels. [*Jūn guì*] is the envoy for various medicinals, because the acrid fragrance is able to separately penetrate the channels and collaterals, [and] therefore governs the hundred diseases. [*Jūn guì*] is distinguished from *mǔ guì* by its severity and the difference [is that *jūn guì* is able to] ascend and descend. Generally [*jūn guì*] is [given] when yīn evils are abundant and resistant to [other] medicinals. Without [*jūn guì*] these [medicinals are] unable to enter.

Jú Pí 橘皮
Peel of Citrus reticulata

氣味苦辛、溫，無毒。主胸中瘕熱逆氣，利水穀。久服去臭，下氣通神。

The qì and flavor are bitter, acrid, warm, and non-toxic. [*Jú pí*] governs heat conglomeration in the chest with counterflow qì, and disinhibits water and food [amassment]. When taken over a long period of time, it eliminates malodor, downbears the qì, and frees the *shén*.

陳修園曰：橘皮氣溫，稟春氣而入肝。味苦入心，味辛入肺。胸中為肺之部位，唯其入肺，所以主胸中之瘕熱逆氣。疏泄為肝之專長，唯其入肝，所以能利水穀。心為君主之官，唯其入心，則君火明而濁陰之臭氣自去。又推其所以得效之神者，皆其下氣之功也。總結上三句，古人多誤解。

Chén Xiūyuán said: *Jú pí*'s qì is warm, inherits the qì of spring, and enters the liver. The bitter flavor enters the heart, [and] the acrid flavor enters the lungs. The chest center is the position of the lungs, and only [*jú pí*] enters the lungs; therefore, [this] governs heat conglomeration in the chest with counterflow qì. Dredging and discharging are the specialties of the liver, and only [*jú pí*] enters the liver; therefore, [this] can disinhibit water and food. The heart is the organ of the sovereign, and only [when *jú pí*] enters the heart, then the sovereign fire clears and the malodorous qì of turbid yīn is spontaneously eliminated. Moreover, to deduce [how *jú pí*] obtains an effect on the *shén*, this in all cases [is because of] the action of downbearing the qì. To summarize the three sentences above: ancient people often misunderstood [this].

又曰：橘皮筋膜似脈絡，皮形似肌肉，宗眼似毛孔。人之傷風咳嗽，不外肺經。肺主皮毛，風之傷人，先於皮毛，次入經絡而漸深。治以橘皮之苦以降氣，辛以發散，俾從脾胃之大絡，而外轉於肌肉毛孔之外，微微從汗而解也。若削去筋膜，衹留外皮，名曰橘紅。意欲解肌止嗽，不知汗本由內而外，豈能離肌肉經絡而直走於外？

[Chén] additionally said: The sinew membranes[162] of *jú pí* resemble the vessels and collaterals, the shape of the peel resembles the flesh, and the "ancestral eyes"[163] resemble the pores. [When a] person [has] wind damage cough, this is nothing more than the lung channel. The lung governs the skin and body hair, [and when there is] damage to a person [from] wind, [then] this first [enters] into the skin and hair, and next enters the channels and collaterals and gradually [progresses] deeper. To treat this, use the bitter of *jú pí* in order to downbear the qì, and the acrid in order to discharge and disperse. This enables the great collateral vessel of the spleen and stomach to shift [the wind] outwards from the muscles to outside of the pores and following a slight sweat, [the wind damage] will resolve. If [one] scrapes and eliminates the sinew membranes [of the peel], only leaving the outer peel, this is called *jú hóng*. The thought is, if one desires to resolve the flesh and stop cough, [but] does not know [whether] the root of the sweating is from the inside to the outside, how can it be [that the sweat] is able to separate [from] the flesh, as well as channels and collaterals, and directly penetrate to the exterior [without passing the sinew membranes first]?

雷斆去白留白之分，東垣因之，何不通之甚也！至於以橘皮製造為醬，更屬無知妄作。查其製法：橘皮用水煮三次極爛，嚼之無辛苦味，晒乾，外用甘草、麥冬、青鹽、烏梅、元明粉、硼砂，熬濃汁浸晒多次，以汁乾為度。以人參、貝母研末拌勻，收貯數月後用之。

Léi Xiào[164] distinguished [between] eliminating the white [parts] and leaving them, and Dōngyuán followed him [with this practice]. What a deep misunderstanding! As for processing *jú pí* to make into a thick paste, this further belongs to the actions of ignorance and absurdity. To examine the processing method: Use water to decoct the *jú pí* three times [until it is] extremely soft, [where when] chewed [it is] without the acrid and bitter flavors, then sun-dry. Additionally use *gān cǎo, mài dōng, qīng yán, wū méi, yuán míng fěn*, and *péng shā* simmered until there is a concentrated liquid, then gradually expose to the sun repeatedly; use the juice [until] dryness is the measure.[165] Additionally, grind *rén shēn* and *bèi mǔ* into a powder, mix [all of the ingredients together] evenly, [then] collect and store [them. This can be] used after several months.

---

162. The whitish inner membrane of a citrus fruit is called the albedo, or is commonly referred to as the pith.

163. *Zōng yǎn* 宗眼 (ancestral eyes) are likely the tiny pores on the surface of the peel.

164. Léi Xiào 雷斆 was a scholar of medicinals who lived during the time of the *Sòng* of the Southern dynasties (420-479). He wrote the three-volume *Páo Zhì Lùn* 《炮炙論》 (Discussion on Processing Medicinals) where he gave a written account of the methods of blast-frying, honey-frying, stir-frying, calcining, drying in the sun, and distilling for seventy different kinds of medicinals. Today Master Léi's content can be found in the book *Léi Gōng Pào Zhì Lùn* 《雷公炮炙論》 (Master Léi's Discussion on Processing of Medicinals).

165. Meaning apply the paste until it is dry.

據云能化痰療嗽，順氣，止渴，生津，而不知全失橘皮之功用。橘皮治嗽，
妙在辛以散之，今以烏梅之酸收亂之。橘皮順氣，妙在苦以降之，今以麥
冬、人參、甘草之甘壅亂之。橘皮妙在溫燥，故能去痰寬脹，今以麥冬、貝
母、元明粉、硼砂、青鹽之鹹寒亂之。

Accordingly, [it is] said [that *jú pí*] is able to transform phlegm and cure cough, normalize the qì, allay thirst, and engender liquids. However, it is not known that [this paste] completely loses the action of *jú pí*. *Jú pí* treats cough, [as it] is excellent at dispersing with acridness. In this case, using [this together with] the sour and astringency of *wū méi* confuses the [*jú pí*]. *Jú pí* normalizes qì, [as it] is excellent at downbearing with bitterness. In this case, using the sweet and cloying of *mài dōng*, *rén shēn*, and *gān cǎo* confuses the [*jú pí*]. *Jú pí* is excellent at warming and drying; therefore, it can eliminate phlegm and ease distention. In this case, using the salty and cold of *mài dōng*, *bèi mǔ*, *yuán míng fěn*, and *qīng yán* confuses the [*jú pí*].

試問橘皮之本色何在乎？余嘗究俗人喜服之由，總由入口之時得甘酸之味，
則滿口生津。得鹹寒之性，則堅痰暫化。一時有驗，彼此相傳，而陰被其害
者不少也。法製半夏，亦用此藥浸造，罨發黃衣收貯，貽害則一。

May I ask where the inherent qualities of *jú pí* are? I tasted [the paste] to investigate the reason why common people like taking it, and generally this is because at the time it enters the mouth, [one] obtains a sweet and sour flavor, [and] then the mouth fills with the engendered fluids. [If one] obtains the nature of salty and cold, then the hard phlegm is temporarily transformed. After a while [if one is] examined, this will be mutually passed on,[166] and those whose yīn is damaged by [*jú pí* paste] are numerous. The method for prepared *bàn xià* also uses this manufacturing [method] of soaking medicinals, covering until fermented, and storing. The harm that [*jú pí* paste and prepared *bàn xià*] leave behind is the same.[167]

---

166. The sweet and sour flavors when combined with the salty and cold flavors will form a vicious circle of engendering liquids and then transforming them, which leads to loss of body fluids.

167. Prepared *bàn xià* 半夏 also has a drying effect.

Gǒu Qǐ 枸杞
Bark of the root of Lycium chinensis

氣味苦、寒，無毒。主五內邪氣，熱中消渴，周痹風濕。久服堅筋骨，輕身不老，耐寒暑。

The qì and flavor are bitter, cold, and non-toxic. [*Gǒu qǐ*] governs evil qì of the five internal organs, heat strike with dispersion-thirst,[168] and generalized impediment with wind and damp.[169] When taken over a long period of time, [*gǒu qǐ*] hardens the sinews and bones, lightens the body, prevents aging, and makes [one] resistant to coldness and summer-heat.

陳修園曰：枸杞氣寒，稟水氣而入腎。味苦無毒，得火味而入心。五內，即五臟。五臟為藏陰之地，熱氣傷陰即為邪氣，邪氣伏於中則為熱中，熱中則津液不足，內不能滋潤臟腑而為消渴，外不能灌溉經絡而為周痹。熱甚則生風，熱鬱則成濕，種種相因，唯枸杞之苦寒清熱可以統主之。

Chén Xiūyuán said: The qì of *gǒu qǐ* is cold, inherits the qì of water, and enters the kidneys. The flavor is bitter and non-toxic, [and] obtains the fire flavor [which] enters the heart. The five internal organs are namely the five viscera. The five viscera are where the yīn is stored. When heat qì damages the yīn, then this becomes evil qì. If evil qì is hidden in the center, then it becomes heat strike. When there is heat strike, then the fluids are insufficient. Internally, [the fluids] are unable to enrich and moisten the viscera and bowels and [this] causes dispersion-thirst. Externally, [the fluids] are unable to irrigate the channels and collaterals, and [this] causes generalized impediment. If the heat is severe, then wind is generated. If the heat is depressed, then damp is formed. All these kinds [of disease] cause each other. Only the bitter and cold of *gǒu qǐ* clears the heat [and] can be used to control and govern this.

---

168. This is any disease characterized by thirst, increased fluid intake, and copious urine. It is often equated with diabetes mellitus. See: Wiseman, 1998, p. 142.

169. Other versions of the text have *zhōu má fēng shī* 周麻風濕 (generalized numbing wind (leprosy) with damp), instead of *zhōu bì fēng shī* 周痹風濕. Because of the text below, "generalized impediment" is preferred.

「久服堅筋骨，輕身不老，耐寒暑」三句，則又申言其心腎交補之功。以腎字從堅，補之即所以堅之也。堅則身健而輕，自忘老態。況腎水足可以耐暑，心火寧可以耐寒，洵為飲食之上劑。然「苦寒」二字，《本經》概根、苗、花、子而言。若單論其子，嚴冬霜雪之中，紅潤可愛，是稟少陰水精之氣兼少陰君火之化，為補養心腎之良藥。但性緩不可以治大病、急病耳。

The three sentences: "When taken over a long period of time, [gǒu qǐ] hardens the sinews and bones, lightens the body, prevents aging and makes [one] resistant to coldness and summer-heat," further declares [gǒu qǐ's] function of supplementing the interaction [between] the heart and kidneys. Because the word kidney follows harden, therefore supplementing [the kidneys] is then what makes them hard. When [the kidneys] are hardened, then the body is strong and light, and one naturally forgets about being elderly. Moreover, [when] the kidney water is sufficient, [one] can be resistant to summer-heat, and [when the] heart fire is calm, [one] can be resistant to cold. [Gǒu qǐ] truly is a high-grade food preparation. So, the two characters of "bitter and cold" are generally [used when] speaking of [the nature and flavor] of roots, sprouts, flowers, and seeds in the *Shén Nóng Běn Cǎo Jīng*. If [one] only discusses the seeds of [gǒu qǐ], in the middle of severe winters with frost and snow, they are lovably tender and rosy. This inherits the qì of shàoyīn water essence [while] simultaneously transforming the shàoyīn sovereign fire; [therefore,] because [of this, gǒu qǐ] is an excellent medicinal for supplementing and nourishing the heart and kidney. However, its nature is moderate; thus [gǒu qǐ] cannot be used to treat extreme or acute diseases, and that is all.

Mù Xiāng 木香
Root of Aucklandia lappa

氣味辛、溫，無毒。主邪氣，辟毒疫瘟鬼，強志，主淋露。久服不夢寤魘寐。

The qì and flavor are acrid, warm, and non-toxic. [*Mù xiāng*] governs evil qì, wards off toxins, epidemics, plague, and ghosts, strengthens the will, and governs strangury dew.[170] When taken over a long period of time, it prevents awaking from dreams and nightmares during a sound sleep.

---

170. *Lìn lù* 淋露, literally "filter, distillation or soak, drip," is a term occurring in the *Huáng Dì Nèi Jīng Líng Shū Jīng · Guān Néng* 《黃帝內經靈樞經·官能》 (Inner Canon of the Yellow Emperor, Spiritual Pivot, The Function of the Inner Organs) Chapter 2, as something like water transported to different places in the body in combination with heat or cold. In the *Jiǔ Gōng Bā Fēng* 《九宮八風》 (The Eight Winds of the Nine Palaces) Chapter 4, it denotes the pathogenic situation as two kinds of repletion together with one kind of vacuity which is called: *lìn lù hán rè* 淋露寒熱 or "soaking dew cold and heat." It is referred to as chronic fatigue, strangury, and sweat dripping like dew, which excretes the body fluids produced by the middle *jiāo*. See: *Zhōng Guo Yī Xuě Dà Cí Diǎn* 《中國醫學大辭典》 (Great Dictionary of Chinese Medicine), 1988, Volume 3, pp. 2546.

張隱庵曰：木香其數五，氣味辛溫，上徹九天，稟手足太陰天地之氣化，主交感天地之氣，上下相通。治邪氣者，地氣四散也。辟毒疫瘟鬼者，天氣光明也。強志者，天生水，水生則腎志強。主淋露者，地氣上騰，氣騰則淋露降。天地交感，則陰陽和、開闔利，故久服不夢寤魘寐。夢寤者，寤中之夢。魘寐者，寐中之魘也。

Zhāng Yǐn'ān said: There are five kinds of *mù xiāng*. The qì and flavor are acrid and warm, penetrate up to the highest of heavens,[171] and inherit the heavenly and earthly qì transformation of hand and foot tàiyīn. [*Mù xiāng*] governs the mutual interaction of the qì of heaven and earth, and the communication [between] the upper and lower [body. *Mù xiāng*] treats evil qì, because the earthly qì is scattered in all directions. It wards off toxins, epidemics, plague, and ghosts, because of the heavenly qì's brightness. [*Mù xiāng*] strengthens the will, because heaven generates water. When water is generated, then the kidney and will are strengthened. [*Mù xiāng*] governs strangury dew, because [if] the earth qì rises upwards, the qì [also] rises upwards, then the strangury dew downbears. When heaven and earth mutually interact, then yīn and yáng are in harmony, and opening and closing are disinhibited. Therefore, [when *mù xiāng*] is taken over a long period of time, it prevents awaking from dreams and nightmares during a sound sleep. To awaken from a dream is to awaken from within a dream. [Having] nightmares during a sound sleep means having nightmares while sleeping soundly.

Dù Zhòng 杜仲
Bark of Eucommia ulmoidis

氣味辛、平，無毒。主腰膝痛，補中益精氣，堅筋骨，強志，除陰下癢濕，小便餘瀝。久服輕身耐老。

The qì and flavor are acrid, neutral, and non-toxic. [*Dù zhòng*] governs lower-back and knee pain, supplements the center, boosts the essence and qì, hardens the sinews and bones, strengthens the will, eliminates itchy dampness below the genitals,[172] and post-void urinary dribbling. When taken over a long period of time, it lightens the body, and makes [one] resistant to old age.

---

171. *Jiǔ tiān* 九天 or the Ninth Heaven is the highest of all heavens, but can as well mean the center of heaven and the eight directions. In ancient Chinese (Warring States Period) belief, there are nine heavens. Here it is also not unlikely he speaks of the nine orifices.

172. *Yīn xià yǎng shī* 陰下癢濕 (itchy damp below the genitals) means at the scrotum or simply on the genitals. The itchy damp is caused by severe kidney qì vacuity with wind, and this leads to the symptoms of urinary dripping.

參張隱庵杜仲氣味辛平，得金之氣味。而其皮黑色而屬水，是稟陽明、少
陰金水之精氣而為用也。腰為腎府，少陰主之。膝屬大筋，陽明主之。杜仲
稟少陰、陽明之氣，故腰膝之痛可治也。補中者，補陽明之中土也。益精
者，益少陰之精氣也。堅筋骨者，堅陽明所屬之筋，少陰所主之骨也。強志
者，腎藏志，腎氣得補而壯，氣壯而志自強也。陽明燥氣下行，故除陰下濕
癢，小便餘瀝也。久服則金水相生，精氣充足，故輕身耐老也。

A comparison by Zhāng Yǐn'ān: Dù zhòng's qì and flavor are acrid and neutral. It obtains the qì and flavor of metal. The bark is black and belongs to water. This [medicinal] inherits the essence and qì of yángmíng and shàoyīn metal and water and is used to [treat these channels]. The lower back is the house of the kidneys, and shàoyīn governs this. The knees belong to the big sinews, and yángmíng governs this. *Dù zhòng* inherits the qì of shàoyīn and yángmíng; therefore, it can treat pain of the lower back and knees. [*Dù zhòng*] supplements the center, because it supplements the center earth of yángmíng. It boosts essence, because it boosts the essence qì of shàoyīn. [*Dù zhòng*] hardens the sinews and bones, because it hardens the sinews belonging to yángmíng, and the bones [which are] governed by shàoyīn. [*Dù zhòng*] strengthens the will, because the kidneys store the will. If the kidney qì receives supplementation and strength, the qì is strengthened, and [then] the will naturally is strengthened. The dry qì of yángmíng circulates downwards, therefore, [*dù zhòng*] eliminates itchy dampness below the genitals and post-void urinary dribbling. When taken over a long period of time, then metal and water will generate one another, the essence and qì [become] full and sufficient, and therefore [they] lighten and make [one] resistant to old age.

Sāng Gēn Bái Pí 桑根白皮
Bark of the root of Morus alba

氣味甘、寒，無毒。主傷中，五勞六極，羸瘦，崩中絕脈，補虛益氣。

The qì and flavor are sweet, cold, and non-toxic. [*Sāng gēn bái pí*] governs damage to the center, the five taxations and the six extremes,[173] marked emaciation, flooding[174] with an expiring pulse; it supplements vacuity, and boosts the qì.

---

173. For the five taxations see Footnote 28 above. The *liù jí* 六極 (six extremes) are six forms of extreme vacuity detriment, and are affecting blood, sinews, flesh, qì, bones, or essence. See: Wiseman, 1998, p. 535.

174. *Bēng zhōng* 崩中 here is the same as *bēng lòu* 崩漏 (flooding). This is abnormal vaginal discharge of blood. See: ibid, p. 211.

舊本列為中品，今從《崇原》。

Formerly, it was classified in middle grade [of the three grades of medicinals]. Today, [I] follow the [classification of the] Chóng Yuán.[175]

葉天士曰：桑皮氣寒，稟水氣而入腎。味甘無毒，得土味而入脾。中者，中州脾也。脾為陰氣之原，熱則中傷，桑皮甘寒，故主傷中。五勞者，五臟勞傷真氣也。六極者，六腑之氣虛極也。

Yè Tiānshì said: *Sāng pí's* qì is cold, inherits the qì of water, and enters the kidneys. The flavor is sweet and non-toxic, obtains the earth flavor, and enters the spleen. The center is the middle region and the spleen. The spleen is the source of the yīn qì, [and when there is] heat, then the center is damaged. *Sāng pí* is sweet and cold; therefore, it governs damage to the center. The five taxations, are the taxation of the five viscera [which] damage the true qì. The six extremes are the extreme qì vacuity of the six bowels.

臟腑俱虛，所以肌肉削而羸瘦也。其主之者，桑皮甘以固脾氣而補不足，寒以清內熱而退火邪，邪氣退而脾陰充，脾主肌肉，自然肌肉豐而勞極愈矣。崩中者，血脫也。脈者，血之府。血脫故脈絕不來也。脾統血而為陰氣之原，甘能益脾，所以主崩中絕脈也。火與元氣勢不兩立，氣寒清火，味甘益氣，氣充火退，虛得補而氣受益矣。

If the viscera and bowels are both vacuous, therefore the flesh is reduced and [there is] marked emaciation. For governing this, use the sweet [flavor] of *sāng pí* to secure the spleen qì, and supplement insufficiency. Use the cold [flavor] to clear the internal heat and abate the fire evil. [When] the evil qì is abated and the spleen yīn is full, the spleen [will] govern the flesh. Naturally, [if] the flesh is plentiful, [there will be] recovery of the taxation and extremes! Flooding is blood desertion.[176] The vessels are the house of blood. [When there is] blood desertion, then the pulse expires and [the pulse wave] does not arrive. The spleen controls the blood, [it] is the source of yīn qì, and sweet is able to boost the spleen. Therefore, [*sāng gēn bái pí*] governs flooding with an expired pulse. Fire and original qì are unable to coexist. [This medicinal's] qì is cold and clears fire; the flavor is sweet and boosts qì. If the qì is full, the fire abates. When vacuity obtains supplementation, [then] the qì receives benefit!

---

175. The *Chóng Yuán* 《崇原》 is an abbreviation for *Běn Cǎo Chóng Yuán* 《本草崇原》 (Honored Originals of the Materia Medica) by Zhāng Yǐn'ān 張隱庵.

176. *Xuè tuō* 血脫 (blood desertion) is depletion of true yīn and emptiness of the sea of blood. See: Wiseman, 1998, p. 27.

陳修園曰：今人以補養之藥，誤認為清肺利水之品，故用多不效。且謂生用大瀉肺氣，宜塗蜜炙之。然此藥忌火，不可不知。

Chén Xiūyuán said: [When] modern people use supplementing and nourishing medicinals, [they] mistakenly believe the medicinals clear the lung and disinhibit water, therefore often the [medicinals] they use are ineffective. Moreover, it is said that freshly used [*sāng gēn bái pí*] greatly drains the lung qì, and it is appropriate to mix-fry [this medicinal] with honey. However, this medicinal is contraindicated [for use with] fire, and one cannot but know this.

張隱庵曰：桑割而復茂，生長之氣最盛，故補續之功如此。

Zhāng Yǐn'ān said: [When the] *sāng* is cut, and the luxuriant [growth] returns, the qì [of this] growth is extremely abundant, therefore its action is to supplement and replenish, and the like.

Sāng Shàng Jì Shēng 桑上寄生
Branches and foliage of Viscum coloratum

氣味苦、平，無毒。主腰痛，小兒背強，癰腫，充肌膚，堅髮齒，長須眉，安胎。

The qì and flavor are bitter, neutral, and non-toxic. [*Sāng shàng jì shēng*] governs lower-back pain, children's stiff back, swollen welling-abscesses, fills the flesh and skin, hardens the hair and teeth, promotes growth of the beard and eyebrows, and quiets the fetus.

張隱庵曰：寄生感桑氣而寄生枝節間，生長無時，不假土力，奪天地造化之神效，故能資養血脈於空虛之地，而取效倍於他藥也。主治腰痛者，腰乃腎之外候，男子以藏精，女子以系胞。寄生得桑精之氣，虛系而生，故治腰痛。小兒腎形未足，似無腰痛之證，應有背強癰腫之疾，寄生治腰痛，則小兒背強癰腫亦能治之。充肌膚，精氣外達也。堅髮齒，精氣內足也。精氣外達而充肌膚，則須眉亦長。精氣內足而堅髮齒，則胎亦安。蓋肌膚者，皮肉之餘。齒者，骨之餘。髮與須眉者，血之餘。胎者，身之餘。以餘氣寄生之物，而治餘氣之病，同類相感如此。

Zhāng Yǐn'ān said: [*Sāng shàng*] jì shēng contracts the qì of mulberry and adheres and grows in the region of the branch segments. It grows at all times without depending on the power of soil. [*Sāng shàng*] jì shēng despoils heaven and earth's divine building and transformation effects. Therefore, it is able to support and nourish the blood vessels out of earth's emptiness and [when] taken increases the effect of other medicinals. [*Sāng shàng jì shēng*] governs the treatment of lower-back pain, because the lower back is the external indicator of the kidneys. In males, [the kidneys] store the essence, [and for] females [the kidneys] connect with the womb. [*Sāng shàng*] *jì shēng* obtains mulberry's qì and essence [through the] hollow [tendrils that] connect and grow, therefore [this] governs lower-back pain. [In] children the form of the kidneys is not yet sufficient, [and] appears without signs of lower-back pain, [but there] should be stiffness of the back and the disease of swollen welling-abscess. [If *sāng shàng*] *jì shēng* [can] treat lower-back pain, then it also is able to treat children's stiff back with swollen welling-abscess. [If] the flesh and skin are full, [then the] essence and qì [are able to] externally outthrust. [If] the hair and teeth [are] hard, [then the] essence and qì are internally sufficient. If the essence and qì externally outthrust and fill the flesh, then the beard and eyebrows also grow. If the essence and qì are internally sufficient, and the hair and teeth are hard, then the fetus is also quiet. Now, flesh and skin are the surplus of the skin and flesh.[177] The teeth are the surplus of the bones. The hair, beard, and eyebrows are surplus of the blood. The fetus is a surplus of the body. Because the substance of [*sāng shàng*] *jì shēng* [has] surplus qì, and treats diseases of surplus qì, [substances which are] alike interact with each other like this.

Huái Shí 槐實
Fruit of Sophora japonica

氣味苦、寒。主五內邪氣熱，止涎唾，補絕傷，五痔，火瘡，婦人乳瘕，子臟急痛。

The qì and flavor are bitter and cold. [*Huái shí*] governs the evil qì and heat of the five internal organs, stops drool and spittle,[178] supplements expiry damage, [governs] the five kinds of hemorrhoids,[179] burns, women's milk conglomeration, and acute pain of the uterus.

---

177. *Pí ròu* 皮肉 (skin and flesh) is a more general term than *jī fū* 肌膚 (flesh and skin).

178. *Xián tuò* 涎唾 (drool and spittle) is caused by either kidney vacuity water flooding (lots of liquid saliva) or kidney yīn vacuity fire flaming upwards (thick, scanty salivation). See: Wiseman, 1998, p.552.

179. For the five kinds of hemorrhoids, see Footnote 12 from Chapter 1.

Bǎi Shí 柏實
Seed of Platycladus orientalis

氣味甘、平。主驚悸，清心經之游火。安五臟，滋潤之功。益氣，壯火食氣，火寧則氣益也。除風濕痹，得秋金之令，能燥濕平肝也。久服令人潤澤美色，耳目聰明，滋潤皮膚及諸竅。不飢不老，輕身延年。柏之性不假灌溉而能壽也。

The qì and flavor are sweet and neutral. [*Bǎi shí*] governs fright-palpitations [by] clearing the wandering fire of the heart channel, [and] quiets the five viscera [because] its action enriches and moistens. [*Bǎi shí*] boosts the qì: [when] vigorous fire consumes the qì, if the fire is tranquilized, then the qì is boosted, eliminates wind-damp impediment [by] obtaining the season of autumn and metal, it is able to dry damp and harmonize the liver. When [*bǎi shí*] is taken over a long period of time, it makes one have a moist and beautiful complexion, sharpens the hearing and brightens the vision [by] enriching and moistening the skin, as well as all the orifices, prevents hunger and aging, lightens the body, and prolongs life. The nature of *bǎi shí* is truly irrigating and is able to [lead to] longevity.

徐靈胎曰：柏得天地堅剛之性以生，不與物變遷，經冬彌翠，故能寧心神，斂心氣，而不為邪風游火所侵剋也。人之生理謂之仁，仁藏於心。物之生機在於實，故實亦謂之仁。凡草木之仁，皆能養心氣，以類相應也。

Xú Língtāi said: *Bǎi* (arborvitae tree) obtains the nature of hardness from heaven and earth, [and] uses [this to] grow; [it] does not take part in the changes [of the seasons like other] things, [but] passes the winter completely green. Therefore, it is able to tranquilize the heart *shén*, constrains the heart qì; [therefore, the heart channel does] not become invaded or restrained by evil wind and wandering fire. The principle of human life is called benevolence,[180] and benevolence is stored in the heart. The mechanism of life for things is located in the seed; therefore, the seed is also called the kernel. Generally, the kernels of herbs and trees are all able to nourish the heart qì. This is because similar [things] correspond with each other.

---

180. With the following sentence, Xú Língtāi draws a parallel between *rén* 仁 (benevolence), which can also be translated as (kernel) being the storage for the basic principle or physiology in human life, and *shí* 實 the (seed) being the basic life mechanism for flora and fauna.

Dà Zǎo 大棗
Mature fruit of Ziziphus jujuba

氣味甘、平，無毒。主心腹邪氣，安中，養脾氣，平胃氣，通九竅，助十二經，補少氣、少津液，身中不足，大驚，四肢重，和百藥。久服輕身延年。

The qì and flavor are sweet, neutral, and non-toxic. [*Dà zǎo*] governs evil qì in the heart and abdomen, quiets the center, nourishes the spleen qì, calms the stomach qì, frees the nine orifices, assists the twelve channels, supplements the shortage of qì,[181] and shortage of liquids. [It governs] insufficiency within the body, great fright, heaviness of the four limbs, and it harmonizes the one hundred medicinals. When taken over a long period of time, it lightens the body and prolongs life.

陳修園曰：大棗氣平入肺，味甘入脾。肺主一身之氣，脾主一身之血，氣血調和，故有以上諸效。

Chén Xiūyuán said: *Dà zǎo's* neutral qì enters the lungs and the sweet flavor enters the spleen. The lungs govern the qì of the whole body; the spleen governs the blood of the whole body. [When the] qì and blood are regulated and harmonized, for this reason [*dà zǎo* has] all the above [mentioned] effects.

Pò Xiāo 朴硝
Impure mirabilite[182]

氣味苦、寒，無毒。主治百病，除寒熱邪氣，逐五臟六腑積聚，固結留癖，能化七十種石。煉餌服之，輕身神仙。

The qì and flavor are bitter, cold, and non-toxic. [*Pò xiāo*] governs the treatment of the one hundred diseases. [It] eliminates cold and heat evil qì, and expels accumulations, gatherings, hard binds, and lodged conglomerations from the five viscera and six bowels. [*Pò xiāo*] is able to transform the seventy kinds of calculi.[183] When [*pò xiāo*] is taken as condensed [little] cakes, it lightens the body and makes [one] immortal.

---

181. *Shǎo qì* 少氣 (shortage of qì) is characterized by weak, short, and hasty breath and weak voice. It is mainly caused by center and lung qì vacuity. See: Wiseman, 1998, p. 529.

182. *Pò xiāo* 朴硝 is also spelled *pǔ xiāo* 朴硝 or *pú xiāo* 朴硝.

183. This is likely a printing mistake. It should be seventy-two kinds of stones.

張隱庵曰：雪花六出，元精石六棱，六數為陰，乃水之成數也。朴硝、硝石，面上生牙，如圭角，作六棱，乃感地水之氣結成，而稟寒水之氣化，是以形類相同。但硝石遇火能焰，兼得水中之天氣。朴硝止稟地水之精，不得天氣，故遇火不焰也，所以不同者如此。

Zhāng Yǐn'ān said: [Like] snowflakes, [*pò xiāo* has] a hexagon shape, [or like] *yuán jīng shí* (selenite) [it has] six corners. The number six is yīn; [this,] therefore, [is] the accomplished number of water.[184] *Pò xiāo* and *xiāo shí* (saltpeter) have tooth-like cusps on the surface, and those are like the protrusion of a jade tablet[185] with six corners; thus [this] contracts the qì of earth and water to [become] formed. [*Pò xiāo* and *xiāo shí*] inherit the qì transformation of cold water. This is because their shape and classification are identical. However, *xiāo shí* is able to burn if ignited and so [*xiāo shí*] simultaneously obtains the heavenly qì within water. *Pò xiāo* only inherits the essence of earth and water, and does not obtain the heavenly qì; therefore, it does not burn if ignited, and the difference is this.

Zhū Shā 朱砂
Mercuric sulfide[186]

氣味甘、微寒，無毒。主身體五臟百病，養精神，安魂魄，益氣明目，殺精魅邪惡鬼。久服通神明不老。

The qì and flavor are sweet, slightly cold, and non-toxic.[187] [*Zhū shā*] governs the hundred diseases of the body and the five viscera, nourishes the essence and spirit, quiets the *hún* and *pò*, boosts the qì, brightens the eyes, and kills the essence of evil spirits and evil ghosts. When taken over a long period of time, [*zhū shā*] frees the *shén míng* and prevents aging.

陳修園曰：朱砂氣微寒入腎，味甘無毒入脾，色赤入心。主身體五臟百病者，言和平之藥，凡身體五臟百病，皆可用而無顧忌也。心者，身之本，神之居也。腎者，氣之源，精之處也。心腎交，則精神交養。隨神往來者謂之魂，並精出入者謂之魄，精神交養則魂魄自安。氣者得之先天，全賴後天之穀氣而昌，朱砂味甘補脾所以益氣。明目者，以石藥凝金之氣，金能鑒物，

---

184. Zhāng Yǐn`ān 張隱庵 is making a comparison of the hexagon mineral shape with the trigram for earth, which has six yīn strokes: ☷. Water is the most extreme yīn, and the most extreme yīn phase of water is ice, which has hexagon crystals.

185. A *guī* 圭 (jade tablet) looks like a miniature obelisk. It was held by the king for ceremonial purposes, and has four or six corners.

186. Other text versions have *dān shā* 丹砂 (mercuric sulfide or cinnabar).

187. Today, this has been proven to be wrong. It is a neurotoxin and listed under the obsolete substances in Bensky. See: Bensky, 2004, p. 1045.

赤色得火之象，火能爍物也。殺精魅邪惡鬼者，具天地純陽之正色，陽能勝陰，正能勝邪也。久服通神明不老者，明其水升火降之效也。

Chén Xiūyuán said: The slightly cold qì of *zhū shā* enters the kidneys, the sweet and non-toxic flavor enters the spleen, and the red color enters the heart. [In regards to *zhū shā's*] governing the hundred diseases of the body and the five viscera, it is said to be a harmonizing and balanced medicinal. Generally it can be used for all of the hundred diseases of the body and the five viscera without considering the contraindications. The heart is the root of the body and is inhabited by the *shén*. The kidneys are the source for qì and the residence of essence. When heart and kidneys interact, then the essence and *shén* are mutually nourished. Following the coming and going of the *shén* is called the *hún*, and the issuing forth and entering of the essence is called the *pò*. When the essence and *shén* are mutually nourished, then the *hún* and *pò* are naturally quieted. The qì [that is] obtained [from] pre-heaven depends entirely on the grain qì of post-heaven [in order to be] prosperous. The flavor of *zhū shā* is sweet and supplements the spleen, therefore boosting the qì. [*Zhū shā*] brightens the eyes, because stonelike medicinals concentrate the qì of metal, and metal is able to reflect things. The red color has the appearance of fire, and fire is able to illuminate things. [*Zhū shā*] kills the essence of evil spirits and evil ghosts, because it possesses the upright color of the pure yáng of heaven and earth. Yáng is able to dominate yīn, and upright is able to dominate evil. When taken over a long period of time [*zhū shā*] frees the *shén míng* and prevents aging. [This is] clearly [because of] its effectiveness in upbearing water and downbearing fire.

Huá Shí 滑石
Talcum

氣味甘、寒，無毒。主身熱泄澼，女子乳難，癃閉。利小便，蕩胃中積聚寒熱，益精氣。久服輕身，耐飢，長年。

The qì and flavor are sweet, cold, and non-toxic. [*Huá shí*] governs generalized heat, diarrhea afflux, difficult lactation in women, [and] dribbling urinary block. [*Huá shí*] disinhibits urine, sweeps away cold and heat accumulations and gatherings within the stomach, and boosts the essence and qì. When taken over a long period of time, it lightens the body, makes [one] resistant to hunger, and prolongs life.

按：滑石氣寒，得寒水之氣，入手足太陽。味甘，入足太陰。且其色白兼入手太陰。所主諸病，皆清熱利水之功也。益精延年，言其性之循不比他種石藥偏之為害也。讀者勿泥。

Commentary: *Huá shí's* qì is cold, obtains the qì of cold water, and enters the hand and foot tàiyáng. The flavor is sweet and enters the foot tàiyīn. Moreover, its color is white, so [*huá shí*] simultaneously enters the hand tàiyīn. [*Huá shí*] governs the various diseases [because it has] both the actions of clearing heat and disinhibiting water. Boosting the essence and prolonging life speaks of [*huá shí*] following its nature, which is unlike other stonelike medicinals, [which] are inclined to cause harm. Reader, do not feel restrained [by conventions].

Zǐ Shí Yīng 紫石英
Purple Fluorite

氣味甘、溫，無毒。主心腹咳逆邪氣，補不足，女子風寒在子宮，絕孕十年無子。久服溫中，輕身延年。

The qì and flavor are sweet, warm, and non-toxic. [*Zǐ shí yīng*] governs counterflow cough evil qì in the heart and abdomen, supplements insufficiency, wind-cold in the uterus, and infertility without [conceiving a] child for ten years. When taken over a long period of time, [*zǐ shí yīng*] warms the center, lightens the body, and prolongs life.

陳修園曰：紫石英氣溫，稟木氣而入肝。味甘無毒，得土味而入脾。咳逆邪氣者，以心腹為脾之部位，人之呼吸，出心肺而入肝腎，脾居中而轉運，何咳逆之有？惟脾虛受肝邪之侮，不能下轉而上衝，故為是病。其主之者，溫能散邪，甘能和中，而其質又重而能降也。

Chén Xiūyuán said: *Zǐ shí yīng's* qì is warm, inherits the qì of wood, and enters the liver. [*Zǐ shí yīng*] is sweet, non-toxic, obtains the earth flavor, and enters the spleen. Regarding the counterflow cough evil qì, [this is] because the heart and abdomen are the position of the spleen. A person's breathing issues forth from the heart and lungs and enters liver and kidneys. The spleen resides in the center and transports. What is counterflow cough? Only [when] the spleen is vacuous, [does] it contract the insult of liver evil; [then] it is not able to shift downwards, but surges upwards, therefore, causing this disease. [*Zǐ shí yīng*] governs the [above mentioned diseases], because warmth is able to disperse evil, sweetness is able to harmonize the center, and the nature [of *zǐ shí yīng*] is heavy, therefore it is able to downbear.

補不足者，氣溫味甘，補肝脾之不足也。風寒入於子宮，則肝血不藏，脾血亦不統，往往不能生育，脾土之成數十，所以十年無子也。紫石英氣溫可以散子宮之風寒，味甘可以補肝脾之血也。久服溫中輕身延年者，夸其補血納氣之力也。

[*Zǐ shí yīng*] supplements insufficiency, because the qì is warm and the flavor is sweet, so it supplements the insufficiency of the liver and spleen. When wind and cold enter into the uterus, then the liver blood is not stored, the spleen blood is also not controlled, [and therefore, in these cases one is] frequently unable to give a birth. The number of the spleen earth is ten; therefore, [there is] infertility for ten years. *Zǐ shí yīng's* qì is warm and can be used to disperse wind-cold in the uterus. The sweet flavor can be used to supplement the blood of the liver and spleen. When taken over a long period of time, [*zǐ shí yīng*] warms the center, lightens the body, and prolongs life. [This is] because its power to supplement the blood and absorb the qì is praiseworthy.

按：白石英治略同，但紫色屬陰，主治衝脈血海，功多在下。白為金色，主治消渴，兼理上焦之燥。

Commentary: *Bái shí yīng* treats approximately the same [diseases]. However, the purple color belongs to yīn, [and therefore, *zǐ shí yīng* is] indicated for the penetrating vessel, the sea of blood,[188] [where] its actions [are] greater for the lower body. White is the color of metal and [*bái shí yīng* is] indicated for dispersion-thirst and simultaneously regulates dryness in the upper *jiāo*.

Chì Shí Zhī 赤石脂
Red Halloysite

氣味甘、平，無毒。主黃膽，泄痢，腸澼膿血，陰蝕下血赤白，邪氣癰腫，疽痔惡瘡，頭瘍疥瘙。久服補髓益氣，肥健不飢，輕身延年。**五色石脂，各隨五色補五臟。**

The qì and flavor are sweet, neutral, and non-toxic. [*Chì shí zhī*] governs jaundice, diarrhea, intestinal afflux[189] with pus and blood, genital erosion with red and white bloody discharge,[190] evil qì with swollen welling-abscess, flat-abscesses, hemorrhoids, malign sores, head sores, and scabies. When taken over a long period of time, [*chì shí zhī*] supplements the marrow, boosts the qì, fattens, strengthens, prevents hunger, lightens the body, and prolongs life. *The five colors of shí zhī each follow [the rules of] the five colors [that] supplement the five viscera.*[191]

---

188. *Chōng mài* 衝脈 (the penetrating vessel) is one of the eight extraordinary vessels. *Xuě hǎi* 血海 (sea of blood) is one of the four seas. Together, these can be seen as a unit, as the penetrating vessel is the sea of blood in the body and influences the uterus.

189. *Cháng pì* 腸澼 (intestinal afflux) is bloody dysentery. See: Wiseman, 1998, p. 317.

190. *Yīn shí* 陰蝕 (genital erosion) is depressed fire that damages the liver and spleen, which causes depressed damp-heat in the lower body with pus, sores, itching and worms, and red or white discharge. See: ibid, p. 241.

191. There are five colors of halloysite: red, green, yellow, brown, and white.

陳修園曰：赤石脂氣平稟金氣，味甘得土味，手足太陰藥也。太陰濕勝，在皮膚則為黃疸，在腸胃則為泄痢，甚則為腸澼膿血。下注於前陰，則為陰蝕，並見赤白濁帶下。注於後陰，則為下血。皆濕邪之氣為害也。

Chén Xiūyuán said: *Chì shí zhī's* qì is neutral, and inherits the qì of metal. The flavor is sweet, obtains the earth flavor, [and] is the hand and foot tàiyīn medicinal. [When] tàiyīn is dominated by damp [that] is located in the skin, then [this] is jaundice. [When damp] is located in the intestines and stomach, then [this] is diarrhea. [If this is] severe, then [there] is intestinal afflux with pus and blood. [When damp] pours down from the anterior yīn, then [this] is genital erosion and [this can] also present [with] red and white turbid vaginal discharge. [When damp] pours from the posterior yīn, then [this] is bloody diarrhea. [These are] all harms caused by the qì of damp evil.

石脂具濕土之質，而有燥金之用，所以主之。癰腫、疽痔，惡瘡、頭瘍，疥瘙等證，皆濕氣鬱而為熱，熱盛生毒之患。石脂能燥濕化熱，所以主之。久服補髓益氣、肥健不飢、延年者，濕去則津生，自能補髓益氣，補髓助精也、益氣助神也。精神交會於中土，故有肥健不飢，輕身延年之效也。

Shí zhī's nature possesses [both] damp and earth, but has a metal and drying effect; therefore, [*chì shí zhī*] governs this. Swollen welling-abscesses, flat-abscesses, hemorrhoids, malign sores, head sores, scabies, and other signs of this kind, always [indicate] damp qì that is depressed and causes heat. [When] heat is abundant, [one] suffers [from the] generation of toxins. *Shí zhī* is able to dry damp and transform heat; therefore, it governs this. When taken over a long period of time, [*chì shí zhī*] supplements the marrow, boosts the qì, fattens, strengthens, prevents hunger. [It also] prolongs life, [because when] damp is eliminated, then the fluids are generated, [and] naturally [these fluids] are able to supplement the marrow and boost the qì. Supplementing the marrow assists the essence, and boosting the qì assists the *shén*. The essence and *shén* gather in center-earth; therefore, [there are] the effects of fattening, strengthening, preventing hunger, lightening the body, and prolonging life.

Yǔ Yú Liáng 禹餘糧
Limonite

氣味甘寒，無毒。主咳逆，補中降氣，不使以逆。寒熱，除脾胃濕滯
之寒熱，非謂可以通治寒熱。煩滿，性寒除熱，即可以止煩。質重降
逆，即可以泄滿。下利赤白，除濕熱之功。血閉，癥瘕，消濕熱所滯之
淤積。大熱，熱在陽明者，熱必甚，此能除之。煉餌服之不飢，其質類
穀粉而補脾土，所以謂之糧而能充飢也。輕身延年。補養後天之效。

The qì and flavor are sweet, cold, and non-toxic. [Yǔ yú liáng] governs counterflow cough, [it does this] by supplementing the center and descending qì; it does not enable this to counterflow. [Governs] cold and heat, [yǔ yú liáng does this] by eliminating stagnant damp cold and heat of the spleen and stomach; this does not mean it can be used to free and treat the cold and heat. Vexation and fullness, [yǔ yú liáng governs this because the] cold nature eliminates heat, then [it] can be used to stop vexation; because the nature is heavy, and downbears counterflow, then it can drain fullness. [Yǔ yú liáng governs] red and white diarrhea because [of it's] action of eliminating damp-heat. [Governs] blood block, concretions, and conglomerations because [it] disperses the siltlike accumulations of the stagnant damp-heat. [Governs] great heat, [because] when heat is located in the yángmíng channels, the heat will be severe; [then] this [mineral] is able to eliminate [the heat]. [Yǔ yú liáng] is taken as refined little cakes to prevent hunger [because] its nature is like grain flour and supplements spleen earth; therefore, it is called grain[192] and is able to satisfy hunger. It lightens the body and prolongs life by the effect of supplementing and nourishing the post-heaven qì.

按：李時珍曰：生池澤者，為禹餘糧。生山谷者，為太一餘糧。《本經》雖
分兩種，而治體則同。

Commentary by Lǐ Shízhēn: [That which] grows in ponds and marshes is yǔ yú liáng; [that which] grows in valleys is tài yī yú liáng. Although the Shén Nóng Běn Cǎo Jīng differentiates the two kinds, nevertheless, the principle of treatment is the same.[193]

---

192. Yǔ yú liáng 禹餘糧 litterally means Yǔ surplus grain.

193. In fact, Lǐ Shízhēn 李時珍 says: yǔ yú liáng 禹餘糧 grows in ponds or on islands by the East China Sea, and tài yī yú liáng 太一餘糧 in valleys of Mount Tài Shān. See: Lǐ Shízhēn Běn Cǎo Gāng Mù 《本草綱目》 (Compendium of the Materia Medica), Chapter 10.

Fà Bì 髮髲
Crinis Carbonisatus Hominis

氣味苦、溫，無毒。主五癃，關格不通，利小便水道，療小兒驚、大人痙，仍自還神化。

The qì and flavor are bitter, warm, and non-toxic. [Fà bì][194] governs the five dribblings [of urine],[195] block and repulsion[196] obstruction; [it] disinhibits the urine and the waterways, treats children's fright [wind[197] and] tetany in adults, and yet naturally still transforms the *shén*.

以皂莢水洗淨，復用甘草水洗、鹽水洗，晒乾，入瓶內，以鹽土固濟，煅存性，謂之血餘灰，研極細用。

Use zào jiá water to wash [the fà bì] clean, again wash using gān cǎo water, wash [again using] salt water, [then] sun dry. Place this into a vase, secure [the lid] with the aid of salt earth[198] and calcine to preserve [fà bì's] nature; this is called xuè yú huī.[199] Grind extremely fine to use.

陳修園曰：心主血，髮者血之餘也，屬手少陰心。《經》云：「腎之合骨也，其榮髮也，」屬足少陰腎。又云：皮毛者，肺之合也。髮亦毛類，屬手太陰肺。肺為水源，小腸為心腑，故主五癃，關格不通、水道不利等症。調肺氣，寧心神，除心肺之痰，故主小兒癇、大人痙等證。

Chén Xiūyuán said: The heart governs the blood. Hair is surplus blood, so [fà bì] belongs to the hand shàoyīn heart [channel]. The [Nèi] Jīng said: "The connection of the kidneys and the bones manifests as the hair,"[200] [therefore fà bì] belongs to the foot shàoyīn kidney [channel. The Nèi Jīng]

---

194. *Bì* 髲 literally means "wig." Here it means "human hair."

195. *Wǔ lóng* 五癃 (the five stranguries) are the same as *wǔ lín* 五淋 (*lóng* 癃 was often exchanged for *lín* 淋 because of an emperor name ban): stone, unctuous, blood, qì and taxation strangury, caused by either damp-heat in the lower burner or spleen and kidney vacuity. See: Wiseman, 1998, p. 207.

196. *Guān gé* 關格 (block and repulsion) means urinary stoppage with continuous vomiting due to spleen and kidney vacuity. See: ibid, p. 24.

197. *Xiǎo ér jīng* [*fēng*] 小兒驚[風] (infantile convulsions). See: ibid, p. 60.

198. The description hints at a medicinal processing technique, where things in pots that have been sealed with clay or the like are heated until red hot.

199. *Xuè yú huī* 血餘灰 literally means "ashed surplus of the blood." It is the same as *xuè yú tàn* 血餘炭 (charred human hair).

200. See: *Huáng Dì Nèi Jīng Sù Wèn·Wǔ Zàng Shēng Chéng* 《黃帝內經素問·五臟生成》 (Inner Canon of the Yellow Emperor Plain Questions · Generation of the Five Viscera), Chapter 10, Line 1.

further says that the skin and hair are connected with the lungs.[201] Hair is also similar to [body] hair[202] and so belongs to the hand tàiyīn lung [channel]. The lungs are the source of water and the small intestine is the bowel of the heart. Therefore, [fà bì] governs the five dribblings, [as well as] block and repulsion obstruction, inhibited waterways, and similar conditions. [Fà bì] regulates the lung qì, tranquilizes the heart and *shén*, eliminates phlegm of the heart and lungs, and therefore governs children's epilepsy, tetany in adults, and similar patterns.

其曰：「仍自還神化」者，謂髮為血餘，乃水精奉心化血所生。今取以煉服，仍能入至陰之臟，助水精而上奉心臟之神，以化其血也。後人感於以人補人之說，每用紫河車增熱為害，十服十死，不如用此藥之驗。

[What is] meant by "yet naturally still transforms the *shén*," is that hair is the surplus of blood; thus, [the blood is] generated [from] the water and essence [that] support the heart [and are] transformed into blood. Now, [when one] applies the use of refining the [fà bì] by fire and takes [this], the [fà bì] is still able to enter the viscus of consummate yīn,[203] [in order to] assist the water and essence, and divinely support the ascent [of the water and essence] to the heart viscus in order to transform this [into] blood. People of later generations confused this with the theory of supplementing humans with human [parts], and with each use of *zǐ hé chē*, they increased the heat, [which] caused harm. In ten dosages, [there were] ten deaths. It is not like using this proven medicinal's [effectiveness.]

Lóng Gǔ 龍骨
Os draconis

氣味甘、平，無毒。主心腹鬼疰精物老魅，咳逆，泄痢膿血，女子漏下，癥瘕堅結，小兒熱氣驚癇。

The qì and flavor are sweet, neutral, and non-toxic. [Lóng gǔ] governs ghost infixation,[204] spirit things and old demons in the heart and abdomen, counterflow cough, diarrhea with pus and blood, women's spotting [of blood],[205] concretions, conglomerations, and hard binds, as well as heat qì and fright epilepsy in children.

---

201. Ibid.

202. *Fà* 髮 and *máo* 毛 both mean hair. The difference is that *fà* 髮 is only used for human hair, whereas *máo* 毛 can be used for hair, fur, and feathers.

203. This is the kidney.

204. *Zhù* 疰 (influx or infixation) also means "contagious deadly disease."

205. *Lòu xià* 漏下 (spotting) is scant non-menstrual bleeding from the uterus. See: Wiseman, 1998, p. 567.

陳修園曰：龍得天地純陽之氣，凡心腹鬼疰精物，皆屬陰氣作祟，陽能制陰也。肝屬木而得東方之氣，肝火乘於上則為咳逆，奔於下則為泄痢膿血，女子漏下。龍骨能斂戢肝火，故皆治之。

Chén Xiūyuán said: The dragon obtains the qì of pure yáng from heaven and earth. In general, ghost infixation and spirit things in the heart and abdomen all belong to yīn qì exerting a disturbing influence. Yáng is able to control yīn. The liver belongs to wood and obtains the qì of the east. If liver fire takes advantage by ascending, then [there] is counterflow cough. If [the liver fire] runs from the lower body, then there is diarrhea with pus and blood and women's spotting [of blood]. Lóng gǔ is able to astringe liver fire; therefore, it always treats [the above mentioned diseases].

且其用變化莫測，雖癥瘕堅結難療，亦能穿入而攻破之。至於驚癇癲痓，皆肝氣上逆挾痰而歸迸入心。龍骨能斂火安神，逐痰降逆，故為驚癇癲痓之聖藥。仲景風引湯，必是熟讀《本經》從此一味悟出全方，而神妙變化，亦如龍之莫測。余今詳注此品，復為點睛欲飛矣。

Furthermore, its use in transmuting and transforming is immense, even if [there are] concretions, conglomerations and hard binds which are difficult to cure. [Additionally, lóng gǔ] is also able to penetrate, attack, and break [up the accumulations]. As for the fright epilepsy and withdrawal and tetany[206] [this] always is liver qì ascending counterflow, complicated by phlegm, which returns to gush into the heart. Lóng gǔ is able to restrain fire, quiet the spirit, expel the phlegm, and downbear counterflow; therefore, it is the sacred medicine for fright epilepsy and withdrawal and tetany. Zhòngjǐng's Fēng Yǐn Tāng must be thoroughly studied [in] the Běn Jīng,[207] and from this single flavor, [one can] comprehend the production of the entire formula and its marvellous transmutation and transformation [effects, which] are also like the immensity of a dragon. Today, I carefully annotated this item, and again it is like adding the finishing touch![208]

痰，水也，隨火而升。龍屬陽而潛於海，能引逆上之火與泛濫之水，而歸其宅。若與牡蠣同用，為治痰之神品。今人祇知其性澀以止脫，何其淺也。

Phlegm is water, so it follows fire and upbears. Dragons belong to yáng and hide in the sea. So they are able to lead the fire of counterflow ascent, as well as excessive flooding of water and return [the water] to its home. If used together with mǔ lì, [lóng gǔ] is a divine medicinal to treat phlegm. The people of today only know that its astringent nature is used to stop desertion–what amateurs they are!

---

206. The term diān 癲 (convulsions or epileptic spasms) can also be translated as "withdrawal disease," which includes depression, abnormal behavior and speech, and indifference. It is identified as binding depression of phlegm and qì. See: Wiseman, 1998, p. 694.

207. This is likely a reference to Jīn Guì Yào Lüè 《金匱要略》 (Essential Prescriptions of the Golden Cabinet), Chapter 5, Line 3.

208. Literally, this passage should be translated as "to [paint] a dot [as] eye [of a painted dragon, to make it] want to fly." Huà lóng diǎn jīng yù fēi 畫龍點睛欲飛。

Ē Jiāo 阿膠
Gelatinous glue produced from Equus asinus

氣味甘、平，無毒。主心腹內崩，勞極灑灑如瘧狀，腰腹痛，四肢酸疼，女子下血，安胎。久服輕身益氣。

The qì and flavor are sweet, neutral, and non-toxic. [Ē jiāo] governs flooding in the heart and abdomen, extreme shivering like in a state of malaria [which is caused by] taxation.[209] [It also governs] lumbar and abdominal pain, soreness and aching of the four limbs, and women's descent of blood, and [it] quiets the fetus. When taken over a long period of time, [ē jiāo] lightens the body and boosts the qì.

陳修園曰：阿膠以阿井之水，入黑驢皮煎煉成膠也。《內經》云：「手少陰外合於濟水，內合於心，」故能入心。又曰：「皮毛者，肺之合也。」以皮煎膠，故能入肺。味甘無毒，得地中正之土氣，故能入脾。

Chén Xiūyuán said: [To make] ē jiāo use water from the Ā wells,[210] add black donkey skin, and process with heat to form the glue. The Nèi Jīng says: "The hand shàoyīn externally unites in the Jì Shuǐ[211] river and [hand shàoyīn] internally unites with the heart."[212] Therefore, [ē jiāo] is able to enter the heart. [The Nèi Jīng] further says: "The skin and hair unite with the lungs,"[213] and because [ē jiāo] is skin boiled into glue, therefore, [it is] able to enter the lungs. [Ē jiāo's] flavor is sweet, non-toxic, [and] obtains the upright earth qì of center-earth; therefore it is able to enter the spleen.

---

209. There is a pattern called láo nüè 勞瘧 (taxation malaria) which is characterized by mild aversion to cold and mild heat effusion. The cause of this is debilitation of the right qì or enduring taxation detriment plus the pathogen malaria. See: Wiseman, 1998, p. 604.

210. The Ā Jǐng 阿井 (Ā wells) are wells in the town Ā Chéng in the north east of the Yánggǔ prefecture in Shāndōng Province, that are famous for their cold, clear, and sweet water.

211. Jì Shuǐ 濟水 is the name of a river in ancient China. It springs in Hénán and flows through Shāndōng, and the estuary mouth is also in Shāndōng. Today, this is the lower course of the Huáng Hé 黃河 (Yellow River).

212. See: Huáng Dì Nèi Jīng Líng Shū Jīng · Jīng Shuǐ 《黃帝內經靈樞經· 經水》 (Inner Canon of the Yellow Emperor Spiritual Pivot · Channels and Rivers), Chapter 12, Line 3. In this chapter, each of the inner vessels (microcosm) is paralleled with a river in the outer world (macrocosm).

213. See: Huáng Dì Nèi Jīng Sù Wèn · Kài Lùn 《黃帝內經素問· 欬論》 (Inner Canon of the Yellow Emperor Plain Questions·Discussion on Cough), Chapter 38, Line 1.

凡心包之血，不能散行經脈，下入於腹，則為崩墮，阿膠入心補血，故能治之。勞極氣虛，皮毛灑灑如瘧狀之先寒。阿膠入肺補氣，故能治之。

Generally, [when] the blood of the pericardium is not able to disperse and circulate in the channels and vessels, [it] descends and enters into the abdomen, resulting in flooding and miscarriage.[214] Ē jiāo enters the heart and supplements the blood, [and] therefore is able to treat this [pattern. In cases of] taxation with extreme qì vacuity, shivering of the skin and [body] hair, like the initial chills in a state of malaria, ē jiāo enters the lungs and supplements the qì; therefore, [it] is able to treat this.

脾為後天生血之本，脾虛則陰血內枯，腰腹空痛，四肢酸疼。阿膠補養脾陰，故能治之。且血得脾以統，所以有治女子下血之效。胎以血為養，所以有安胎之效。血足氣亦充，所以有輕身益氣之效也。

The spleen is the root of post-heaven and the generation of blood. If [the spleen] is vacuous, then the yīn and blood are internally desiccated, the lower back and abdomen have empty pain, and [there is] soreness and aching of the four limbs. Ē jiāo supplements and nourishes the spleen yīn; therefore it is able to treat this. Moreover, the blood is controlled by the spleen, and therefore [ē jiāo] is effective at treating women's descent of blood. The fetus is nourished by blood; therefore [ē jiāo] is effective at quieting the fetus. If the blood is sufficient, the qì also is full; therefore [ē jiāo] is effective at lightening the body and boosting the qì.

東阿井，在山東兗州府陽谷縣，東北六十里，即古之東阿縣也。此清濟之水，伏行地中，歷千里而發於此井，其水較其旁諸水，重十之一、二不等。

Dōng Ā Jǐng[215] 東阿井 is located sixty lǐ[216] northeast of Yánggǔ county 陽谷縣 in the Duìzhōu prefecture 兗州府 in Shāndōng [province] 山東; this equates to the ancient Dōng'ā county 東阿縣. The water [of this well] is clear and flows hidden underground, passes through [the earth] for a thousand lǐ,[217] and springs up in this well. The water, compared with all the waters nearby, is so heavy, that one or two out of ten do not equal it.[218]

---

214. The term bēng duò 崩墮 (flooding and miscarriage) can also mean abortion of the fetus.

215. A place name, literally: eastern Ā well. See Footnote 210 above.

216. Lǐ 里 (a Chinese mile), which equals approximately 0.5 kilometers.

217. This simply means a long distance.

218. Zhòng shuǐ 重水 (heavy water) is sweet and rich in minerals, but this can also mean "valuable water," since in the eighteenth century minerals in water were yet unknown.

104

人之血脈，宜伏而不宜見，宜沉而不宜浮。以之制膠，正與血脈相宜也。必用黑皮者，以濟水合於心，黑色屬於腎，取水火相濟之義也。所以妙者，驢亦馬類，屬火而動風。肝為風臟而藏血，今借驢皮動風之藥，引入肝經。又取阿水沉靜之性，靜以制動。俾風火熄而陰血生，逆痰降。此《本經》性與天道之言，得聞文章之後，猶難語此，況其下乎？

It is appropriate for the blood vessels of humans to be hidden and inappropriate [for them] to be visible. It is appropriate for [the pulse] to be deep and inappropriate [for it] to be superficial. When using manufactured glue, the right and the blood vessels will suit each other. [One] must use black [donkey] skin, because [this] aids the water to combine in the heart. The black color belongs to the kidneys, so this applies the significance of water and fire aiding each other. What is wonderful about this is that donkeys also are in the horse species and belong to fire and stirring wind. The liver is the viscus of the wind and stores the blood. In this case, by making use of the donkey skin, the medicinal [for] stirring wind is conducted into the liver channel. We also take the tranquil nature of Ā [well] water; as tranquility is used to control stirring. This enables the wind and fire to be extinguished, and the yīn and blood to be generated, [and, therefore, the] counterflow phlegm is downborne. These are the words of the *Shén Nóng Běn Cǎo Jīng's* nature and the natural laws. After hearing the writing of this chapter, it is still difficult to speak of the condition below; what more can be said?

Bái Jiāo 白膠
Glue produced from Cervus nippon

氣味甘、平，無毒。主傷中勞絕，腰痛羸瘦，補中益氣，婦人血閉無子，止痛安胎。久服輕身延年。

The qì and flavor are sweet, neutral, and non-toxic. [*Bái jiāo*] governs damage to the center, taxation expiry, lower-back pain, and marked emaciation. [*Bái jiāo*] supplements the center, boosts the qì, [governs] women's blood block infertility, stops pain, and quiets the fetus. When taken over a long period of time, it lightens the body, and prolongs life.

陳修園曰：白膠即鹿角煎熬成膠。何以《本經》白膠列為上品、鹿茸列為中品乎？蓋鹿茸溫補過峻，不如白膠之甘平足貴也。功用略同，不必再釋。其主婦人血閉、止痛安胎者，皆補衝脈血海之功也。輕身延年者，精足血滿之效也。

Chén Xiūyuán said: *Bái jiāo* is namely *lù jiāo* that has been boiled until it becomes glue. Why is *bái jiāo* classified as a highest grade medicinal in the *Shén Nóng Běn Cǎo Jīng,* whereas *lù róng* is classified as middle grade medicinal? [This is] because *lù róng's* [capacity] to warmly supplement is excessively drastic. [*Lù róng*] is not as good as the sweet and neutral of *bái jiāo* [which is] sufficiently valued. The action is about the same, [and one] need not explain it again. The governing of women's blood block, stopping pain, and fetus quieting, are in all cases [because of] the action of [*bái jiāo* in] supplementing the penetrating vessel and sea of blood. Lightening of the body and prolonging life are the effects of essence sufficiency and blood fullness.

Niú Huáng 牛黃
Bezoar of Bos taurus domesticus

氣味苦 、平 。主驚癇，寒熱，熱盛狂痙，除邪逐鬼 。

The qì and flavor are bitter and neutral. [*Niú huáng*] governs fright epilepsy, cold and heat, abundant heat with mania and tetany; [it] eliminates evils and expels ghosts.

Shè Xiāng 麝香
Dried secretion from the musk pod of Moschus moschiferus[219]

氣味辛 、溫，無毒 。主辟惡氣 、殺鬼精物，去三蟲蠱毒，溫瘧驚癇 。久服除邪，不夢寤魘寐 。

The qì and flavor are acrid, warm, and non-toxic. [*Shè xiāng*] governs the repelling of malign qì, kills ghosts and spirit things, eliminates the three parasites[220] and *gǔ* venoms, [and] governs warm malaria[221] with fright epilepsy. When taken over a long period of time, it eliminates evils and prevents awakening with dreams and nightmares from a sound sleep.

【參】麝食柏葉 、香草及蛇蟲，其香在臍，為諸香之冠 。香者，天地之正氣也，故能辟惡而殺毒 。香能通達經絡，故能逐心竅凝痰，而治驚癇 。驅募原邪氣，以治溫瘧 。而魘寐之症，當熟寐之頃，心氣閉塞而成 。麝香之香氣最盛，令閉者不閉，塞者不塞，則無此患矣 。孕婦忌之 。

---

219. The musk deer is listed in appendices I and II of CITES.

220. See Footnote 41 from Chapter 1.

221. *Wēn nüè* 溫瘧 (warm malaria) is malaria with generalized heat but less pronounced aversion to cold caused by malaria. See: Wiseman, 1998, p. 664.

神農本草經讀・卷二

Comparison: The musk deer consumes arborvitae leaves, aromatic herbs, as well as snakes and insects.[222] Its fragrance is located at the navel, and [*shè xiāng*] is the best of all the fragrant [medicinals]. Fragrance is the right qì of heaven and earth, therefore [*shè xiāng*] is able to repel malign [evil], kill [ghosts, and *gǔ*] venoms. Fragrance is able to freely penetrate the channels and collaterals; therefore, [*shè xiāng*] is able to expel congealed phlegm from the heart orifices and treat fright epilepsy. [One can] expel evil qì from the membrane source[223] by treating warm malaria. The condition of awakening from a nightmare develops when, just at the moment of deep sleep, the heart qì becomes blocked. The fragrant qì of *shè xiāng* is most abundant, and causes [what is] blocked [to become] unblocked, and [what is] congested [to become] decongested. Then [the patient] will not suffer from this anymore! [*Shè xiāng*] is contraindicated for pregnant women.

Shí Mì 石蜜
Crystalized honey of Apis cerana[224]

氣味甘、平，無毒。主心腹邪氣，諸驚癇痙，安五臟諸不足，益氣補中，止痛解毒，除眾病，和百藥。久服強志輕身，不飢不老。

The qì and flavor are sweet, neutral, and non-toxic. [*Shí mì*] governs evil qì of the heart and abdomen, as well as the various [kinds of] fright epilepsy and tetany, quiets the various insufficiencies of the five viscera, boosts the qì, supplements the center, stops pain, resolves toxins, eliminates a multitude of diseases, and harmonizes the hundred medicinals. When taken over a long period of time, it strengthens the will, lightens the body, and prevents hunger and aging.

陳修園曰：石蜜氣平，稟金氣而入肺。味甘無毒，得土味而入脾。心腹者，自心下以及大小腹與脅肋而言也。邪氣者，六淫之氣自外來。七情之氣自內起，非固有之氣，即邪氣也。其主之者，甘平之用也。諸驚癇痙者，厥陰風木之為病也。其主之者，養胃和中，所謂厥陰不治，取之陽明是也。

Chén Xiūyuán said: The qì of *shí mì* is neutral, inherits the qì of metal, and enters the lungs. The flavor is sweet, non-toxic, obtains the earth flavor, and enters the spleen. The heart and abdomen are said to be [the region] from below the heart to the greater and smaller abdomen and the ribsides. The evil qì are the qì of the six excesses,[225] [where the qì is] from the outside [of the body].

---

222. The musk deer is an herbivore.

223. *Mó/mù yuán* 募原 (membrane source) is a not clearly defined membrane of the chest or diaphragm, and denotes a location between interior and exterior. See: Wiseman, 1998, p. 389.

224. Rock honey here simply means honey. It can also be fermented honey that looks similar to candied sugar.

225. *Liù yín* 六淫 (the six excesses) are the excess of the six qì (wind, cold, summer-heat, dryness, damp, and fire). See: Wiseman, 1998, p. 535.

The qì of the seven affects[226] rise from the inside [of the body; therefore, when] the qì is not stable, then [there is] evil qì. Apply [*shí mì's*] sweet and neutral [nature] to govern this. The various kinds of fright epilepsy and tetany are diseases of juèyīn wind and wood. [*Shí mì*] governs this [by] nourishing the stomach and harmonizing the center, and this is what is called: "When juèyīn is not be treated, apply yángmíng [to treat this]."

脾為五臟之本，脾得補而安，則五臟俱安，而無不足之患矣。真氣者，得於天而充於穀，味甘益脾，即所以益氣而補中也。止痛者，味甘能緩諸急。解毒者，氣平能勝諸邪也。諸花之精華，采取不遺，所以能除眾病。諸花之氣味，醞釀合一，所以能和百藥也。久服強志輕身、不飢不老者，皆調和氣血，補養精神之驗也。

The spleen is the root of the five viscera, [and if] the spleen is supplemented and quieted, then the five viscera are all quiet and do not suffer from insufficiency! The right qì is obtained from heaven and is filled by grain. The sweet flavor boosts the spleen; then as a result [this] boosts the qì and supplements the center. [*Shí mì*] stops pain, because the sweet flavor is able to moderate the various tensions. [*Shí mì*] resolves toxins, because the neutral qì is able to dominate all evils. The essence and bloom of all flowers are gathered without exception; therefore [*shí mì*] is able to eliminate a multitude of diseases. The qì and flavors of all flowers are united and brewed into [*shí mì*]; therefore, [it is] able to harmonize the hundred medicinals. When taken over a long period of time, it strengthens the will, lightens the body, prevents hunger and aging; in all cases [this is because *shí mì*] harmonizes the qì and blood, [and] supplements and nourishes the essence and spirit.

Guī Bǎn 龜板
Shell of Chinemys reevesii

氣味甘、平，無毒。主漏下赤白，破癥瘕痎瘧，五痔陰蝕，濕痹四肢重弱，小兒囟不合。久服輕身不飢。

The qì and flavor are sweet, neutral, and non-toxic. [*Guī bǎn*] governs red and white spotting, and breaks up concretions and conglomerations with malaria. [It treats] the five kinds of hemorrhoids, genital erosion, damp impediment with heaviness and weakness of the four limbs, and lack of closure of the fontanel in children. When taken over a long period of time, it lightens the body and prevents hunger.

---

226. *Qī qīng* 七情 (the seven affects) are joy, anger, anxiety, thought, sorrow, fear, and fright. See: Ibid, p. 526.

神農本草經讀・卷二

陳修園曰：龜甲諸家俱說大補真水，為滋陰第一神品，而自余視之，亦不盡然。大抵介蟲屬陰，皆能除熱。生於水中，皆能利濕。其甲屬金，皆能攻堅，此外亦無他長。

Chén Xiūyuán said: The various kinds of *guī jiǎ* are unanimously said to greatly supplement the true water,[227] [and] are the number-one medicinal for nourishing yīn, but from my point of view, this is not completely [correct. It is] greatly supported that reptiles with carapaces belong to yīn, and in all cases are able to eliminate heat. [Animals] that live in the water, in all cases are able to dis-inhibit dampness. The carapace [of *guī*] belongs to metal and in all cases is able to attack hardness. In addition to this there are no other chief [points of discussion].

《本經》云：主治漏下赤白者，以濕熱為病。熱勝於濕則漏下赤色，濕勝於熱則漏下白色，龜甲專除濕熱，故能治之。破癥瘕者，其甲屬金，金能攻堅也。痎瘧，老瘧也，瘧久不愈，濕熱之邪痼結陰分，唯龜甲能入陰分而攻之也。

The *Shén Nóng Běn Cǎo Jīng* says, [*guī bǎn*] governs and treats red and white spotting, because damp-heat causes disease. If heat is dominated by damp, then the spotting is red in color. If damp is dominated by heat, then the spotting is white in color. *Guī jiǎ* specifically eliminates damp-heat; therefore it is able to treat this. [*Guī jiǎ*] breaks concretions and conglomerations; [this is because] the carapace belongs to metal, and metal is able to attack hardness. Malaria is old malaria. If malaria has not been cured for a long period of time, the evil of damp-heat is intractably bound in the yīn aspect. Only *guī jiǎ* is able to enter the yīn aspect and attack this.

火結大腸則生五痔，濕濁下注則患陰蝕，肺合大腸，腎主陰戶，龜甲性寒以除其熱，氣平以消其濕也。脾主四肢，因濕成痺以致重弱，龜居水中，性能勝濕，甲屬甲冑，質主堅強，故能健其四肢也。小兒囟骨不合，腎虛之病。龜甲主骨，故能合之也。久服輕身不飢者，言陰精充足之效也。

If fire is bound in the large intestine, then [this] generates the five kinds of hemorrhoids. If damp turbidity downpours, then [the patient] suffers from genital erosion. The lungs connect with the large intestine and the kidneys govern entrance to the vagina. The cold nature of *guī jiǎ* [is] used to eliminate heat and its neutral qì [is] used to disperse damp. The spleen governs the four limbs, and [when] dampness causes the formation of impediment, as a result [there is] heaviness and weakness. Turtles live in the water, [and therefore their] nature is able to dominate dampness. The carapace is affiliated with armor and helmets, and its quality governs hardness and strength; therefore, [*guī*] is able to strengthen the four limbs. Lack of closure of the fontanel in children is a disease of kidney vacuity. *Guī jiǎ* governs the bones; therefore, it is able to close the [fontanels]. When taken over a long period of time, [*guī jiǎ*] lightens the body and prevents hunger; this is said to be the effect of abundant yīn essence.

---

227. From the text below, it is deduced that these are necessary body liquids.

Mǔ Lì 牡蠣
Shell of Ostrea rivularis

氣味鹹、平、微寒，無毒。主傷寒寒熱，溫瘧灑灑，驚恚怒氣，除拘緩，鼠瘻，女子帶下赤白，久服強骨節，殺邪鬼，延年。

The qì and flavor are salty, neutral, slightly cold, and non-toxic. [Mǔ lì] governs cold and heat due to cold damage, shivering [during] warm malaria, fright, rage, and anger; [it] eliminates hypertonicity and slackening, mouse fistulae,[228] and women's red or white vaginal discharge. When taken over a long period of time, it strengthens the bones and joints, kills evil ghosts, and prolongs life.

按：補陰則生搗用，若煅過則成灰，不能補陰矣。方書注云：煅用者皆取粉，外治之法。荒經者誤收，遂相沿不改矣。

Commentary: [In order to] supplement the yīn, then use fresh and pound. [If mǔ lì] is calcined excessively, then it becomes ash, and this is not able to supplement the yīn! The annotations in formula books say: "[Those who] use [mǔ lì] calcined, always take [this as a] powder, [and this is a] method of external treatment." Without cultivating the classics, [one] mistakenly accepts this, and consequently, [this has been practiced] year after year without [being] corrected!

陳修園曰：牡蠣氣平者，金氣也，入手太陰肺經。微寒者，寒水之氣也，入膀胱經。味鹹者，真水之味也，入足少陰腎經。此物得金水之性。凡病起於太陽，皆名曰傷寒。傳入少陽之經，則為寒熱往來。其主之者，借其得秋金之氣，以平木火之游行也。

Chén Xiūyuán said: *Mǔ lì's* neutral qì [is] metal qì, and enters the hand tàiyīn lung channel. The slight coldness is the qì of cold and water, and enters the urinary bladder channel. The salty flavor is the flavor of true water, and enters the foot shàoyīn kidney channel. This substance obtains the nature of metal and water. Generally, when a disease rises in tàiyáng, [it is] always called cold damage. [If the disease] transmits to enter the channel of shàoyáng, then it becomes alternating cold and heat. [Mǔ lì] governs this by obtaining the qì of autumn and metal in order to calm the wandering movement of wood and fire.

---

228. See Footnote 12 in Chapter 1.

溫瘧者，但熱不寒之瘧疾，為陽明經之熱病。灑灑者，即陽明白虎證中背微寒、惡寒之義，火欲發而不能徑達也。主以牡蠣者，取其得金之氣，以解炎暑之苦。白虎湯命名，亦同此意也。驚恚怒氣，其主在心，其發在肝。牡蠣氣平，得金之用以制木。味鹹，得水之用以濟火也。拘者筋急，緩者筋緩，為肝之病。

Warm malaria, is malaria with only heat but no chills, and is a heat disease of the yángmíng channel. Shivering then signifies a yángmíng *bái hǔ* pattern[229] with slight cold in the center of the back, or aversion to cold [in the center of the back]. The fire desires to manifest but is not able to [find] a way to outthrust. [What] governs the use of *mǔ lì* is it's ability to apply the qì of metal in order to resolve the severity of blazing summer-heat. *Bái Hú Tāng's* name also has the same meaning. The fright, rage, and anger are [all] governed in the heart and manifest in the liver. *Mǔ lì's* qì is neutral, [and] it is able to use metal in order to control wood. [*Mǔ lì's*] flavor is salty, [and] it is able to use water in order to aid fire. Hypertonicity is tension of the sinews, slackening is slackness of the sinews, and [these] are diseases of the liver.

鼠瘻即瘰癧之別名，為三焦膽經火鬱之病，牡蠣之平以制風，寒以勝火，鹹以頓堅，所以鹹主之。止「帶下赤白」與「強骨節」二句，其義互見於龜板注中，不贅。殺鬼邪者，補肺而申其清肅之威。能延年者，補腎而得其益精之效也。

Mouse fistulae is another name for scrofula. [This] is a disease of depressed fire in the sānjiāo and gallbladder channels. The neutral [qì] of *mǔ lì* is used to control wind, the cold [qì] is used to dominate fire, and the salty [flavor] softens hardness; therefore, the salty [flavor] governs [mouse fistulae]. Stopping [with] the two phrases "red and or white vaginal discharge" and "strengthens the bones and joints," the significance [of these phrases] was presented within the commentary on *guī bǎn*; [therefore this does not have to be] redundantly [repeated. *Mǔ lì*] kills ghost evils, because it supplements the lungs and extends its clearing and depurating power. [*Mǔ lì*] is able to prolong life, because it supplements the kidneys and effectively is able to boost the essence.

---

229. *Bái hǔ* 白虎 patterns are yángmíng patterns characterized by great heat, great thirst, great sweating, abdominal fullness, generalized heaviness, dry tongue, enuresis, etc., and a large, surging, or floating and slippery pulse, which can be cured by *Bái Hǔ Tāng* 白虎湯 (White Tiger Decoction). See: Mitchell et al., 1999, p. 317.

Sāng Piāo Xiāo 桑螵蛸
Cocoon-like egg capsules of Paratenodera sinensis

氣味鹹、平。主傷中，疝瘕，陰痿，益精生子，女子血閉腰痛，通五淋，利小便水道。

The qì and flavor are salty and neutral. [*Sāng piāo xiāo*] governs damage to the center, mounting-conglomeration,[230] and impotence. [It] boosts essence for bearing children, [governs] women's blood block with lumbar pain, frees the five stranguries,[231] and disinhibits the urine and waterways.

陳修園曰：螵蛸，螳螂之子也。氣平屬金，味鹹屬水。螳螂於諸蟲中，其性最剛。以其具金性，能使肺之治節申其權，故主疝瘕，女子血閉、通五淋、利小便水道也。又具水性，能使腎之作強得其用，故主陰痿、益精生子、腰痛也。其主傷中者，以其生於桑上，得桑氣而能續傷也。今人專取其縮小便，雖曰能開而亦能闔，然要其本性，在此而不在彼。

Chén Xiūyuán said: [*Sāng*] *piāo xiāo* are the larvae of praying mantis. The neutral qì belongs to metal and the salty flavor belongs to water. Among all the insects, the praying mantis has the hardest nature. Because [*sāng piāo xiāo*] possesses the nature of metal, [it is] able to employ the management and regulation of the lung to extend its authority, [and] therefore governs mounting-conglomeration, women's blood block, and the five stranguries, as well as disinhibiting the urine and waterways. Moreover [*sāng piāo xiāo*] possesses the nature of water: [it is] able to employ the kidney's holding the office of labor[232] and receives its usefulness. Therefore, [*sāng piāo xiāo*] governs impotence, boosts essence for bearing children, and [governs] lower-back pain. [*Sāng piāo xiāo*] governs damage to the center, because it grows on mulberry trees, and so obtains the mulberry qì and is able to replenish [what has been] damaged. The people of today specifically apply this to reduce the urine. Although it is said [that *sāng piāo xiāo*] is able to open, but [it] is also able to close. So, the importance of [*sāng piāo xiāo's*] original nature is in the former [action], and not in the latter.

---

230. *Shàn jiǎ* 疝瘕 (mounting-conglomeration) is either heat-pain in the smaller abdomen with sticky white discharge from the urethra, attributed to wind evil transforming to heat and combining with damp in the lower abdomen, or swollen painful abdomen stretching to the back, attributed to wind-cold qì and blood bind in the abdomen. See: Wiseman, 1998, p. 400.

231. See Footnote 195 in this chapter.

232. *Shèn zuò qiáng* [*zhī guān*] 腎作強[之官] (the kidney holds the office of labor). This means that the kidney governs agility. Mental and physical agility are dependent upon kidney qì, essence, and marrow. See: Wiseman, 1998, p. 327.

卷之三

Chapter Three

閩吳航陳念祖修園甫著
男 元豹道彪古愚元犀道照靈石 同挍字

Written by Chén Niànzǔ Xiūyuán from Mǐn Wúháng.
Revised by Yuánbào Dàobiāo Gǔyú and Yuánxī Dàozhào Língshí.

中品

Medicinals of the Middle Grade

Gān Jiāng 乾薑
Dried root of Zingiber officinale

氣味辛、溫，無毒。主胸滿咳逆上氣，溫中止血，出汗，逐風濕痺，腸澼下
痢。生者尤良。

The qì and flavor are acrid, warm, and non-toxic. [*Gān jiāng*] governs chest fullness, cough with counterflow qì ascent, warms the center, stops bleeding, and promotes sweating. [It also] expels wind-damp-impediment, intestinal afflux, and dysentery. *When it is fresh, [gān jiāng] is especially good.*

陳修園曰：乾薑氣溫，稟厥陰風木之氣，若溫而不烈，則得衝和之氣而屬土
也。味辛，得陽明燥金之味，若辛而不偏，則金能生水而轉潤矣，故乾薑為
臟寒之要藥也。

Chén Xiūyuán said: *Gān jiāng's* qì is warm, and inherits the qì of juèyīn wind and wood. If [*gān jiāng*] is warm but not intense, then it obtains the qì of harmonious flow[233] and belongs to earth. The flavor is acrid, [and] obtains the flavor of yángmíng dry metal. If [*gān jiāng*] is acrid but not one-sided, then metal is able to generate water and transport moisture! Therefore *gān jiāng* is an important medicinal for cold in the viscera.

胸中者，肺之分也，肺寒則金失下降之性，氣壅於胸中而滿也，滿則氣上，
所以咳逆上氣之症生焉。其主之者，辛散溫行也。中者，土也，土虛則寒，
而此能溫之。止血者，以陽虛陰必走，得暖則血自歸經也。

The chest center is an aspect of the lungs. If the lungs are cold, then metal loses its nature to descend and downbear. The qì congests in the chest center, and [there is] fullness. If there is fullness, then the qì ascends, [and] therefore this is how the pattern of counterflow cough qì ascent is born! [*Gān jiāng*] governs this by acrid dispersion and warm movement. The center is the earth. If earth is

---

233. *Chōng hé zhī qì* 衝和之氣 (qì of harmonious flow) means that a forceful qì leads to harmony. It stands for true qì or original qì.

vacuous, then [there is] cold, and this [medicinal] is able to warm [the cold. *Gān jiāng*] stops bleeding, because when yáng is vacuous, the yīn will leave. [When this condition] obtains warmth, then the blood naturally returns to the channels.

出汗者，辛溫能發散也。逐風濕痹者，治寒邪之留於筋骨也。治腸澼下痢者，除寒邪之陷於腸胃也。以上諸治皆取其雄烈之用，如孟子所謂剛大浩然之氣，塞於天地之間也。生則辛味渾全，故又申言曰：生者尤良。

[*Gān jiāng*] promotes sweating, because the acrid and warm [qì and flavor] are able to discharge and disperse. [*Gān jiāng*] expels wind-damp-impediment, because it treats cold evils lodged in the sinews and bones. [*Gān jiāng*] treats intestinal afflux and dysentery, because it eliminates cold evils trapped in the intestines and stomach. For the various treatments above, all of the applications of [*gān jiāng*] use its intensity and robustness. This resembles what Mèngzǐ called an unyielding, large, and vast qì squeezed between heaven and earth.[234] If [*gān jiāng*] is fresh, then the acrid flavor is [still] intact. Therefore, [Shén Nóng] further declared: "The fresh one is especially good."

即《金匱》治肺痿用甘草乾薑湯自注炮用，以肺虛不能驟受過辛之味，炮之使辛味稍減，亦一時之權宜。非若後世炮黑、炮灰，全失薑之本性也。葉天士亦謂炮黑入腎，何其陋歟？

Hence the *Jīn Guì* [says]: "To treat lung wilting[235] use *Gān Cǎo Gān Jiāng Tāng* [and] naturally [one must] pay attention to using the [*gān jiāng*] blast-fried," because the lungs [are] vacuous, [they] are not able to suddenly receive the excessive flavor of acrid. [By] employing blast-frying, the acrid flavor is somewhat reduced, and this is also [merely is] a temporary expedient. It is not like the blast-frying until black or blast-frying to ash of later generations, which [leads to a] complete loss of the original nature of ginger. Yè Tiānshì also said that when [*gān jiāng*] is blast-fried until black, it enters the kidneys–how can he be so ignorant?

---

234. This is an indirect quotation of the great philosopher Mèngzǐ 孟子 (372~289 B.C.) in: *Mèngzǐ, Gōng Sūn Chǒu Shàng* 《孟子・公孙丑上》 (Mencius, First Part of Gōng Sūn Chǒu [a follower of Mèngzǐ]), Chapter 3, Line 2.

235. This is dryness or fluid damage in the lungs with hot or cold phlegm. See: Wiseman, 1998, p. 379.

Shēng Jiāng 生薑
Fresh root of Zingiber officinale

氣味辛、微溫，無毒。久服去臭氣，通神明。

The qì and flavor are acrid, slightly warm, and non-toxic. When [*shēng jiāng*] is taken over a long period of time, it eliminates malodor and frees the *shén míng*.

陳修園曰：凡藥氣溫屬厥陰風木。大溫為熱，屬少陰君火。微溫稟春初之木氣，則專入足少陽膽經也。味辛屬陽明燥金，大辛屬手太陰肺、手陽明大腸，微辛為土中之金，則專入足陽明胃經也。

Chén Xiūyuán said: Generally, if a medicinal's qì is warm, it belongs to juèyīn wind and wood. If [a medicinal's qì] is greatly warm, it is hot, and belongs to shàoyīn sovereign fire. If [a medicinal's qì] is slightly warm, and inherits the wood qì of the beginning of spring, then it specifically enters the foot shàoyáng gallbladder channel. The acrid flavor belongs to yángmíng dry metal. If [the flavor] is greatly acrid, it belongs to the hand tàiyīn lung and hand yángmíng large intestine [channels]. Slightly acrid is the metal [aspect] of center-earth; then [this] specifically enters the foot yángmíng stomach channel.

仲景桂枝湯等，生薑與大棗同用者，取其辛以和肺衛，得棗之甘以養心營，合之能兼調營衛也。真武湯、茯苓桂枝湯用之者，以辛能利肺氣，氣行則水利汗止，肺為水之上源也。

In Zhòngjǐng's *Guì Zhī Tāng* and others' [formulas], *shēng jiāng* and *dà zǎo* are used together. [This is] because [Zhòngjǐng] applies the acridness of [*shēng jiāng*] in order to harmonize the defense [qì] of the lung, and obtains the sweetness of [*dà*] *zǎo* in order to nourish the construction [qì] of the heart. When united, [*shēng jiāng* and *dà zǎo*] are simultaneously able to regulate the construction and defense. [*Shēng jiāng*] is used in *Zhēn Wǔ Tāng* and *Fú Líng Guì Zhī Tāng*, because the acridness is able to disinhibit the lung qì. If the qì moves, then water is disinhibited and sweating stops, [this is because] the lungs are the upper source of water.

大小柴胡湯用之者，以其為少陽本經之藥也。吳茱萸湯用之者，以其安陽明之氣，陽明之氣以下行為順，而嘔自止矣。少陰之氣，上交於陽明中土，而利亦止矣。凡此之類，《本經》雖未明言，而仲景於氣味中獨悟其神妙也。

[*Shēng jiāng*] is used in *Dà* and *Xiǎo Chái Hú Tāng*, because it is a medicinal of the root channel of shàoyáng.[236] [*Shēng jiāng*] is used in *Wú Zhū Yú Tāng*, because it quiets the qì of yángmíng. If the qì of yángmíng moves downwards, this is the normal [flow] and retching naturally stops! The qì of shàoyīn ascends to intersect with yángmíng center-earth[237] and when disinhibited, [this] also stops! Generally things of this kind are not yet clearly spoken of in the *Shén Nóng Běn Cǎo Jīng*, but Zhòngjīng alone hits the mark of [understanding] the qì and flavor, and comprehends [*shēng jiāng's*] divine mystery.

久服去臭氣通神明者，以臭氣為濁陰之氣，神明為陽氣之靈，言其有扶陽抑陰之效也。今人祇知其散邪發汗，而不知其有匡正止汗之功，每於真武湯，近效白朮湯，輒疑生薑而妄去之，皆讀書死於句下過也。又病家每遇方中有生薑，則曰素有血疾，或曰曾患眼赤及喉痹等症，不敢輕服。是亦自置死地也，又何怨哉？

When taken over a long period of time, it eliminates malodor and frees the *shén míng*, because malodor qì is the qì of turbid yīn and the *shén míng* is the spirit of yáng qì. This means [*shēng jiāng*] has the effect of supporting the yáng and restraining the yīn. People of today only know that [*shēng jiāng*] disperses evils and promotes sweating, but they do not know that its action corrects the right and stops sweating. Whenever [*shēng jiāng* is used] in *Zhēn Wǔ Tāng*, the effect is close to that of *Bái Zhú Tāng*. [The people of today] often suspect *shēng jiāng* and rashly remove this; [therefore] these are all students who died under the sentences.[238] Furthermore, when a patient's family encounters *shēng jiāng* within a formula, then they will say [the patient] suffered from blood disease or they will say he previously suffered from red eyes or a throat impediment and other similar patterns, and so they do not dare to recklessly take [the formula]. This also naturally places [the patient] into the field of death, and who is to be blamed for that?!

---

236. The gallbladder.

237. This means the heart channel continues along the spleen channel in the channel circuit.

238. This means that these people read too little without thinking about what they had read, and did not draw the appropriate conclusions.

Cōng Bái 蔥白
Stalk of Allium fistulosum

氣味辛、平，無毒。作湯，治傷寒寒熱，中風面目浮腫，能出汗。

The qì and flavor are acrid, neutral, and non-toxic. When made into a decoction, [*cōng bái*] treats cold and heat in cold damage, as well as wind strike with puffy swelling[239] of the face and [around] the eyes, and is able to promote sweating.

陳修園曰：蔥白辛平發汗。太陽為寒水之經，寒傷於表則發熱惡寒，得蔥白之發汗而解矣。風為陽邪，多傷於上。風勝則面目浮腫，得蔥白之發汗而消矣。此猶人所易知也。

Chén Xiūyuán said: *Cōng bái* is acrid, neutral, and promotes sweating. Tàiyáng is the channel of cold water, and if cold damages the exterior, then [there is] heat effusion and aversion to cold. Obtain the promotion of sweating with *cōng bái* and [this will] resolve! Wind is a yáng evil, [and it] often damages the upper [body]. If wind dominates, then [there is] puffy swelling of the face and [around] the eyes. Obtain the promotion of sweating with *cōng bái* and [this will] disperse! This also is [something] people easily understand.

至於仲景通脈四逆湯，面赤者加蔥，非取其引陽氣以歸根乎？白通湯以之命名者，非取其葉下之白，領薑、附以入腎宮，急救自利無脈，命在頃刻乎？二方皆回陽之神劑，回陽先在固脫。仲師豈反用發汗之品？學者不參透此理，總屬誤人之庸醫。

As for Zhòngjǐng's *Tōng Mài Sì Nì Tāng*, [where he] added *cōng* [*bái*] if the face was red: is this not applying [*cōng bái's* ability to] guide the yáng qì in order to return [the yáng qì] to its root? When the name of *Bái Tōng Tāng* is used, is this not applying the white [part] below the leaves plus *lǐng jiāng*[240] and *fù* [*zǐ*] in order to [assist the yáng] to enter the kidney palace.[241] [Where *Bái Tōng Tāng* is used] in order to quickly save [cases of] spontaneous diarrhea without [a palpable] pulse, where death may come in an instant? These two formulas are divine preparations for returning the yáng, and returning the yáng first consists in securing desertion. How could it be that master Zhòng[242] conversely uses [*cōng bái*] as a medicinal for promoting sweating? Scholars who do not thoroughly understand this principle are always categorized as vulgar healers who harm people.

---

239. *Fú zhǒng* 浮腫 (puffy swelling) is vacuity water swelling caused by debilitation of the lungs, spleen, and kidneys. See: Wiseman, 1998, p. 469.

240. *Lǐng jiāng* 領薑 here means "dry ginger."

241. *Shèn gōng* 腎宮 (kidney palace) is the organ kidney.

242. Zhāng Zhòngjǐng 張仲景.

Dāng Guī 當歸
Root of Angelica sinensis

氣味苦、溫，無毒。主咳逆上氣，溫瘧，寒熱洗洗在皮膚中，婦人漏中絕子，諸惡瘡瘍，金瘡。煮汁飲之。

The qì and flavor are bitter, warm, and non-toxic. [*Dāng guī*] governs cough with counterflow qì ascent, warm malaria, shivering from [alternating] cold and heat[243] inside the skin, women's spotting with infertility, and all kinds of malign sores and incised wounds. *Cook the juice and drink this.*

參各家說：當歸氣溫，稟木氣而入肝。味苦無毒，得火味而入心。其主咳逆上氣者，心主血、肝存血，血枯則肝木挾心火而刑金。當歸入肝養血，入心清火，所以主之也。

Comparison of the doctrine of each philosophical school: *Dāng guī's* qì is warm, inherits the qì of wood, and enters the liver. The flavor is bitter, non-toxic, obtains the fire flavor, and enters the heart. It governs cough with counterflow qì ascent, because the heart governs the blood and the liver preserves the blood. If the blood is desiccated, then the liver wood coerces the heart fire and punishes the metal. *Dāng guī* enters the liver and nourishes the blood, enters the heart and clears the heat, and therefore is used to govern these [patterns].

肝為風，心為火，風火為陽，陽盛則為但熱不寒之溫瘧，而肺受風火之邪，肺氣怯不能為皮毛之主，故寒熱洗洗在皮膚之中。當歸能令肝血足而風定，心血足而火息，則皮膚中之寒熱可除也。

The liver is wind, the heart is fire, and the wind and fire are yáng. If yáng is abundant, then there is warm malaria and heat but without chills. However, [if] the lungs contract the evil of wind and fire, the lung qì is timid, and is unable to govern the skin and hair. Therefore, there is trembling from chills and heat within the skin. *Dāng guī* is able to make the liver blood sufficient and stabilize the wind, [as well as make] the heart blood sufficient and the [vacuity] fire cease. Then the cold and heat within the skin can be eliminated.

---

243. The meaning of *xǐ xǐ* 洗洗 is "tidal trembling."

肝主藏血，補肝即所以止漏也。手少陰脈動甚為有子，補心即所以種子也。瘡瘍皆屬心火，血足則心火息矣。金瘡無不失血，血長則金瘡瘳矣。「煮汁飲之」四字，別言，先聖大費苦心，謂「中焦受氣，取汁變化而赤是謂血」，當歸煮汁，滋中焦之汁，與地黃作湯同義。可知時傳炒燥，土炒，反涸其自然之汁，大失經旨。

The liver governs the storage of blood, and [because *dāng guī*] supplements the liver, [it] therefore stops spotting. If the hand shàoyīn pulse is severely stirred, this is pregnancy, [and *dāng guī*] supplements the heart, [thereby producing] descendants. Sores all belong to the category of heart fire. If the blood is sufficient, then the heart fire ceases! There are no incised wounds without loss of blood, and if the blood is increased, then the incised wounds heal! "Decoct the juice and drink this"– these four additional characters [caused] the sages of former times great pain and bitterness. [It is] said: "The middle *jiāo* receives the qì, takes the juice, [then] changes and transforms it into the red, [and] this is called blood."[244] The decocted juice of *dāng guī*, enriches the juice of the middle *jiāo*. This acts the same as making a decoction out of *dì huáng*. It is evident that the current conduct of dry-roasting and earth-frying[245] on the contrary dries up [*dāng guī's*] natural juice, and this greatly misses the point of the classic.

Chuān Xiōng 川芎
Root of Ligusticum wallichii[246]

氣味辛、溫，無毒。主中風入腦，頭痛，寒痹，筋攣緩急，金瘡，婦人血閉無子。

The qì and flavor are acrid, warm, and non-toxic. [*Chuān xiōng*] governs wind-stroke that enters the brain, headache, cold impediment, hypertonicity of the sinews, and slackening and tensing [of the sinews. It also governs] incised wounds and women's blood block with infertility.

陳修園曰：川芎氣溫，稟春氣而入肝。味辛無毒，得金味而入肺。風為陽邪，而傷於上，風氣通肝，肝經與督脈會於顛頂而為病，川芎辛溫而散邪，所以主之。

Chén Xiūyuán said: *Chuān xiōng's* qì is warm, inherits the qì of spring, and enters the liver. [It's] flavor is acrid, non-toxic, obtains the metal flavor, and enters the lungs. Wind is a yáng evil and

---

244. See: *Huáng Dì Nèi Jīng Líng Shū Jīng · Jué Qì* 《黃帝內經靈樞經· 決氣》 (Inner Canon of the Yellow Emperor Spiritual Pivot · The Determination of the Qì), Chapter 30, Line 2.

245. *Tù chǎo* 土炒 (earth-frying) is a method in which finely powdered Terra flava usta is heated and then the *dāng guī* is fried with it. Once it turns brown, the earth is sifted out. This method reduces the oil in the *dāng guī* and leads it directly to the spleen and stomach. See: Bensky 2004, p. 753.

246. In other text versions it is written *xiōng qióng* 芎藭.

[causes] damage in the upper [part of the body]. Wind qì is connected to the liver. The liver channel and the governing vessel meet at the vertex of the head and [there, the wind] causes disease. *Chuān xiōng* is acrid and warm, and disperses evil; therefore, it governs this.

血少不能熱膚，故生寒而為痺。血少不能養筋，故筋結而為攣，筋縱而為緩，筋縮而為急。川芎辛溫而活血，所以主之。治金瘡者，以金瘡從皮膚以傷肌肉。

If blood is scant, it is unable to heat the skin, [which] therefore generates cold and causes impediment. If blood is scant, it is unable to nourish the sinews; therefore, the sinews bind and [there] is hypertonicity. When the sinews are free,[247] [there] is slackening. When the sinews are contracted, [there] is tensing. *Chuān xiōng* is acrid, warm, and quickens the blood; therefore, it governs this. [*Chuān xiōng*] treats incised wounds, because the incised wounds [pass] through the skin to damage the flesh.

川芎稟陽明金氣，能從肌肉而達皮膚也。婦人以血為主，血閉不通，則不生育。川芎辛溫，通經而又能補血，所以治血閉無子也。

Chuān xiōng inherits the yángmíng metal qì, and so it is able to [pass] through the flesh and reach the skin. Women are governed by blood, [but] when blood is blocked and not free, then they [are] not [able to] give birth. *Chuān xiōng* is acrid, warm, frees the channels, and also is able to supplement the blood; therefore, it treats blood block with infertility.

Yín Yáng Huò 淫羊藿
Foliage of Epimedium brevicornum

氣味辛、寒，無毒。主陰痿絕傷，莖中痛，利小便，益氣力，強志。羊脂拌炒。

The qì and flavor are acrid, cold, and non-toxic. [*Yín yáng huò*] governs yīn-wilting, expiry damage, and pain in the penis. [It also] disinhibits the urine, boosts the qì and power, and strengthens the will. *Stir-fry with goat fat.*

---

247. Free as in let go, or not tight. The sinews are loose, the opposite of rigid.

陳修園曰：淫羊藿氣寒，稟天冬水之氣而入腎。味辛無毒，得地之金味而入肺。金水二臟之藥，細味經文，俱以補水臟為主。陰者，宗筋也，宗筋屬於肝木。木遇烈日而痿，一得氣寒之羊藿，即如得甘露而挺矣。

Chén Xiūyuán said: *Yín yáng huò's* qì is cold, inherits the heavenly qì of winter and water, and enters the kidneys. [It's] flavor is acrid, non-toxic, obtains the metal flavor of earth, and enters the lungs. Therefore [*yín yáng huò*] is the medicinal of the two viscera of metal and water. [When one] carefully considers the writing of the classics, [it appears that they] all [say] the use of [*yín yáng huò*] mainly supplements the viscus of water. The yīn is the ancestral sinew,[248] and the ancestral sinew belongs to liver wood. When wood encounters intense sun and wilts, [but] once it obtains the cold qì of [*yín*] *yáng huò*, then it is like obtaining sweet dew and [the ancestral sinew can] stand firm!

絕傷者，絡脈絕而不續也。《金匱》有云：絡脈者，陰精陽氣所往來也。羊藿氣寒味辛，具水天之氣環轉運行而能續之也。莖，玉莖也，火鬱於中則痛，熱者清之以寒，鬱者散之以辛，所以主莖中痛也。

Expiry damage is when the collaterals and vessels expire and are not replenished. The *Jīn Gùi [Yào Lüè]* said: "The collaterals and vessels are where the yīn essence and the yáng qì come and go."[249] [*Yín*] *yáng huò's* qì is cold and the flavor is acrid. It possesses the qì of heavenly water, which circulates, moves, and is able to replenish [the collaterals and vessels]. The "stalk" is the "jade stalk,"[250] and if fire is depressed in the center, then [there is] pain. The heat is cleared by the cold [qì]. The depression is dispersed by the acrid [flavor]. Therefore [*yín yáng huò*] governs pain in the penis.

小便主於膀胱，必假三焦之氣化而出，三焦之火盛，則孤陽不化而為溺短、溺閉之證。一得羊藿之氣寒味辛，金水相涵，陰氣濡布，陽得陰而化，則小便利矣。

Urine is governed by the urinary bladder. It must borrow the transformation qì of the sānjiāo and issue forth. If the fire of the sānjiāo is abundant, then the solitary yáng [can] not transform and causes short voidings of urine, or signs of urinary block. Once [the solitary yáng] obtains the cold qì and acrid flavor of [*yín*] *yáng huò*, metal and water contain each other; [then the] yīn qì moistens and spreads throughout. [When] the yáng obtains the yīn and transforms, then the urine is disinhibited!

---

248. The penis.

249. In fact, this quotation stems from a commentary of Chapter 14 of the *Jīn Gùi Yào Lüè* 《金匱要略》 (Essential Prescription's of the Golden Cabinet) entitled *Jīn Gùi Yào Lüè Lùn Zhù* 《金匱要略論注》 (Treatise on the Essential Prescriptions of the Golden Cabinet) by Xú Bīn 徐彬 compiled in 1671. *Luò mài* 絡脈 (collateral vessel) here refers to the conception vessel.

250. The penis.

肺主氣，腎藏志。孟夫子云：「夫志，氣之帥也」。潤肺之功歸於補腎，其益氣力強志之訓，即可於孟夫子善養剛大之訓悟之也。第此理難與時醫道耳！

The lung governs the qì and the kidneys store the will. Master Mèng said: "The will is the commander-in-chief of the qì."[251] The action of moistening the lungs results in supplementing the kidneys. This pattern boosts the qì and power, and strengthens the will; then [one] can comprehend the pattern of master Mèng's tendency to nourish the strong and large [qì]. However, this principle is difficult [to be integrated] in the modern way of healing, and that is all!

葉天士云：淫羊藿浸酒治偏風不遂，水潤腰痛。

Yè Tiānshì said: *Yín yáng huò* soaked in wine treats hemilateral wind and paralysis, desiccated water, and lower-back pain.

Jīng Jiè 荊芥
Foliage, stem, or flower buds of Schizonepeta tenuifolia

氣味辛、溫，無毒。主寒熱，鼠瘻，瘰癧，生瘡，破結聚氣，下瘀血，除濕疸。

The qì and flavor are acrid, warm, and non-toxic. [*Jīng jiè*] governs cold and heat, mouse fistulae, scrofula, and fresh sores. [It] breaks binds and qì gatherings, purges blood stasis, and eliminates damp jaundice.

【參】荊芥氣溫，稟木氣而入肝膽。味辛無毒，得金味而入肺。氣勝於味，以氣為主，故所主皆少陽相火、厥陰風木之症。寒熱往來，鼠瘻、瘰癧、生瘡等症，乃少陽之為病也。荊芥辛溫以發相火之鬱，則病愈矣。

Comparison: *Jīng jiè's* qì is warm, inherits the qì of wood, and enters the liver and gallbladder. [*Jīng jiè's*] flavor is acrid, non-toxic, obtains the metal flavor, and enters the lungs. When the qì dominates [that] of the flavor, [this is] because the qì is the governor; therefore, [*jīng jiè*] governs all conditions of shàoyáng ministerial fire and juèyīn wind wood. Alternating cold and heat, mouse fistulae, scrofula, fresh sores, and similar conditions are diseases of the shàoyáng. *Jīng jiè's* acrid warmth is used to discharge the depressed ministerial fire—then the disease [will] recover!

---

251. See: *Mèngzǐ · Gōng Sūn Chǒu Shàng* 《孟子·公孙丑上》 (Mencius, First Part of Gōng Sūn Chǒu), Chapter 3, Line 2.

飲食入胃，散精於肝，肝不散精，則氣滯而為積聚。肝臟主血，血隨氣而運行。肝氣一滯，則血亦滯而為瘀，乃厥陰之為病也。荊芥辛溫以達肝木之氣，則病愈矣。

[When] food and drink enter the stomach, it disperses the essence into the liver. If the liver does not disperse the essence, then the qì stagnates and this causes accumulations and gatherings. The liver viscus governs the blood, and the blood follows the qì and circulates. If liver qì is completely stagnant, then the blood also is stagnant, and [this] causes stasis; therefore, [this] is a disease of juèyīn. *Jīng jiè's* acrid warmth is used to outthrust the qì of liver wood–then the disease [will] recover!

其除濕疸者，以疸成於濕。荊芥溫而兼辛，辛入肺而調水道，水道通則濕疸除矣。今人炒黑，則變為燥氣而不能達，失其辛味而不能發，且謂為產後常用之品，昧甚！

[*Jīng jiè*] eliminates damp jaundice, because jaundice is formed from damp. *Jīng jiè* is warm and concurrently acrid; the acrid enters the lungs and regulates the waterways. [When] the waterways are free [flowing], then damp jaundice is eliminated! The people of today stir-fry [*jīng jiè*] until it is black; then the qì changes to become drying and is unable to outthrust. [Therefore, *jīng jiè*] loses the acrid flavor, and is unable to discharge. Further, it is said [that this] medicinal is commonly used after birth. This is extremely ignorant!

Má Huáng 麻黃
Stalk of Ephedra sinica

氣味苦、溫，無毒。主中風傷寒頭痛，溫瘧，發表出汗，去邪熱氣，止咳逆上氣，除寒熱，破癥堅積聚。**去節根。**

The qì and flavor are bitter, warm, and non-toxic. [*Má huáng*] governs wind strike and cold damage with headache, as well as warm malaria. [It also] effuses the exterior. [It] promotes sweating, eliminates evil heat qì, stops cough with counterflow qì ascent, eliminates cold and heat, and breaks concretions, hardenings, accumulations, and gatherings. *Remove the nodes and roots.*

陳修園曰：麻黃氣溫，稟春氣而入肝。味苦無毒，得火味而入心。心主汗，肝主疏泄，故為發汗上藥。其所主皆繫無汗之症。太陽證中風傷寒頭痛、發熱、惡寒、無汗而喘，宜麻黃以發汗。

Chén Xiūyuán said: *Má huáng*'s qì is warm, inherits the qì of spring, and enters the liver. [It's] flavor is bitter, non-toxic, obtains the fire flavor, and enters the heart. The heart governs sweat[252] and the liver governs free coursing. Therefore, [*má huáng*] is a superb herb for effusing sweat. [*Má huáng*] always governs conditions [that are] tied to absence of sweating. For tàiyáng patterns of wind strike and cold damage with headache, fever, aversion to cold, and absence of sweating with panting, it is appropriate to effuse sweating with *má huáng*.

但熱不寒，名曰溫瘧。熱甚無汗、頭痛，亦宜麻黃以發汗。咳逆上氣，為手太陰之寒證。發熱惡寒，為足太陽之表證，亦宜麻黃以發汗。即藏堅積聚為內病，亦繫陰寒之氣凝聚於陰分之中，日積月累而漸成。得麻黃之發汗，從陰出陽，則藏堅積聚自散。凡此皆發汗之功也。

Fever without cold is called warm malaria. When the heat is severe, with absence of sweating and headache, it is also appropriate to effuse sweat with *má huáng*. Cough with counterflow qì ascent is a cold sign of hand tàiyīn. [When there is] heat effusion with aversion to cold, [this] is an exterior sign of foot tàiyáng, [and] it is also appropriate to effuse sweat with *má huáng*. Accordingly, concretions, hardenings, accumulations, and gatherings are an internal disease, and also the qì of yīn cold congeals and gathers within the yīn aspect. This accumulates over a long period of time and gradually is formed. If this obtains effusion of sweat by *má huáng*, it follows the yīn and issues forth from the yáng, then the concretions, hardenings, accumulations, and gatherings naturally disperse. Generally, all these are the actions of effusing sweat.

根節古云止汗，是引止汗之藥，以達於表而速效，非麻黃根節自能止汗，舊解多誤。

The ancient [authors] say that the roots and nodes stop sweating. This medicinal [acts as a] guide [to] stop sweating because [it] outthrusts to the exterior and is immediately effective. It is not that the roots and nodes of *má huáng* are able to stop sweat by themselves, so old explanations are often wrong.

252. *Xīn zhǔ hàn* 心主汗 (heart governs sweat) is a quotation from the *Huáng Dì Nèi Jīng Líng Shū Jīng · Jiǔ Zhēn Lùn* 《黃帝內經靈樞經· 九鍼論》 (Inner Canon of the Yellow Emperor Spiritual Pivot · Theory of the Nine Needles), Chapter 78, Line 20. In this section, the five liquids and their source viscera are discussed.

Gé Gēn 葛根
Root of Pueraria lobata

氣味甘、辛、平，無毒。主消渴，身大熱，嘔吐，諸痹，起陰氣，解諸毒。

The qì and flavor are sweet, acrid, neutral, and non-toxic. [*Gé gēn*] governs dispersion-thirst, great heat of the [whole] body, vomiting, and all kinds of impediment. It raises the yīn qì and resolves all toxins.

Gě Gǔ 葛穀
Seeds of Pueraria lobata

氣味甘、平，無毒。主下痢十歲以上。

The qì and flavor are sweet, neutral, and non-toxic. [*Gě gǔ*] governs dysentery in [people who are] above ten years old.

葉天士曰：葛根氣平，稟天秋平之金氣，入手太陰肺經。味甘辛無毒，得地金土之味，入足陽明燥金胃。其主消渴者，辛甘以升騰胃氣，氣上則津液生也。其主身大熱者，氣平為秋氣，秋氣能解大熱也。

Yè Tiānshì said: *Gé gēn's* qì is neutral, inherits the metal qì of heaven, autumn, and balance, [and] enters the hand tàiyīn lung channel. [*Gé gēn's*] flavor is sweet, acrid, and non-toxic, obtains the earth flavor of metal and earth, [and] enters the foot yángmíng dry metal stomach. [*Gé gēn*] governs dispersion-thirst, because the acrid and sweet [are] used to upbear the stomach qì. If the qì ascends, then fluids are generated. [*Gé gēn*] governs great heat of the [whole] body; [this is] because the qì [is] neutral [and] acts as autumn qì. Autumn qì is able to resolve great heat.

脾有濕熱，則壅而嘔吐，葛根味甘，升發胃陽，胃陽鼓動，則濕熱下行而嘔吐止矣。諸痹皆起於氣血不流通，葛根辛甘和散，氣血活，諸痹自愈也。陰者從陽者也，人身陰氣，脾為之原，脾與胃合，辛甘入胃，鼓動胃陽，陽健則脾陰亦起也。甘者，土之沖味。平者，金之和氣。所以解諸毒也。

When the spleen has damp-heat, it results in congestion and vomiting. *Gé gēn's* flavor is sweet, [which] upbears and effuses stomach yáng. If stomach yáng is stirred up, then damp-heat moves downwards and the vomiting stops! All impediments rise from the lack of circulation of qì and blood. *Gé gēn's* acrid and sweet [flavors] harmonize and disperse, invigorating the qì and blood, [so that] all impediments are naturally cured. Yīn follows yáng; the yīn qì in the human body has its origin in the spleen. [When] the spleen and the stomach combine, the acrid and sweet [flavors] enter the stomach [and] stir up the stomach yáng. When the yáng is strengthened, then the spleen yīn also rises. Sweet is the [most] intense flavor of the earth. Neutral is the harmonious qì of metal. Therefore, [*gé gēn*] resolves all toxins.

張隱庵曰：「元人張元素謂：葛根為陽明仙藥，若太陽初病用之，反引邪入陽明」等論，皆臆說也。余讀「仲祖《傷寒論》方，有葛根湯治「太陽病項背幾幾。」又治太陽與陽明合病。若陽明本病，祇有白虎、承氣諸湯，並無葛根湯證，況葛根主宣通經脈之正氣以散邪，豈反引邪內入耶？前人學不明經，屢為異說，李時珍一概收錄，不加辨正，學者看本草發明，當合經論參究，庶不為前人所誤。」

Zhāng Yǐn'ān said: "Zhāng Yuánsù[253] of the *Yuán* dynasty[254] said: *Gé gēn* is a yángmíng immortality medicinal. If in the beginning of a tàiyáng disease [this medicinal] is used, [it will] adversely draw the evil inward to yángmíng, [but] this is all a speculation. I have studied the formulas of ancestor Zhòng's[255] *Shāng Hán Lùn* and there, *Gé Gēn Tāng* treats "tàiyáng diseases with stiff neck and [when] the back is like a bird unable to stretch its wings to fly."[256] Further [it] treats tàiyáng and yángmíng combination disease.

If [the evil in] yángmíng is the root disease, this is only a *bái hǔ* pattern or one for various kinds of *Chéng Qì Tāng*, and absolutely is not a *Gé Gēn Tāng* pattern. Moreover, *gé gēn* governs the [ability of the] right qì to diffuse and free the channels and vessels in order to disperse the evils; how could it instead guide the evils to enter into the interior, eh? Our predecessors did not clearly study the classics, and often act on different theories. Lǐ Shízhēn categorically collected and recorded [these disparate theories] refusing to distinguish the right [from the wrong]. When scholars observe this invention of the materia medica, they should compare it carefully to the classical theories, so that they do not make the mistakes of their predecessors.

253. Zhāng Yuánsù 張元素 is Zhāng Jiégǔ 張潔古 (1151-1234). See Footnote 31 of the introduction.

254. This is the Mongol *Yuán* dynasty (1279-1368), but actually, Zhāng Yuánsù lived in the *Jīn* dynasty (1115-1234).

255. Zhāng Zhòngjǐng's 張仲景.

256. This is Line 14 of *Shāng Hán Lùn* 《傷寒論》 (Discussion on Cold Damage) *Tàiyáng bìng xiàng bèi [qiáng] shū shū* 「太陽病項背[強]幾幾」 "In tàiyáng diseases with a stiff neck and back, like a bird unable to stretch its wings to fly." See: Mitchell, 1999, p.79.

Huáng Qín 黃芩
Root of Scutellaria baicalensis

氣味苦 、寒 、無毒 。主諸熱，黃疸，腸澼泄痢，逐水，下血閉，惡瘡，疽
蝕，火瘍 。

The qì and flavor are bitter, cold, and non-toxic. [*Huáng qín*] governs all heat, jaundice, intestinal afflux, and diarrhea. [It] expels water and precipitates blood block, malign sores, flat-abscesses, and fire-ulcers.[257]

陳修園曰：黃芩與黃連 、黃柏皆氣寒味苦而色黃，主治大略相似 。大抵氣寒
皆能除熱，味苦皆能燥濕，色黃者皆屬於土，黃而明亮者則屬於金，金借土
之色以為色，故五金以黃金為貴也 。但黃芩中空似腸胃，腸為手陽明，胃為
足陽明 。其主諸熱者，指腸胃諸熱病而言也 。

Chén Xiūyuán said: *Huáng qín, huáng lián,* and *huáng bǎi* all have cold qì, bitter flavor, yellow color, and their indications are generally the same. Generally [speaking, medicinals] with a cold qì all are able to eliminate heat. [Medicinals] with a bitter flavor are all able to dry damp, and those [with] a yellow color all belong to earth. The [medicinals] that are brightly yellow then belong to metal. Metal depends on the color of earth in order to have its own color; of the five metals[258] gold is the most precious. However, only *huáng qín* is hollow inside, resembling the intestines and stomach. The [large] intestine is hand yángmíng, and the stomach is foot yángmíng. [*Huáng qín*] governs all heat; this indicates all heat diseases of the intestine and stomach.

黃疸為大腸經中之鬱熱 。腸澼泄痢者，為大腸腑中之鬱熱 。逐水者，逐腸中
之水 。下血閉者，攻腸中之蓄血 。惡瘡，疽蝕，火瘍者，為肌肉之熱毒 。陽
明主肌肉，瀉陽明之火即所以解毒也 。《本經》之言主治如此，仲景於少陽
經用之：於心下悸易茯苓，於腹痛易芍藥，又於《本經》言外別有會悟也 。

Jaundice is depressed heat in the large intestine channel. Intestinal afflux and diarrhea are depressed heat in the large intestine bowel. Expels water [means] expelling water from within the intestine. Precipitates blood block [means] attacking blood amassment within the intestine. Malign sores, flat-abscesses, and fire-ulcers are heat toxins of the flesh. Yángmíng governs the flesh, [and when] the fire of yángmíng is drained, then as a result this resolves the toxins. It is written in the *Shén Nóng*

---

257. *Huǒ yáng* 火瘍 (fire-ulcers) are various kinds of heat ulcerations and sores mostly caused by fire toxin pathogens that encroach upon the white eyeballs. See: Wiseman, 1998, p. 236 under the heading *Gān* 疳 "*Gān* disease." The *gān* disease of the eyeballs equates to episcleritis in Western medicine.

258. *Wǔ jīn* 五金 (the five metals) are: gold, silver, iron, copper, and tin.

Běn Cǎo Jīng, that the main treatment is like this. [However,] Zhòngjǐng uses this for the shàoyáng channel: if there are palpitations below the heart, [he] exchanges [*huáng qín*] for *fú líng*. If there is abdominal pain, [he] exchanges [*huáng qín*] for *sháo yào*. Moreover, these words go beyond the understanding of the *Shén Nóng Běn Cǎo Jīng*.

Xuán / Yuán Shēn 玄 / 元參
Root of Scrophularia ningpoensis

氣味苦、微寒，無毒。主腹中寒熱積聚，女子產乳餘疾，補腎氣，令人明目。

The qì and flavor are bitter, slightly cold, and non-toxic. [*Xuán shēn*] governs cold or heat accumulations and gatherings in the abdomen, women's postpartum residual disease; [it] supplements the kidney qì and [also] causes the eyes to brighten.

陳修園曰：玄參所以治腹中諸疾者，以其啟腎氣上交於肺，得水天一氣，上下環轉之妙用也。張隱庵注解甚妙，詳於丹參注中。其云主產乳餘疾者，以產後脫血則陰衰，而火無所制。治之以寒涼既恐傷中，加之以峻補又恐拒隔，惟元參清而帶微補，故為產後要藥。令人目明者，黑水神光屬腎，補腎自能明目也。

Chén Xiūyuán said: *Xuán shēn* therefore treats all diseases within the abdomen; [this is] because it initiates the kidney qì's ascent and interaction in the lungs. [Because *xuán shēn*] obtains the qì of yīn and yáng, water and heaven, it is ingeniously used to circulate the upper and the lower [parts of the body]. Zhāng Yǐn'ān commented on and explained [*xuán shēn's*] extreme ingenuity in detail in the commentary on *dān shēn* [right below]. This says that [*xuán shēn*] governs postpartum residual diseases, because if the blood is deserted after giving birth, then the yīn is debilitated, and the fire is without control. When [one] uses cold and cool [medicinals] to treat, then [one must] fear damage to the center; additionally, if using drastic supplementation [medicinals], again one [must] fear refusal against obstruction. Only *xuán shēn* both clears and slightly supplements. Therefore, it is an important medicinal for postpartum [conditions. *Xuán shēn*] causes the eyes to brighten because the pupil[259] belongs to the kidneys and if the kidneys are supplemented, naturally this is able to brighten the eyes.

---

259. The term *hēi shuǐ shén guāng* 黑水神光 (black water spirit light) must refer to the pupil, which is attributed to the kidneys.

Dān Shēn 丹參
Root of Salvia miltiorrhiza

氣味苦、微寒，無毒。主心腹邪氣，腸鳴幽幽如走水，寒熱積聚，破癥除瘕，止煩滿，益氣。

The qì and flavor are bitter, slightly cold, and non-toxic. [*Dān shēn*] governs evil qì in the heart and abdomen, intestinal rumbling like the gurgling of swift water, [as well as] cold and heat accumulations and gatherings. [*Dān shēn* also] breaks concretions and eliminates conglomerations, stops vexation and fullness, and boosts the qì.

張隱庵曰：丹參、玄參皆氣味苦寒，而得少陰之氣化。但玄參色黑，稟少陰寒水之精而上通於天。丹參色赤，稟少陰君火之氣而下交於地。上下相交，則中土自和。故玄參下交於上，而治腹中寒熱積聚。丹參上交於下，而治心腹寒熱積聚。

Zhāng Yǐn'ān said: The qì and flavor of both *dān shēn* and *xuán shēn* are bitter, cold, and obtain the qì transformation of shàoyīn. However, *xuán shēn's* color is black; [therefore, it] inherits the essence of shàoyīn cold water, and ascends to communicate with heaven. *Dān shēn's* color is red; [therefore, it] inherits the qì of shàoyīn sovereign fire, and descends to interact with the earth. If the upper and lower [body] interact with each other, then the center-earth naturally is harmonized. Therefore *xuán shēn* descends to interact with the upper [body], and treats cold or heat accumulations and gatherings in the abdomen. *Dān shēn* ascends to interact with the lower [body], and treats cold or heat accumulations and gatherings in the heart and abdomen.

君火之氣下交，則土溫而水不泛溢，故治腸鳴幽幽如走水。破癥除瘕者，治寒熱之積聚也。止煩滿益氣者，治心腹之邪氣也。夫止煩而治心邪，止滿而治腹邪，益正氣，所以治邪氣也。

When the qì of sovereign fire descends to interact, then the earth warms and water does not flood and overflow. Therefore [*dān shēn*] treats intestinal rumbling like the gurgling of swift water. [*Dān shēn*] breaks concretions and eliminates conglomerations, because it treats accumulations and gatherings of cold and heat. [It] stops vexation and fullness, and boosts the qì, because it treats the evil qì of the heart and abdomen. [*Dān shēn*] stops vexation and treats heart evils. It stops fullness and treats abdominal evils, and boosts the right qì; therefore, [it] treats the evil qì.

陳修園曰：今人謂一味丹參，功兼四物湯，共認為補血行血之品，為女科之專藥，而丹參之真功用掩矣。

Chén Xiūyuán said: Nowadays people say that the single ingredient of *dān shēn's* action is twice that of *Sì Wù Tāng*, and it is commonly believed that this medicinal supplements and circulates the blood. [Therefore, it] is a special medicinal for gynecology. However, the true action of *dān shēn's* use [is then] concealed!

[Mǔ] Dān Pí [牡]丹皮
Bark of the root of Paeonia suffruticosa

氣味辛、寒，無毒。主寒熱，中風瘛瘲，驚癇邪氣，除癥堅瘀血留舍腸胃，安五臟，療癰瘡。

The qì and flavor are acrid, cold, and non-toxic. [*Mǔ dān pí*] governs cold and heat, wind strike with tugging and slackening,[260] and fright epilepsy evil qì, eliminates concretions and hard static blood lodging in the intestines and stomach, quiets the five viscera, and cures welling-abscesses and sores.

陳修園曰：丹皮氣寒，稟水氣而入腎。味辛無毒，得金味而入肺。心火具炎上之性，火鬱則寒，火發則熱。丹皮稟水氣而制火，所以主之。肝為風臟，中風而害其筋則為瘛瘲，中風而亂其魂則為驚癇。

Chén Xiūyuán said: [*Mǔ*] *dān pí's* qì is cold, inherits the qì of water, and enters the kidneys. The flavor is acrid, non-toxic, obtains the metal flavor, and enters the lungs. Heart fire possesses the nature of flaming upward; [when] fire is depressed, this results in cold. If fire is discharged, this results in heat. [*Mǔ*] *dān pí* inherits the qì of water, and controls fire; therefore it governs this. The liver is the viscus of wind. [When] wind strikes [the liver] and harms the sinews, then there is tugging and slackening. If [there is] wind strike and [the patient's] *hún* is confused, then there is fright epilepsy.

丹皮得金味以平肝，所以主之。邪氣者，風火之邪也，邪氣動血，留舍腸胃，瘀積癥堅。丹皮之寒能清熱，辛能散結，可以除之。肺為五臟之長，肺安而五臟俱安。癰瘡皆屬心火，心火降而癰瘡可療。

[*Mǔ*] *dān pí* obtains the metal flavor in order to harmonize the liver; therefore, [*mǔ dān pí*] governs this. The evil qì [here] are the evils of wind and fire. The evil qì stirs the blood, lodges and abides

---

260. *Zhòng fēng chì zòng* 中風瘛瘲 (wind strike with tugging and slackening) is convulsions with alternating tensing and relaxation of the sinews often caused by wind phlegm or pathogenic heat. In Western medicine, this would be equal to clonic spasms. See: Wiseman, 1998, p. 631.

in the intestines and stomach, and [forms] static accumulations and hard concretions. The cold of [*mǔ*] *dān pí* is able to clear heat, and the acrid is able to disperse binds, so [*mǔ dān pí*] can be used to eliminate this. The lungs act as the chief of the five viscera, [and if] the lungs are quiet, all the five viscera are quiet as well. Welling-abscesses and sores all belong to heart fire. [When one uses *mǔ dān pí*], the heart fire downbears and the welling-abscesses and sores can be cured.

Fáng Jǐ 防己
Root of Aristolochia fangchi/ Root of Stephaniae tetrandrae[261]

氣味辛 、平，無毒 。主風寒溫瘧，熱氣諸癇，除邪，利大小便 。

The qì and flavor are acrid, neutral, and non-toxic. [*Fáng jǐ*] governs wind-cold, warm malaria, heat qì, and the various epilepsies. [It also] eliminates evil and disinhibits the stool and urine.

述：防己氣平，稟金之氣 。味辛無毒，得金之味，入手太陰肺經 。風寒溫瘧者，感風寒而患但熱不寒之瘧也 。熱氣諸癇者，心有熱而患牛 、馬 、豬 、羊 、雞 、諸癇也 。溫熱皆為陽邪，癇瘧皆屬風木，防己辛平可以統治之 。除邪者，又申言可除以上之邪氣也 。然肺為水之上源，又與大腸為表裏，防己之辛平調肺氣，則二便利矣 。

Commentary: *Fáng jǐ's* qì is neutral, [and] inherits the qì of metal. The flavor is acrid, non-toxic, obtains the flavor of metal, and enters the hand tàiyīn lung channel. Wind-cold and warm malaria is contraction of wind-cold [where the patient] suffers from malaria and fever without chills. Heat qì and the various epilepsies [are because the] heart has heat, and [the patient] suffers from the various epilepsies of cow, horse, pig, sheep, or chicken epilepsy.[262] Warmth and heat are both yáng evils; epilepsy and malaria both belong to wind and wood; [because] *fáng jǐ* is acrid and neutral, [it] can be used to govern this. Eliminates evil: this [sentence merely] further expands, that [*fáng jǐ*] can eliminate the above-mentioned evil qì. So, the lungs are the upper source of water and together with the large intestine act [as having an] exterior-interior [relationship. Therefore, when] the acrid and neutral [flavors] of *fáng jǐ* regulate the lung qì, then the stool and urine are disinhibited!

261. There are two different species: *hàn fáng jǐ* 漢防己 (Stephaniae tetrandrae Radix) and *guǎng fáng jǐ* 廣防己 (Aristolochiae fangchi Radix). The latter is nowadays obsolete, because it is toxic. It is not really clear, which one is meant here. However, in the decoctions listed below, this is *guǎng fáng jǐ* 廣防己 (Aristolochiae fangchi Radix).

262. *Niú, mǎ, zhū, yáng,* [*quǎn*], *jī, zhū xián* 牛 、馬 、豬 、羊 、[犬] 、雞 、諸癇 are the various epilepsies of cow, horse, pig, sheep, [dog], or chicken. The six animal epilepsies are seizures classified according to the sound the patient makes at the onset of the disease. See: *Bèi Jí Qiān Jīn Yào Fāng*《備急千金要方》 (Essential Prescriptions Worth a Thousand in Gold for Every Emergency), Chapter 5.

張隱庵曰：《經》云：水道不行則形消氣索。是水有隨氣而運行於膚表者，有水火上下之相濟者，如氣滯而水不行則為水病、痰病矣。防己生於漢中者，破之紋如車輻，莖藤空通，主通氣行水，以防己土之制，故有防己之名。

Zhāng Yǐn'ān said: The classic says: "If the waterways do not circulate, then the body disperses the qì and is exhausted."[263] This water [which] exists, follows qì and moves into the skin and exterior; [this is because of] the existence of the mutual aid of water and fire [in the] upper and lower. For example, [if] the qì stagnates and water does not circulate, this results in water and phlegm diseases! *Fáng jǐ* grows in Hànzhōng.[264] When it is broken, [one can see] linear markings like the spokes of a wheel, and the stalks are hollow and continuous. [*Fáng jǐ*] governs the free [flow] of qì and circulates the water; [this is] because [*fáng jǐ*] restrains earth, [and] therefore it has the name *fáng jǐ*.[265]

《金匱》方治水病有防己黃耆湯、防己茯苓湯。治痰病有木防己湯、防己加茯苓芒硝湯。《千金方》治遺尿、小便澀，有三物木防己湯。蓋氣運於上，而水能就下也。

In the *Jīn Guì*, the formulas for treating water disease are *Fáng Jǐ Huáng Qí Tāng* and *Fáng Jǐ Fú Líng Tāng*. [The formulas that] treat phlegm diseases are *Mù Fáng Jǐ Tāng* and *Fáng Jǐ Jiā Fú Líng Máng Xiāo Tāng*. In the *Qiān Jīn Fāng*, there is *Sān Wù Mù Fáng Jǐ Tāng* for treating enuresis and rough urination. Now, if the qì is transported to the upper [body], consequently the water is able to [move] downwards at once.

而李東垣有云：「防己乃下焦血分之藥，病在上焦氣分者禁用。」又云：「如險健之人，幸災樂禍，首為亂階，若善用之亦可敵凶突險。此瞑眩之藥，故聖人存而不廢。」噫！如此議論，不知從何處參出？夫氣化而後水行，防己乃行氣利水之品，反云上焦氣分不可用，何不通之甚乎？防己能運行去病，是運中有補。

Accordingly, Lǐ Dōngyuán said: "*Fáng jǐ* is a medicinal of the lower *jiāo* and blood aspect. If the disease is located in the upper *jiāo* or qì aspect, it is contraindicated." He further said: "[*Fáng jǐ*] is like a mean and crafty person, who takes pleasure in others' misfortune and whose chief [concern] is to confuse the ranks, [but] if it is used skillfully, [*fáng jǐ*] can match the inauspicious and sudden dan-

---

263. This is a quotation from the *Huáng Dì Nèi Jīng Sù Wèn · Shì Cóng Róng Lùn* 《黃帝內經素問・示從容論》 (Inner Canon of the Yellow Emperor Plain Questions · Discussion on Revealing the Unhurried), Chapter 76, Line 2.

264. Hànzhōng 漢中 is an old name for the eastern Shǎnxī 陝西 province of today.

265. *Fáng jǐ* 防己 literally means "self-protecting."

ger. This is a confusing medicinal.[266] Therefore, the sages preserved [*fáng jǐ*] and did not abandon it."[267] Alas, when the discussion is like this, it is unknown from where to start the investigation! The qì transforms and after the water moves, *fáng jǐ* then is a medicinal which moves qì and disinhibits water. Conversely, [Lǐ Dōngyuán] said: This cannot be used for the the upper *jiāo* of the qì aspect. What an extreme lack of thorough understanding! *Fáng jǐ* is able to eliminate disease by moving; within this moving [quality], there is supplementation.

《本經》列於中品之前，奚為存而不廢？緣其富而貪名，無格物實學，每為臆說，使後人遵之如格言，畏之若毒藥，非古人之罪乎？李時珍乃謂千古而下，惟東垣一人誤矣。嗟嗟！安得伊黃人再世，更將經旨復重宣。

The *Shén Nóng Běn Cǎo Jīng* arranges [*fáng jǐ*] prior to the middle grade [of medicinals], why was it preserved and not abandoned? The reason is that [Lǐ Dōngyuán,] was wealthy and coveted his name, [so he wanted this] without investigating matters, and truly studying each assumption and theory. [When] later generations employed and obeyed his investigations and words, if [they] fear toxic medicinals, is this not the fault of [Lǐ Dōngyuán]? Lǐ Shízhēn therefore said: Through the ages, only the single person of [Lǐ] Dōngyuán was mistaken! Alas! How can he be reborn as a yellow person, and generally change the use and aim of the classics, yet repeatedly declare [the changes]?

Gǒu Jǐ 狗脊
Rhizome of Cibotium barometz

氣味苦、平。主腰背強，關機緩急，風痹寒濕膝痛，頗利老人。

The qì and flavor are bitter and neutral. [*Gǒu jǐ*] governs lower-back and back stiffness, relaxes joint[268] tension, [relieves] wind impediment with cold-damp knee pain, and is rather advantageous for old people.

---

266. *Miàn xuàn yào* 瞑眩藥 (confusing, dizzying medicinal) is a term from *Mèngzǐ · Téngwén Gōng Shàng* 《孟子·滕文公上》(Mencius · First Part of Duke Tengwen), Chapter 5, Line 1. Here, it is said that if a medicinal does not cause confusion and dizziness, it does not cure the disease. The confusion and dizziness are an external sign of the medicinal's benefit.

267. See Lǐ Gǎo's 李杲 *Yī Xuě Fā Míng* 《醫學發明》(Inventions of Medicine).

268. *Guān jǐ* 關機 means the joints in the human body.

神農本草經讀・卷三

Qín Jiāo 秦艽
Root of Gentiana macrophylla

氣味苦、平，無毒。主寒熱邪氣，寒濕風痺，肢節痛，下水，利小便。

The qì and flavor are bitter, neutral, and non-toxic. [*Qín jiāo*] governs the evil qì of cold and heat, cold-damp-wind impediment, and limb and joint pain. [It also] purges water and disinhibits the urine.

張隱庵曰：秦艽氣味苦平，色如黃土，羅紋交紏，左右旋轉，稟天地陰陽交感之氣。蓋天氣左旋右轉，地氣右旋左轉，左右者，陰陽之道路。

Zhāng Yǐn'ān said: *Qín jiāo's* qì and flavor are bitter and neutral. The color is like yellow earth, with a ribbed and entangled pattern that revolves around it on both sides. [*Qín jiāo*] inherits the qì of heaven and earth, mutual interacting as yīn and yáng. Now, the heavenly qì[269] revolves to the left and circles to the right, the earthly qì[270] revolves to the right and circles to the left. Left and right are the pathways of yīn and yáng.

主治寒熱邪氣者，地氣從內以出外，陰氣外交於陽，而寒熱邪氣自散矣。治寒濕風痺，肢節痛者，天氣從外以入內，陽氣內交於陰，則寒濕風三邪合而成痺以致肢節痛者，可愈也。地氣運行則水下，天氣運行則小便利。

[*Qín jiāo*] governs the evil qì of cold and heat, because the earthly qì from the interior issues forth to the exterior. The yīn qì of the exterior interacts in the yáng, and the evil qì of cold and heat naturally disperse! [*Qín jiāo*] treats cold-damp-wind impediment and limb joint pain, because the heavenly qì from the exterior enters the interior, and the yáng qì of the interior interacts in the yīn. As a result, the three evils of cold, damp, and wind, that combine forming the impediment and cause the limb and joint pain, can [then] be healed. When the earthly qì moves, then water is purged. When the heavenly qì moves, then urine is disinhibited.

---

269. Yáng qì.
270. Yīn qì.

Zǐ Wǎn 紫菀
Root and rhizome of Aster tataricus

氣味苦、溫，無毒。主咳逆上氣，胸中寒熱結氣，去蠱毒，痿蹷，安五臟。

The qì and flavor are bitter, warm, and non-toxic. [*Zǐ wǎn*] governs cough with counterflow qì ascent, [as well as] cold or hot bound qì in the chest center; [it] expels *gǔ* venoms, crippling wilt,[271] and quiets the five viscera.

張隱庵曰：紫者，黑赤之間色也。黑赤，水火之色也。紫菀氣味苦溫，稟火氣也。其質陰柔，稟水氣也。主治咳逆上氣者，啟太陽寒水之氣從皮毛而合肺也。治胸中寒熱結氣者，助少陰火熱之氣，通利三焦而上達也。蠱毒在腹屬土，火能生土，故去蠱毒。痿蹷在筋屬木，水能生木，故去痿蹷。水火者，陰陽之徵兆也，水火交則陰陽合，故安五臟。

Zhāng Yǐn'ān said: Purple is a color between black and red. Black and red are the colors of water and fire. *Zǐ wǎn's* qì and flavor are bitter and warm, and it inherits the qì of fire. [*Zǐ wǎn's*] yīn and soft quality inherits the qì of water. [*Zǐ wǎn*] governs cough with counterflow qì ascent because it initiates the qì of tàiyáng cold water from the skin and [body] hair and [these] combine in the lungs. [*Zǐ wǎn*] treats cold or hot bound qì in the chest center because it assists the qì of shàoyīn fire and heat fire to freely disinhibit the sānjiāo and outthrust upwards. *Gǔ* venoms located in the abdomen belong to earth. Fire is able to generate earth; therefore, [*zǐ wǎn*] expels *gǔ* venoms. Crippling wilt is located in the sinews and belongs to wood. Water is able to generate wood; therefore, [*zǐ wǎn*] expels crippling wilt. Water and fire are the signs of yīn and yáng. If water and fire interact, then yīn and yáng combine, therefore quieting the five viscera.

Zhī Mǔ 知母
Root of Anemarrhena asphodeloides

氣味苦、寒，無毒。主消渴熱中，除邪氣，肢體浮腫，下水，補不足，益氣。

The qì and flavor are bitter, cold, and non-toxic. [*Zhī mǔ*] governs dispersion-thirst, heat strike, and eliminates evil qì. [It also governs] puffy swelling of the limbs and body, purges water, supplements insufficiency, and boosts the qì.

---

271. The term *bì* 蹷 (cripple, lame) denotes a spastic paralysis of the lower extremities.

葉天士曰：知母氣寒，稟水氣而入腎。味苦無毒，得火味而入心。腎屬水，心屬火，水不制火，火爍津液，則病消渴。火熏五內，則病熱中。其主之者，苦清心火，寒滋腎水也。

Yè Tiānshì said: *Zhī mǔ's* qì is cold, inherits the qì of water, and enters the kidneys. The flavor is bitter, non-toxic, obtains the fire flavor, and enters the heart. The kidneys belong to water, the heart belongs to fire; if water does not control fire, the fire scorches the fluids, resulting in disease of dispersion-thirst. If fire fumes the five viscera, this results in disease of heat strike. [*Zhī mǔ*] governs this, because bitter clears heart fire and cold enriches kidney water.

除邪氣者，苦寒之氣味能除燥火之邪氣也。熱勝則浮，火勝則腫。苦能清火，寒能退熱，故主肢體浮腫也。腎者水臟，其性惡燥，燥則開合不利而水反蓄矣。知母寒滑，滑利關門而水自下也。補不足者，苦寒補寒水之不足也。益氣者，苦寒益五臟之陰氣也。

[*Zhī mǔ*] eliminates evil qì, because the qì and flavor of bitter and cold are able to eliminate the evil qì of dryness-fire. If heat dominates, then [there is] puffiness; if fire dominates, then [there is] swelling. Bitter is able to clear fire, cold is able to abate heat, therefore [*zhī mǔ*] governs puffy swelling of the limbs and body. The kidneys are the water viscus, the nature [of the kidney is to be] averse to dryness. If [there is] dryness, the opening and closing are inhibited, and water is instead amassed! *Zhī mǔ* is cold and slippery. [When] the slippery disinhibits closed doors, then water is naturally purged. [*Zhī mǔ*] supplements insufficiency, because bitter and cold supplement the insufficiency of cold water.[272] [*Zhī mǔ*] boosts the qì, [because] the bitter and cold boost the yīn qì of the five viscera.

愚按：《金匱》有桂枝芍藥知母湯，治肢節疼痛、身體尪羸、腳腫如脫，可知長沙諸方，皆從《本經》來也。

My humble comments: In the *Jīn Guì* there is *Guì Zhī Sháo Yào Zhī Mǔ Tāng* [which] treats limb and joint pain, weakness and emaciation of the body, and swelling of the legs like in desertion. [From this we] can know, that all the formulas of Chángshā[273] derive from the *Shén Nóng Běn Cǎo Jīng*.[274]

---

272. This means insufficiency of the kidneys.

273. Zhāng Zhòngjǐng.

274. This annotation was either written by Chén Xiūyuán's 陳修園 nephew Fèng Téng 鳳騰 or Chén Xiūyuán 陳修園.

Bèi Mǔ 貝母
Bulb of Fritillaria cirrhosa

氣味辛、平，無毒。主傷寒煩熱，淋瀝邪氣，疝瘕，喉痹，乳難，金瘡，風痓。

The qì and flavor are acrid, neutral, and non-toxic. [*Bèi mǔ*] governs cold damage vexation heat, strangury and urinary dripping evil qì, mounting-conglomeration, throat impediment, difficult lactation, incised wounds, and wind tetany.

陳修園曰：貝母氣平味辛，氣味俱屬於金，為手太陰、手陽明藥也。其主傷寒煩熱者，取西方之金氣以除酷暑。《傷寒論》以白虎湯命名，亦此意也。其主淋瀝邪氣者，肺之治節行於膀胱，則邪熱之氣除，而淋瀝愈矣。

Chén Xiūyuán said: *Bèi mǔ's* qì is neutral and its flavor is acrid, so the qì and flavor both belong to metal. [*Bèi mǔ*] is a medicinal of hand tàiyīn and hand yángmíng. [*Bèi mǔ*] governs cold damage vexation heat, because it uses the metal qì of the west[275] to eliminate scorching summerheat. The name of *Bái Hǔ Tāng* in the *Shāng Hán Lùn* also has this same meaning.[276] [*Bèi mǔ*] governs strangury and urinary dripping evil qì, [because when] the lung manages and regulates the movement of the bladder, then the evil heat qì is eliminated, and the strangury and urinary dripping are healed!

疝瘕為肝木受病，此則金平木也。喉痹為肺竅內閉，此能宣通肺氣也。乳少為陽明之汁不通，金瘡為陽明之經脈受傷，風痓為陽明之宗筋不利，貝母清潤而除熱，所以統治之。今人以之治痰嗽，大失經旨。且李士材謂：貝母主燥痰，半夏主濕痰，二物如冰炭之反，皆臆說也。

Mounting conglomeration is contraction of disease in liver wood. When this [medicinal is taken], then metal calms wood. Throat impediment is an internal block of the orifice of the lung, and this [medicinal] is able to diffuse and free the lung qì. Scant breast milk is obstruction of the juice of yángmíng. Incised wounds are contraction of damage of the channel and vessel of yángmíng. Wind tetany is inhibition of the ancestral sinews[277] of yángmíng. *Bèi mǔ* clears, moisturizes, and eliminates

---

275. The west is associated with the element of metal, the north with water, the east with wood, the south with fire and the center with earth. See: *Huáng Dì Nèi Jīng Sù Wèn · Jīn Guì Zhēn Yán Lùn* 《黃帝內經素問·金匱真言論》 (Inner Canon of the Yellow Emperor Plain Questions · Discussions of True Words from the Golden Cabinet), Chapter 4, Line 3.

276. This is because *Bái Hǔ Tāng* 白虎湯 means *White Tiger Decoction*, and white is the color of metal.

277. Here, *zōng jīn* 宗筋 (ancestral sinews) means the gathering point of the three yīn and three yáng channels in the pubic region in women. Because of this term, it becomes clear that he is speaking of childbed wind or postpartum wind strike. See: Wiseman, 1998, pp. 60 and 468.

heat; therefore, it governs these [conditions]. People of today use [*bèi mǔ*] for treating phlegm cough, but this greatly loses the intention of the classic. Further, Lǐ Shìcái said: *Bèi mǔ* governs dry phlegm and *bàn xià* governs damp phlegm. The two plants are opposites like ice and charcoal, [but these are] all [Lǐ Shìcái's] theoretical opinions.

Guā Lóu Gēn 栝蔞根
Root of Trichosanthes kirilowii

氣味苦、寒，無毒。主消渴，身熱，煩滿大熱，補虛安中，續絕傷。

The qì and flavor are bitter, cold, and non-toxic. [*Guā lóu gēn*] governs dispersion-thirst, generalized heat, vexation and fullness with great heat; [it] supplements vacuity, calms the center, and replenishes expiry damage.

陳修園曰：栝蔞根氣寒，稟天冬寒之水氣而入腎與膀胱。味苦無毒，得地南方之火味而入心。火盛爍液則消渴，火浮於表則身熱，火盛於裏則煩滿大熱，火盛則陰虛，陰虛則中失守而不安，栝蔞根之苦寒清火，可以統主之。

Chén Xiūyuán said: *Guā lóu gēn's* qì is cold, inherits the heavenly water qì of winter and cold, and enters the kidneys and urinary bladder. [*Guā lóu gēn's*] flavor is bitter, non-toxic, obtains the fire flavor of earth and south, and enters the heart. If fire is abundant, it scorches the humor, and then [there is] dispersion-thirst. If fire floats in the exterior, then [there is] generalized heat. If fire is abundant in the interior, then [there is] vexation and fullness with great heat. If fire is abundant, then yīn is vacuous. If yīn is vacuous, then the center loses its defense and is disquieted. The bitter and cold of *guā lóu gēn* clears fire; [therefore,] it is able to govern these [diseases].

其主續絕傷者，以其蔓延能通陰絡而續其絕也。實名栝蔞，《金匱》取治胸痹，《傷寒論》取治結胸，蓋以能開胸前之結也。

[*Guā lóu gēn*] replenishes expiry damage, because its spreading is able to free the yīn collaterals and replenish their expiry. The seeds are called *guā lóu*, and in the *Jīn Guì* they are taken to treat chest impediment. In the *Shāng Hán Lùn* [the seeds] are taken to treat chest bind. So, possibly they are able to open binds in the front of the chest.

張隱庵曰：半夏起陰氣於脈外，上與陽明相合而成火土之燥。花粉起陰津於脈中，天癸相合而能滋其燥金。《傷寒》、《金匱》諸方，用半夏以助陽明之氣，渴者燥熱太過，即去半夏易花粉以滋之。聖賢立方加減，必推物理所以然。

Zhāng Yǐn'ān said: *Bàn xià* raises the yīn qì from outside of the vessels, and the upper [body] and yángmíng combine with each other and become the dryness of fire and earth. *Huā fěn*[278] raises the yīn liquids from within the vessels, [and] the original yīn[279] combine with each other, and is able to enrich the dry metal. All the formulas from the *Shāng Hán* and the *Jīn Guì* use *bàn xià* to assist the qì of yángmíng. Thirst [is when] dryness and heat are greatly excessive; then remove *bàn xià* and exchange it with *huā fěn* in order to enrich this [dryness]. When the sage [Zhāng Zhòngjǐng] established the modifications [of his] formulas, he must have inferred that the principles of this plant are like this.

Sháo Yào 芍藥
Root of Paeonia rubra

氣味苦、平，無毒。主邪氣腹痛，除血痹，破堅積，寒熱疝瘕，止痛，利小便，益氣。

The qì and flavor are bitter, neutral, and non-toxic. [*Sháo yào*] governs the evil qì of abdominal pain, eliminates blood impediment, breaks hard accumulations, cold and heat mounting-conglomeration, stops pain, disinhibits urine, and boosts the qì.

陳修園曰：芍藥氣平，是夏花而稟燥金之氣。味苦，是得少陰君火之味。氣平下降，味苦下泄而走血，為攻下之品，非補養之物也。

Chén Xiūyuán said: *Sháo yào's* qì is neutral; it is a summer flower, and inherits the qì of dry metal. [*Sháo yào's*] flavor is bitter, [and] obtains the flavor of shàoyīn sovereign fire. [*Sháo yào's*] qì is neutral, descending, and downbearing, the bitter flavor drains the lower [body] and moves the blood. [This is] because [it is a] medicinal for offensive purgation; it is not a plant that supplements or nourishes.

---

278. *Tiān huā fěn* 天花粉 is another name for *guā lóu gēn* 栝蔞根 (trichosanthes root).

279. *Tiān guǐ* 天癸 (heavenly tenth) is another name for the original yīn; this is the kidney essence. See: Wiseman, 1998, p. 286.

邪氣腹痛、小便不利及一切諸痛，皆氣滯之病，其主之者，以苦平而泄其氣也。血痺者，血閉而不行，甚則為寒熱不調。堅積者，積久而堅實，甚則為疝瘕滿痛者，皆血滯之病，其主之者，以苦平而行其血也。

The evil qì of abdominal pain, inhibited urination, as well as the various kinds of pain are all diseases of qì stagnation. [*Sháo yào*] governs this, because the bitter and neutral discharge the [patient's stagnant] qì. Blood impediment is blood block that does not move, [and when] severe, then [there] is disharmony of cold and heat. Hard accumulations are chronic accumulations that are hard and solid, [and when] severe, then [there] is mounting-conglomeration with fullness and pain. These are all diseases of blood stagnation, [and *sháo yào*] governs these, because it is bitter and neutral and moves the [stagnant] blood.

又云：益氣者，謂邪氣得攻而淨，則元氣自然受益，非謂芍藥能補氣也。今人妄改聖經，以酸寒二字易苦平，誤認為斂陰之品，殺人無算。試取芍藥而嚼之，酸味何在乎？張隱庵云：赤芍，白芍花異而根無異。今肆中一種赤芍藥，不知何物之根，為害殊甚。

Moreover, it is said that [*sháo yào*] boosts the qì; this means [that when] the evil qì [which is] contracted, is attacked and cleansed, then the original qì naturally receives a boost. It does not mean, that *sháo yào* [itself] is able to supplement the qì. Today, people rashly alter the sage's classic, and exchange the two characters "bitter and neutral" for "sour and cold." They falsely believe [*sháo yào*] to be a medicinal [that] constrains the yīn, [thus] killing an incalculable [number] of people. [I] tested *sháo yào* and chewed it. Where is the sour flavor? Zhāng Yǐn'ān said: The flowers of *sháo yào* and *bái sháo* are different, but the root cannot be distinguished. Nowadays, within the market [there is] one kind of red *sháo yào*, but without knowing which kind of root it is, [it can] cause extraordinary harm.

Mù Tōng 木通
Stalk of Akebia quinata

氣味辛、平，無毒。主除脾胃寒熱，通利九竅，血脈，關節，令人不忘，去惡蟲。

The qì and flavor are acrid, neutral, and non-toxic. [*Mù tōng*] governs and eliminates cold and heat of the spleen and stomach; unblocks the nine orifices, the blood vessels and the joints; prevents people's forgetfulness; and expels malign *gǔ*.

木通，《本經》名通草。陳士良撰《食性本草》，改為木通。今復有
所謂通草，即古之通脫木也，與此不同。

In the Shén Nóng Běn Cǎo Jīng, mù tōng is called tōng cǎo. When Chén Shìliáng[280] compiled his Shí Xìng Běn Cǎo, he altered it to mù tōng. Today, there is yet [a plant] that is called tōng cǎo, [but] this is the ancient tōng tuō mù, and this is not the same.

張隱庵曰：木通藤蔓空通，其色黃白，氣味辛平，稟土金相生之氣化，而為
通關利竅之藥也。稟土氣，故除脾胃之寒熱。藤蔓空通，故通利九竅、血
脈、關節。血脈通而關竅利，則令人不忘。稟金氣，故去惡蠱。

Zhāng Yǐn'ān said: Mù tōng's vine is hollow and continuous, and the color is yellowish-white. [Mù tōng's] qì and flavor are acrid, neutral, and inherit the qì transformation of earth and metal [which] generate each other. So [mù tōng] is a medicinal for opening gates and disinhibiting orifices. [Mù tōng] inherits the earth qì; therefore, [it] eliminates the cold and heat from the spleen and stomach. The vine is hollow and continuous; therefore, it unblocks the nine orifices, the blood vessels, and the joints. If the blood vessels are free [flowing], and the joints and orifices are disinhibited, then this prevents people's forgetfulness. [Mù tōng] inherits the metal qì; therefore, [it] expels malign gǔ.

防己、木通，皆屬空通蔓草。防己取用在下之根，則其性自下而上，從內而
外。木通取用在上之莖，則其性自上而下，自外而內，此根升梢降，一定不
易之理。後人用之主利小便，須知小便之利，亦必上而後下，外而後內也。

Fáng jǐ and mù tōng both belong to the hollow and continuous creepers. With fáng jǐ, [one] uses the roots from under [the ground]; as a result, its nature is [directed] from the lower to upper, and from the inside to the outside. With mù tōng, [one] uses the stalks from above [the ground]; as a result, its nature is [directed] from the upper to the lower, and from the outside to the inside. This [is because] the roots upbear and the tips downbear; this surely [is an] unchanging principle. The people of later generations mainly used [mù tōng] to disinhibit the urine, [so they] should have known that to disinhibit the urine, [this] must also ascend and then descend, from the outside and then to the internal [body].

---

280. Chén Shìliáng 陳士良, also written 陳仕良 (tenth century), author of the *Shí Xìng Běn Cǎo* 《食性本草》 (Materia Medica on the Nature of Food) is a physician of the Later *Táng* from the city of Kāifēng. See: Lǐ, 1985, p. 314.

神農本草經讀・卷三

Bái Zhǐ 白芷
Root of Angelica dahurica

氣味辛、溫。主女人漏下，赤白，血閉，陰腫，寒熱，風侵頭目淚出，長肌膚，潤澤，可作面脂。

The qì and flavor are acrid and warm. [*Bái zhǐ*] governs women's spotting, red and white [vaginal discharge], blood block, genital swelling, cold and heat, wind invading the head and eyes [causing] tearing; it grows the skin [and flesh], moisturizes, and can be used as a facial cream.

Kǔ Shēn 苦參
Root of Sophora flavescens

氣味苦、寒。主心腹結氣，癥瘕積聚，黃膽，溺有餘瀝。逐水，除癰腫，補中，明目止淚。

The qì and flavor are bitter and cold. [*Kǔ shēn*] governs bound qì in the heart and abdomen, concretions, conglomerations, accumulations, and gatherings, jaundice, and dripping after urination. [*Kǔ shēn*] expels water, eliminates swollen welling-abscesses, supplements the center, brightens the eyes, and stops tearing.

徐靈胎曰：此以味為治也。苦入心，寒除火，故苦參專治心經之火，與黃連功用相近，但黃連似去心臟之火為多，苦參似去心腑小腸之火為多，則以黃連之氣味清，而苦參之氣味濁也。

Xú Língtāi said: This [medicinal] uses the flavor to treat. Bitter enters the heart, cold eliminates fire, and therefore *kǔ shēn* specifically treats fire in the heart channel. The action is similar to *huáng lián*, but *huáng lián* appears to remove fire [which] is copious from the heart viscus. *Kǔ shēn* appears to remove fire [which] is copious from the bowel of the small intestine. Therefore the qì and flavor of *huáng lián* are clear, but the qì and flavor of *kǔ shēn* are turbid.

按：「補中」二字，亦取其苦以燥脾之義也。

Comment: The two characters "supplement the center," also mean: [when one] applies the bitter of [kǔ shēn, this can be] used to dry the spleen.

Shuǐ Píng 水萍
Whole plant of Spirodela polyrhiza

氣味辛、寒。主暴熱，得水之氣，故能除熱。身癢，濕熱在皮膚。下水氣萍入水不濡，故能滌水。勝酒，水氣勝則酒氣散矣。長須發，益皮毛之血氣。主消渴。得水氣之助。久服輕身。亦如萍之輕也。

The qì and flavor are acrid and cold. [*Shuǐ píng*] governs fulminant heat *by obtaining the qì of water, therefore it is able to eliminate heat.* [It governs] generalized itching *because damp-heat is located in the skin.* [It] purges water qì *[because shuǐ píng enters the water without [becoming] moist; therefore, it is able to sweep water away.* [It] dominates alcohol *[because when] water qì dominates, then the alcohol qì is dispersed.* [It] grows the beard and hair *[because it] boosts the blood and qì of the skin and hair.* [It] governs dispersion-thirst *by obtaining assistance from water qì,* and when taken over a long period of time, it lightens the body, *this also is like the lightness of [shuǐ] píng.*

徐靈胎曰：水萍生於水中，而能出水上，且其葉入水不濡，是其性能敵水者也。故凡水濕之病皆能治之。其根不著土而上浮水面，故又能主皮毛之疾。

Xú Língtái said: *Shuǐ píng* grows within water and is able to grow out of the water [and onto the] surface. Further, its leaves are in the water, but do not become moist. This means that [*shuǐ píng's*] nature is able to resist water. Therefore, generally all kinds of diseases of water and damp are able to be treated with this. [*Shuǐ píng's*] root does not touch the earth and it floats on the water surface; therefore, [*shuǐ píng*] has the ability to govern diseases of the skin and hair.

Kuǎn Dōng Huā 款冬花
Flower of Tussilago farfara

氣味辛、溫，無毒。主咳逆上氣善喘，喉痹，諸驚癇，寒熱邪氣。

The qì and flavor are acrid, warm, and non-toxic. [*Kuǎn dōng huā*] governs cough with counterflow qì ascent and a tendency to pant, throat impediment, the various fright epilepsies, as well as cold and heat evil qì.

張隱庵曰：款冬生於水中，花開紅白，氣味辛溫，從陰出陽，蓋稟水中之生陽，而上通肺金之藥也。太陽寒水之氣，不從皮毛外交於肺，則咳逆上氣而善喘。款冬稟水氣而通肺，故可治也。

Zhāng Yǐn'ān said: *Kuǎn dōng* grows within the water; its blossoms are pink. The qì and flavor are acrid and warm, so it is yáng issuing forth from yīn. Therefore, it inherits the generative yáng within water, and is a medicinal which ascends to the lung-metal. When the qì of tàiyáng cold water does not [flow] from outside the skin and [body] hair to interact in the lungs, then [there is] cough with counterflow qì ascent, and a tendency to pant. *Kuǎn dōng* inherits the water qì and frees the lungs; therefore, it can treat this.

厥陰、少陽木火之氣結於喉中，則為喉痹。款冬得金水之氣，金能平木，水能制火，故可治也。驚癇，寒熱邪氣，為病不止一端，故曰諸驚癇寒熱邪氣。款冬稟太陽寒水之氣，而上行外達，則陰陽水火之氣自相交會，故可治也。

If the qì of juèyīn or shàoyáng wood or fire bind in the throat, then [this] is throat impediment. *Kuǎn dōng* obtains the qì of metal and water, the metal is able to calm wood, and water is able to control fire; therefore, [*kuǎn dōng huā*] can treat this. Fright epilepsy and evil cold and heat qì are incessant diseases; therefore, [the *Shén Nóng Běn Cǎo Jīng*] said: "the various fright epilepsies, as well as cold and heat evil qì." *Kuǎn dōng* inherits the qì of tàiyáng cold water and ascends to circulate and outthrust to the exterior. As a result, the qì of yīn and yáng, as well as water and fire, naturally converge and meet with each other. Therefore, [*kuǎn dōng*] can treat [the diseases above].

Hòu Pò 厚朴
Bark of Magnolia officinalis

氣味苦、溫，無毒。主中風，傷寒，頭痛，寒熱，驚悸，氣血痹，死肌，去三蟲。生用則解肌而達表，炙香則運土而助脾。

The qì and flavor are bitter, warm, and non-toxic. [*Hòu pò*] governs wind strike, cold damage, headache, cold and heat, fright palpitations, qì and blood impediment, and dead flesh;[281] [it also] eliminates the three worms.[282] *When used fresh, then [hòu pò] resolves the flesh and outthrusts to the exterior. When used honey-fried, then [hòu pò] transports the earth[283] and assists the spleen.*

---

281. Necrosis of the flesh.

282. See Footnote 41 from Chapter 1.

283. This means the stomach qì.

陳修園曰：厚朴氣溫，稟木氣而入肝。味苦無毒，得火味而入心。然氣味厚而主降，降則溫而專於散，苦而專於泄，故所主皆為實症。

Chén Xiūyuán said: *Hòu pò's* qì is warm, inherits the wood qì, and enters the liver. [*Hòu pò's*] flavor is bitter, non-toxic, obtains the fire flavor, [and] enters the heart. This being so, the qì and flavor are rich and govern downbearing. The downbearing then warms and is especially [good at] dispersing; the bitter [is especially good] at discharging. Therefore, [*hòu pò*] always governs conditions caused by repletion.

中風有便溺阻隔症，傷寒有下之微喘症，有發汗後腹脹滿症、大便硬症，頭痛有濁氣上衝症，俱宜主以厚朴也。至於溫能散寒，苦能泄熱，能散能泄，則可以解氣逆之驚悸。

[When there] is wind strike with the condition of stool and urine obstruction; [or] cold damage with the condition of slight panting from purging; or the condition [where] after promotion of sweating, there is abdominal distention and fullness; or the condition [where there is] hardness of the stool; [or] headaches with the condition of turbid qì surging upwards: in each case, it is appropriate to govern by using *hòu pò*. As to warmth [being] able to disperse cold, [and] bitter [being] able to discharge heat, [because *hòu pò*] is able to disperse and discharge, then [this] can resolve the fright palpitations of qì counterflow.

能散則氣行，能泄則血行，故可以治氣血痹及死肌也。三蟲本濕氣所化，厚朴能散而泄之，則三蟲可去也。寬脹下氣，經無明文，仲景因其氣味苦溫而取用之，得《本經》言外之旨也。

[*Hòu pò* is] able to disperse; [thus] as a result, the qì moves. [*Hòu pò* is] is able to discharge; [and] as a result, the blood moves. Therefore, [*hòu pò*] can treat qì and blood impediment, as well as dead flesh. The root of the three parasites is the influence of damp qì; [when] *hòu pò* is able to disperse and discharge [the damp qì], then the three worms can be eliminated. [Regarding *hòu pò's* ability] to ease distention and descend the qì, the writing of the classics is not clear. [It seems that] Zhòngjǐng applied [*hòu pò*] because its qì and flavor are bitter and warm, and so this goes beyond the intention and words of the *Shén Nóng Běn Cǎo Jīng*.

Zhī Zǐ 梔子
Fruit of Gardenia jasminoides

氣味苦寒，無毒。主五內邪氣，胃中熱氣，面赤，酒皰齇鼻，白癩，赤癩，瘡瘍。

The qì and flavor are bitter, cold, and non-toxic. [*Zhī zǐ*] governs the evil qì of the five viscera, heat qì in the stomach, red face, alcohol pimples on the nose,[284] white *lài*,[285] red *lài*,[286] and sores.

陳修園曰：梔子氣寒，稟水氣而入腎。味苦，得火味而入心。五內邪氣，五臟受熱邪之氣也。胃中熱氣，胃經熱煩，懊憹不眠也。心之華在面，赤則心火盛也。鼻屬肺，酒皰齇鼻，金受火剋而色赤也。

Chén Xiūyuán said: *Zhī zǐ's* qì is cold, inherits the qì of water, and enters the kidneys. [*Zhī zǐ's*] flavor is bitter, obtains the fire flavor, and enters the heart. The evil qì of the five viscera is the qì of the five viscera [that] contracts evil heat. Heat qì in the stomach is heat vexation of the stomach vessel with anguish and sleeplessness. The bloom of the heart is in the face;[287] [if the face] is red, then the heart fire is abundant. The nose belongs to the lungs; [if there are] alcohol pimples on the nose, [then] metal is subjected to fire's control and [the nose becomes] red colored.

白癩為濕，赤癩為熱，瘡瘍為心火。梔子下稟寒水之精，上結君火之實，能起水陰之氣上滋，復導火熱之氣下行，故統主之。以上諸症，唯生用之，氣性尚存，若炒黑則為死灰，無用之物矣。仲景梔子豉湯用之者，取其交媾水火、調和心腎之功。加香豉以引其吐，非梔子能涌吐也。俗本謂梔子生用則吐，炒黑則不吐，何其陋歟？按：仲景云：舊有微溏者，勿用。

White *lài* is damp, red *lài* is heat, and sores are heart fire. The lower part of the *zhī zǐ* [plant] inherits the essence of cold water, and the upper part, [which] bears the fruit and seeds, [inherits] sovereign fire. [*Zhī zǐ*] is able to raise the qì of water yīn to enrich the upper [body], yet guides the qì of fire heat to move [in the] lower [body]; therefore, [*zhī zǐ*] governs this. For the various conditions above, [*zhī zǐ*] is only used raw, so that the qì and nature are still preserved. If [the *zhī zǐ*] is stir-fried until black, then it is burnt to ashes and becomes a useless thing! The use of Zhòngjǐng's *Zhī Zǐ*

284. *Jiǔ pào zhā bí* 酒皰齇鼻 (alcohol blisters and pimples on the nose) is the same as *bí chì* 鼻赤 (red nose), and means drinker´s nose or rosacea.

285. *Bái lài* 白癩 (white leprosy) is a disease characterized by gradual whitening of skin areas, numbness of the limbs, etc. In Western terms, this would be tuberculoid leprosy. See: Wiseman, 1998, p. 675.

286. In accordance, *bái lài*, must be leprosy with red skin areas.

287. *Xīn zhī huà zài miàn* 心之華在面 (the bloom of the heart is in the face) means that the health of the heart is reflected in the face, and shows the state of qì and blood. See: Wiseman, 1998, p. 264.

Chǐ Tāng applies the action of the intercourse of water and fire, or the harmonization of heart and kidneys. *Xiāng chǐ* is added in order to guide the vomiting, as *zhī zǐ* [itself] is not able to [cause the] ejection. In vulgar books, it is written [that when] *zhī zǐ* is used raw, then [there is] vomiting; and if stir-fried until black, then [there is] no vomiting–how ignorant is this? *Comment: Zhòngjǐng said: For old [patients] with slightly sloppy stool,[288] do not use [zhī zǐ].*

Zhǐ Shí 枳實
Unripe fruit of Poncirus trifoliata

氣味苦、寒，無毒。主大風在皮膚中如麻豆苦癢，除寒熱結，止痢，長肌肉，利五臟，益氣。

The qì and flavor are bitter, cold, and non-toxic. [*Zhǐ shí*] governs great wind located within the skin like the bitter itching of measles,[289] eliminates cold and heat binds, stops dysentery, grows the flesh, disinhibits the five viscera, and boosts the qì.

張隱庵曰：枳殼氣味苦寒，冬不落葉，稟少陰標本之氣化。臭香形圓，花白多刺，瓤肉黃白，又得陽明金土之氣化。主治大風在皮膚中，如麻豆苦癢者，得陽明金氣而制風，稟少陰水氣而清熱也。

Zhāng Yǐn'ān said: *Zhǐ shí's* qì and flavor are bitter and cold; in winter it does not lose its leaves. [*Zhǐ shí*] inherits the qì transformation of shàoyīn's root and tip. The smell is fragrant, the shape is round, [and there are] white blossoms and many thorns. The pulp [of the fruit] and flesh are yellowish-white, and it obtains the qì transformation of yángmíng metal and earth. [*Zhǐ shí*] governs and treats great wind located within the skin like the bitter itching of measles; [this is because] it obtains the yángmíng metal qì and controls wind. [*Zhǐ shí* also] inherits the shàoyīn water qì and clears heat.

除寒熱結者，稟少陰本熱之氣而除寒，標陰之氣而除熱也。止痢、長肌肉者，得陽明中土之氣也。五臟發原於先天之少陰，生長於後天之陽明，故主利五臟。得少陰之陰，故益氣，得陽明之氣，故輕身。仲祖本論，有大承氣湯，用炙厚朴、炙枳實。小承氣湯，用生厚朴、生枳實。生熟之間，有意存焉，學者不可不參。

[*Zhǐ shí*] eliminates cold and heat binds; [this is because] it inherits the qì shàoyīn [where the] root is heat and eliminates cold. The qì of the tip is yīn and eliminates heat. It stops dysentery and grows

288. See: *Shāng Hán Lùn · Biàn Tài Yáng Bìng Mài Zhèng Bìng Zhì* 《傷寒論·辨太陽病脈證并治》 (On Cold Damage · Symptoms and Treatment of Tàiyáng Diseases), Chapter 6, Line 71.
289. Literally *má dòu* 麻豆 (hemp beans).

the flesh; [this is because] it obtains the qì of yángmíng center-earth. The five viscera originate in pre-heaven shàoyīn, and grow in post-heaven yángmíng; therefore, [*zhǐ shí*] governs disinhibiting the five viscera. [*Zhǐ shí*] obtains the yīn of shàoyīn; therefore, it boosts the qì. It obtains the qì of yángmíng; therefore, it lightens the body. In ancestor Zhòng's original discussion, there is the *Dà Chéng Qì Tāng* which uses honey-fried *hòu pò* and honey-fried *zhǐ shí*. *Xiǎo Chéng Qì Tāng* uses raw *hòu pò* and raw *zhǐ shí*.[290] The differentiation into raw and cooked is intended! Scholars cannot but consider this.

按《本經》有枳實，無枳殼，唐《開寶》始分之。然枳殼即枳實之大者，性宣發而氣散，不如枳實之完結，然既是一種，亦不必過分。

Comment: The *Shén Nóng Běn Cǎo Jīng* contains *zhǐ shí*, but not *zhǐ ké*. [These can only] begin to be distinguished in the *Kāi Bǎo* [*Chóng Dìng Běn Cǎo*][291] of the *Táng* dynasty. It is correct that *zhǐ ké* is just the fully grown *zhǐ shí*, and its nature diffuses and disperses the qì; the completed [entry] is inferior to *zhǐ shí*. So, since this is the same kind, it also will not be excessively different.

Huáng Niè [Bǎi] 黃蘗[柏][292]
Bark of Phellodendron amurense

氣味苦寒，無毒。主五臟腸胃中結熱，黃疸，腸痔，止泄痢，女子漏下赤白，陰傷蝕瘡。

The qì and flavor are bitter, cold, and non-toxic. [*Huáng bǎi*] governs bound heat in the five viscera, intestines, and stomach, [as well as] jaundice and intestinal hemorrhoids. [It also] stops diarrhea, women's spotting, red and white vaginal discharge, and genital damage with erosion and sores.

陳修園曰：黃蘗氣寒，稟天冬寒之水氣。味苦無毒，得地南方之火味。皮厚色黃，得太陰中土之化。五臟為陰，凡經言主五臟者，皆主陰之藥也。治腸胃中熱結者，寒能清熱也。

Chén Xiūyuán said: *Huáng bǎi's* qì is cold, and inherits the water qì of heaven, winter, and cold. [*Huáng bǎi's*] flavor is bitter, non-toxic, and obtains the fire flavor of earth and the southern direc-

---

290. This is not truly the case. In both of these formulas, they are used fried.

291. *Kāi Bǎo Chóng Dìng Běn Cǎo* 《開寶重定本草》 (Kāi Bǎo Revised Materia Medica).

292. Pronounced *bǎi*, it is commonly written *huáng bǎi* 黃柏; this is an abbreviation error. For the rest of this monograph, this medicinal will be referred to as *huáng bǎi*, but I have chosen to leave the Chinese paragraph in its original form.

tion. The skin is thick, yellow, and obtains the transformation of tàiyīn center-earth. The five viscera are yīn. Generally when the classic writes "governs the five viscera," it always governs medicinals of yīn. [*Huáng bǎi*] treats bound heat in the intestines and stomach; [this is because] cold is able to clear heat.

治黃疸、腸痔者，苦能勝濕也。止泄利者，濕熱泄痢，唯苦寒能除之，而且能堅之也。女子胎漏下血，因血熱妄行。赤白帶下，及陰戶傷蝕成瘡，皆因濕熱下注。黃蘗寒能清熱，苦可燥濕，所以主之。然皆正氣未傷，熱毒內盛，有餘之病，可以暫用，否則，不可姑試也。

[*Huáng bǎi*] treats jaundice and intestinal hemorrhoids [because] bitter is able to dominate damp. [*Huáng bǎi*] stops diarrhea, [because it stops] damp-heat diarrhea, [as] only bitter and cold are able to eliminate this. Moreover, [*huáng bǎi*] is able to harden [the stool]. Women's fetal bleeding[293] is caused by frenetic movement of blood due to heat. Red and white vaginal discharge, as well as genital damage with erosion and sores, are always caused by damp-heat pouring downwards. The cold of *huáng bǎi* is able to clear heat, the bitter can dry damp, and it therefore governs these [diseases]. So, in all cases where the right qì has not yet been damaged, [and] heat toxins are internally abundant [or] there is a disease of surplus, [then *huáng bǎi*] can be temporarily used; [but for other conditions, *huáng bǎi*] cannot be temporarily experimented with.

凡藥之燥者，未有不熱。而寒者，未有不濕。黃蘗於清熱之中，而兼燥濕之效。

Of all the drying medicinals, there is none that does not have heat, and [amongst] the cold [medicinals], there is none that does not have damp. Within [*huáng bǎi*] are the concurrent effects of [both] clearing heat and drying damp.

---

293. *Nǔ zǐ tāi lòu* 女子胎漏 (women's fetal bleeding) is spotting and bleeding during pregnancy due to qì-blood vacuity, kidney vacuity, or blood-heat. See: Wiseman, 1998, p. 198.

Shān Zhū Yú 山茱萸
Fruit of Cornus officinalis

氣味酸、平，無毒。主心下邪氣，寒熱，溫中，逐寒濕痹，去三蟲，久服輕身。去核。

The qì and flavor are sour, neutral, and non-toxic. [*Shān zhū yú*] governs evil qì below the heart, and cold and heat. [It] warms the center, expels cold-damp impediment, and removes the three worms. When taken over a long period of time, it lightens the body. *Remove the kernels.*

陳修園曰：山萸色紫赤而味酸平，稟厥陰、少陽木火之氣化。手厥陰心包、足厥陰肝，皆屬於風木也。手少陽三焦、足少陽膽，皆屬於相火也。心下巨闕穴，乃手厥陰心包之募，又心下為脾之分。

Chén Xiūyuán said: *Shān [zhū] yú's* color is purplish-red. The flavor is sour, neutral, and inherits the qì transformation of juèyīn and shàoyáng wood and fire. The hand juèyīn pericardium and the foot juèyīn liver both belong to wind wood. The hand shàoyáng sānjiāo and foot shàoyáng gallbladder both belong to ministerial fire. The Great Tower Gate (CV 14) below the heart is the alarm point of the hand juèyīn pericardium,[294] and the region below the heart is the aspect of the spleen.

曰邪氣者，脾之邪實為肝木之邪也。足厥陰肝木，血少氣亢則剋脾土，並於陽則熱，並於陰則寒也。又寒熱往來，為少陽之病。山萸稟木火之氣化，故咸主之。山萸味酸收斂，斂火歸於下焦。火在下謂之少火，「少火生氣」，所以溫中。

[What is] called evil qì is repletion evil of the spleen [which] causes the evil of liver wood. When foot juèyīn liver wood has scant blood and hyperactive qì, then this controls spleen earth. If [the evil qì] combines in the yáng, then [there is] heat. If [the evil qì] combines in the yīn, then [there is] cold. Moreover, [when there is] alternating chills and fever, [this] is a disease of the shàoyáng. *Shān [zhū] yú* inherits the qì transformation of wood and fire; therefore it governs all of these [patterns]. *Shān [zhū] yú's* flavor is sour, astringent, restrains fire, [and] returns it to the lower *jiāo*. The fire [which is] located in the lower [body] is called lesser fire. "The lesser fire generates qì,"[295] [and] therefore warms the center.

---

294. The Great Tower Gate (CV 14) is the alarm point for the heart. The alarm point for the pericardium is CV 17.

295. This is a quotation from the *Huáng Dì Nèi Jīng Sù Wèn · Yīn Yáng Yìng Xiàng Dà Lùn* 《黃帝內經素問·陰陽應象大論》 (Inner Canon of the Yellow Emperor Plain Questions · Great Discussion on the Correspondence and Phenomenon of Yīn and Yáng), Chapter 5, Line 4, where it is mentioned as the opposite of *zhuāng huǒ* 壯火 (strong fire).

山萸味酸入肝，肝主藏血，血能充膚熱肉，所以逐周身寒濕之痺。三蟲者，厥陰風木之化也。仲景烏梅丸之酸，能治蛔厥，即此物悟出。肝者，敢也，生氣生血之臟也。孫真人生脈散中，有五味之酸，能治倦怠而輕身，亦從此物悟出。

Shān [zhū] yú's sour enters the liver, and the liver governs the storage of blood. The blood is able to fill the skin and heat the flesh; therefore, [shān zhū yú] expels cold-damp impediment from the entire body. The three worms are the transformation of juèyīn wind and wood. [When one considers that] the sour of Zhòngjǐng's Wū Méi Wán is able to treat roundworm reversal, then [one can] comprehend this medicinal's [function]. The liver is bold, and is the viscus of generating qì and blood. The immortal Sūn[296] within Shēng Mài Sǎn had the sourness of wǔ wèi, [because it is] able to treat fatigue and lighten the body; [thus one can] also from this comprehend [this] medicinal's [function].

張隱庵曰：仲祖八味丸，用山茱萸，後人去桂、附改為六味丸，以山茱萸為固精補腎之藥，此外並無他用，皆因安於苟簡，不深討故也。今詳觀《本經》，山茱萸之功能如此，學人能於《本經》之內會悟而廣其用，庶無拘隘之弊。

Zhāng Yǐn'ān said: Ancestor Zhòng's Bā Wèi Wán used shān zhū yú, [but] later generations removed guì and fù, transforming [this] to make Liù Wèi Wán; [this is] because shān zhū yú is a medicinal [that] secures the essence and supplements the kidneys. Apart from this, [these people thought shān zhū yú] had no other use, all because they felt contented with carelessness and did not deeply study this. Today, through detailed observation of the Shén Nóng Běn Cǎo Jīng the action of shān zhū yú's is like this. Students are able to comprehend [shān zhū yú] from the content of the Shén Nóng Běn Cǎo Jīng and spread its use, so that there will be no more inflexible and narrow-minded malpractices.

---

296. This is another name for Sūn Sīmiǎo 孫思邈 (581-682), the famous physician, Daoist and author of the Bèi Jí Qiān Jīn Yào Fāng《備急千金要方》(Essential Prescriptions Worth a Thousand in Gold for Every Emergency).

Wú Zhū Yú 吳茱萸
Unripe fruit of Evodia rutaecarpa

氣味辛、溫，有小毒。主溫中，下氣，止痛，又除濕血痺，逐風邪，開腠
理，咳逆，寒熱。泡[一次]用。

The qì and flavor are acrid, warm, and slightly toxic. [*Wú zhū yú*] governs warming the center, downbears the qì, stops pain, and eliminates damp and blood impediment; [it] expels wind evils, opens the interstices, counterflow cough, and cold and heat. *[Only] use [this] for one steeping.*

陳修園曰：吳萸氣溫，稟春氣而入肝。味辛有小毒，得金味而入肺。氣溫能
袪寒，而大辛之味，又能俾肺令之獨行而無所旁掣。故中寒可溫，氣逆可
下，胸腹諸痛可止。皆肺令下行，坐鎮而無餘事。仲景取治陽明食穀欲嘔
症，及乾嘔吐涎沫症，從《本經》而會悟於言外之旨也。

Chén Xiūyuán said: *Wú [zhū] yú's* qì is warm, inherits the spring qì, and enters the liver. [It's] flavor is acrid, slightly toxic, obtains the metal flavor, and enters the lungs. The warm qì is able to dispel cold, and the extremely acrid flavor further enables the solitary order of the lungs without hindrances from the sides. Therefore, cold strike can be warmed, qì counterflow can be precipitated, [and] the various pain of the chest and abdomen can be stopped. In all cases the lung causes downward movement, [and the lungs can then] attend to their duty without extra work. Zhòngjǐng applied [*wú zhū yú*] to treat yángmíng conditions with desire to retch upon eating, as well as for conditions of dry vomiting with foaming at the mouth. [When one] follows the *Shén Nóng Běn Cǎo Jīng*, one can comprehend the intent beyond the words.

肺喜溫而惡寒，一得吳萸之大溫大辛，則水道通調而濕去。肝藏血，血寒則
滯而成痺，一得吳萸之大辛大溫，則血活而痺除。風邪傷人，則腠理閉而為
寒熱，咳逆諸症，吳萸大辛大溫，開而逐之，則咳逆，寒熱諸證俱平矣。然
猶有疑者，仲景用藥悉遵《本經》，而「少陰病吐利，手足逆冷，煩燥欲死
者，吳茱萸湯主之」二十字，與《本經》不符。而不知少陰之臟，皆本陽明
水穀以資生，而復交於中土。

The lungs like warmth and are averse to cold.[297] Upon obtaining the great warmth and great acridity of *wú [zhū] yú*, then the waterways are regulated and damp is removed. The liver stores the blood. If the blood is cold, then it will stagnate and form impediment. Upon obtaining the

---

297. This is a partial quotation from the *Huáng Dì Nèi Jīng Sù Wèn · Xuān Míng Wǔ Qì* 《黃帝內經素問·宣明五氣》 (Inner Canon of the Yellow Emperor Plain Questions · Explaining the Five Qì), Chapter 23, Line 4.

great warmth and great acridity of *wú* [*zhū*] *yú*, then the blood is invigorated and the impediment eliminated. [When] wind evil damages a person, then the interstices are blocked and this causes the various conditions of cold or heat and counterflow cough. The great warmth and great acridity of *wú* [*zhū*] *yú* opens and expels this; as a result, the various signs of cold or heat and counterflow cough are entirely calmed! So, there might be those who still have doubts that Zhòngjǐng used medicinals that are known to be observed [within] the *Shén Nóng Běn Cǎo Jīng*, but the twelve characters: "in shàoyīn disease with vomiting and diarrhea, counterflow cold of the hands and feet, vexation and agitation with desire for death, then *Wú Zhū Yú Tāng* governs this,"[298] are not consistent with the *Shén Nóng Běn Cǎo Jīng*. However, [skeptics] are ignorant of the fact, that the viscera of shàoyīn are both rooted in yángmíng water and grains [that are] used to supplement life, and [then] return to intersect in center-earth.

若陰陽之氣不歸中土，則上吐而下利。水火之氣不歸中土，則下燥而上煩。中土之氣內絕，則四肢逆冷而過肘膝，法在不治。仲景取吳茱萸大辛大溫之威烈，佐人參之衝和，以安中氣。薑、棗之和胃，以行四末，專求陽明，是得絕處逢生之妙。張隱庵、葉天士之解俱淺。

If the qì of yīn and yáng do not return to center-earth, then there is vomiting in the upper [body] and diarrhea in the lower [body]. If the qì of water and fire do not return to center-earth, then there is agitation in the lower [body] and vexation in the upper [body]. If the qì of center-earth internally expires, then there is counterflow cold of the four limbs, [which reaches] beyond the elbows and knees, [and] as a rule this is not treatable. Zhòngjǐng applies the fierceness of *wú zhū yú's* great acridity and warmth to assist the harmonious flow of *rén shēn* in order to quiet the center qì. *Jiāng* and *zǎo,* [which] harmonize the stomach, [are] used to move the four extremities, specifically seeking yángmíng, [and] this obtains the effect of returning [one] from death's door. The explanations of Zhāng Yǐn'ān and Yè Tiānshì are both shallow.

Xìng Rén 杏仁
Dried seed of Prunus armeniaca

氣味甘、苦、溫，冷利，有小毒。主咳逆上氣，雷鳴喉痹，下氣產乳，金瘡，寒心奔豚。

The qì and flavor are sweet, bitter, warm, beneficially cold,[299] and slightly toxic. [*Xìng rén*] governs cough with counterflow qì ascent, throat impediment with thunderous sounds, downbears qì and breast-milk, incised wounds, and running piglet due to cold in the heart.

---

298. This passage is from the *Shāng Hán Lùn*, Line 309.

299. Moist.

湯泡去皮尖。雙仁者，大毒勿用。

Soak the kernels in hot water and remove the skin and tips. Double kernels are greatly toxic; do not use them.

陳修園曰：杏仁氣味甘苦，其實苦重於甘，其性帶濕，其質冷利冷利者，滋潤之意也。「下氣」二字，足以盡其功用。肺實而脹，則為咳逆上氣。雷鳴喉痺者，火結於喉為痺痛，痰聲之響如雷鳴也。杏仁下氣，所以主之。氣有餘便是火，氣下即火下，故乳汁可通，瘡口可合也。

Chén Xiūyuán said: *Xìng rén's* qì and flavor are sweet and bitter. Its seeds are more bitter than sweet, and their nature contains dampness; their quality is beneficially cold [where] *"beneficially cold," means moistening.* The two characters "downbears the qì" sufficiently exhaust its action.[300] When the lungs are full and distended, then [there is] cough with counterflow qì ascent. Throat impediment with thunderous sounds, is fire bound in the throat, causing impediment and pain, [where] the noise of the phlegm sounds like thunder. *Xìng rén* downbears the qì; therefore, it governs this. When there is surplus qì, this is ordinarily fire. When the qì descends, then the fire also descends; therefore, breast milk can free [flow], and the openings of sores can close.

心陽虛，則寒水之邪自下上奔，犯於心位。杏仁有下氣之功，伐寒水於下，即所以保心陽於上也。凡此皆治有餘之症，若勞傷咳嗽之人，服之必死。時醫謂產於叭噠者，味純甘可用，而不知純甘非杏仁之正味。既無苦降之功，徒存其濕以生痰，甘以壅氣，陰受其害，至死不悟，惜哉！

If there is heart yáng vacuity, then the evil of cold water spontaneously runs down and up, invading the position of the heart. *Xìng rén's* action downbears the qì, by attacking cold water in the lower [body]; as a result, it safeguards the heart yáng in the upper [body]. Generally, this always treats conditions of surplus; if a patient with taxation damage cough were to take [*xìng rén*, they would] die. Contemporary physicians say [that when] produced in Bā Dā,[301] [*xìng rén's*] flavor is purely sweet and can be used, but they are ignorant that purely sweet is not the right flavor of *xìng rén*. Since without the action of bitter and downbearing,[302] [*xìng rén*] merely preserves damp in order to generate phlegm. [Therefore, when] sweet is used, [it] congests the qì, the yīn contracts the harm [from the qì congestion, which] is not realized until [the patient's] death. What a pity!

---

300. Meaning, these words explain its action.

301. Bā Dā 叭噠 is not really a place-name; the two characters are simply onomatopoeic and are used as another name for almonds in southern China, so it should rather be written here: *chǎn yú nán fāng zhī bā dā* 產於南方之叭噠 (almonds produced in the south). This also implies that there are two different products, which leads to confusion, as both apricot kernels and almonds are called *xìng rén* 杏仁 in Chinese.

302. That is, if *xìng rén* was purely sweet, without the bitter and downbearing qualities, then ....

Wū Méi 烏梅
Unripe fruit of Prunus mume

氣味酸、溫、平、澀，無毒。主下氣，除熱，煩滿，安心，止肢體痛，偏枯不仁，死肌，去青黑痣，蝕惡肉。

The qì and flavor are sour, warm, neutral, astringent, and non-toxic. [*Wū méi*] governs descending the qì, [and] eliminates heat, vexation, and fullness. [It] calms the heart and stops generalized limb pain, hemilateral withering and numbness,[303] **and** dead flesh.[304] [It] eliminates blue-green or black moles and consumes malign flesh.[305]

陳修園曰：烏梅氣平，稟金氣而入肺。氣溫，稟木氣而入肝。味酸無毒，得木味而入肝。味澀即酸之變味也。味勝於氣，以味為主。梅得東方之味，花放於冬，成熟於夏，是稟冬令之水精，而得春生之氣而上達也。

Chén Xiūyuán said: *Wū méi's* qì is neutral, inherits the qì of metal, and enters the lungs. The qì is [also] warm, inherits the qì of wood, and enters the liver. [*Wū méi's*] flavor is sour, non-toxic, obtains the wood flavor, and enters the liver. The astringent flavor is namely the transformation of sourness. [*Wū méi's*] flavor dominates the qì; [this is] because the flavor is the most important. *Wū méi* obtains the flavor of the east, releases blossoms in winter, and ripens in summer. It inherits the water and essence of the winter season, and obtains the qì of spring and growth, and outthrusts upwards.

主下氣者，生氣上達，則逆氣自下矣。熱煩滿、心不安，《傷寒論》厥陰症，以「氣上撞心，心疼熱」等字概之，能下其氣，而諸病皆愈矣。脾主四肢，木氣剋土，則肢體痛。肝主藏血，血不灌溉，則偏枯不仁，而為死肌。烏梅能和肝氣，養肝血，所以主之。去青黑痣及蝕惡肉者，酸收之味，外治能消痣與肉也。

[*Wū méi*] governs descent of qì. [When] qì grows, it outthrusts upward; then counterflow qì naturally descends! When there is heat vexation and fullness, the heart is not calm. This is [the same as in] the juèyīn condition from the *Shāng Hán Lùn,* which approximately [said] these words: "[there is] qì ascent dashing against the heart, and aching heat of the heart."[306] [*Wū méi*] is able to

---

303. *Piān kū bù rén* 偏枯不仁 (hemilateral withering and numbness) is wind hemiplegia with gradual emaciation. See: Wiseman, 1998, p. 289.

304. This can also mean numbness; see Footnote 19 from Chapter 1 above as well.

305. *È ròu* 惡肉 (malign flesh) can be verruca (plantar warts), warts, or keloid. See: ibid, p. 384.

306. See: *Shāng Hán Lùn* 《傷寒論》 (Discussion on Cold Damage), Line 326. However, in the *Shāng Hán Lùn* the line is slightly different: 厥陰之為病，消渴，氣上撞心，心中疼熱，饑而不欲食，食則吐蚘。下之利不止。

descend this qì, so it cures all of these diseases entirely! The spleen governs the four limbs; if wood qì restrains the earth, then [there is] generalized limb pain. The liver governs storing the blood; if the blood is not irrigated, then [there is] hemilateral withering, numbness, and dead flesh. *Wū méi* is able to harmonize the liver qì and nourish the liver blood; therefore, it governs these [patterns. *Wū méi*] removes blue-green or black moles, as well as consumes malign flesh; [this is] because the sour flavor contracts, [and] as an external treatment, it is able to disperse moles and [malign] flesh.

張隱庵云：後人不體經義，不窮物理，但以烏梅為酸斂收澀之藥，而春生上達之性未之講也。惜哉！

Zhāng Yǐn'ān said: People of later generations were not familiar with the meaning of the classics and did not study thoroughly the intrinsic order of things. [So they] only used *wū méi* as a sour, restraining, and astringent medicinal, but did not explain its nature of spring growth outthrusting upwards. What a pity!

Xī Jiǎo 犀角
Horn of Rhinoceros

氣味苦、酸、鹹、寒，無毒。主百毒蠱疰、邪鬼瘴氣，解鉤吻、鴆羽、蛇毒，除邪，不迷惑魘寐。久服輕身。

The qì and flavor are bitter, sour, salty, cold, and non-toxic. [*Xī jiǎo*] governs the hundred toxins, *gǔ* infixations,[307] evil ghosts, and miasmic qì. [It] resolves [the toxins of] yellow jessamine, poisoned wine,[308] and snake toxins; eliminates evils; and prevents [one] from having confusing nightmares [while] sleeping soundly. When taken over a long period of time, it lightens the body.

陳修園曰：犀角氣寒，稟水之氣也。味苦酸鹹無毒，得木火水之味也。主百毒蠱疰、邪鬼瘴氣者，以犀為靈異之獸，借其靈氣以辟邪也。解鉤吻、鴆羽、蛇毒、除邪者，以牛屬土而犀居水，得水土之精，毒物投水土中而俱化也。不迷惑魘寐、輕身者，言水火既濟之效也。今人取治血症，與經旨不合。

---

307. *Zhù* 疰 (infixation) means infection with and permanent lodging of a pathogen. See: Wiseman, 1998, p. 300.

308. *Zhèn yǔ* 鴆羽 (feathers of the legendary bird *zhèn*). The feathers of this bird are said to be venomous and can be used to poison wine for killing people, so this term also stands for poisoned wine in general.

Chén Xiūyuán said: *Xī jiǎo's* qì is cold and inherits the qì of water. The flavor is bitter, sour, salty, non-toxic, [and] obtains the flavors of wood, fire, and water. It governs the hundred toxins, *gǔ* infixations, evil ghosts, and miasmic qì; this is because the rhinoceros is a magical animal, and [*xī jiǎo*] makes use of this mystical qì in order to ward off evil. [*Xī jiǎo*] resolves [the toxins of] yellow jessamine, poisoned wine, [and] snake toxins. [It also] eliminates evils, because cows belong to earth and rhinoceroses reside in the water[309] [and therefore] obtains the essence of water and earth. Toxic substances [that] are thrown into water and earth all are transformed [into non-toxic substances]. Saying that [*xī jiǎo*] prevents [one] from having confusing nightmares [while] sleeping soundly, and lightens the body, speaks of the effect of water and fire, [which] have already been aided.[310] People today take [*xī jiǎo*] to treat blood conditions, [but] this does not conform to the intentions of the classics.

Líng Yáng Jiǎo 羚羊角
Horn of the male Saiga tatarica

氣味鹹、寒，無毒。主明目，益氣，起陰，去惡血，注下，辟蠱毒，惡鬼不祥，常不魘寐。俗作羚羊。

The qì and flavor are salty, cold, and non-toxic. [*Líng yáng jiǎo*] governs brightness of the eyes, boosts the qì, raises yīn, eliminates malign blood,[311] and downpour diarrhea. [It also] wards off *gǔ* venoms, malign ghosts, [and things that are] inauspicious, and permanently prevents nightmares [while] sleeping soundly. *It is commonly written as líng yáng.*

參：羚羊角氣寒味鹹無毒，入腎與膀胱二經。主明目者，鹹寒以補水，水足則目明也。益氣者，水能化氣也。起陰者，陰器為宗筋而屬於肝，肝為木，木得烈日而菱，得雨露而挺也。

Comparison: *Líng yáng jiǎo's* qì is cold and the flavor is salty and non-toxic. It enters both the kidney and urinary bladder channels. [*Líng yáng jiǎo*] governs brightness of the eyes, [this is] because salty and cold [are] used to supplement water. If water is sufficient, then [there is] brightness of the eyes. [*Líng yáng jiǎo*] boosts qì; [this is] because water is able to transform the qì. [*Líng yáng jiǎo*] raises the yīn; [this is] because the genitals are the ancestral sinew,[312] and belong to the liver. The liver is

309. It seems that Chén Xiūyuán categorizes rhinoceroses as a sort of cow.

310. *Jì jì* 既濟 (accomplished aid, completion) is the 63rd hexagram of the *Yì Jīng* 《易經》 (Book of Changes) and contains fire above and water below. It looks like ䷾.

311. *È xuè* 惡血 (malign blood) refers to blood that has spilled out and formed stasis or swelling. See: Wiseman, 1998, p. 384.

312. The penis.

wood. [When] wood obtains the fierce [rays of the] sun, it withers, [and when] it obtains rain and dew, it is straight and stiff.

味鹹則破血，故主去惡血。氣寒則清熱，故止注下也。蟲毒為濕熱之毒也，鹹寒可以除之。辟惡鬼不祥、常不夢魘寐者，夸其靈異通神之妙也。

[Líng yáng jiǎo's] flavor is salty; as a result it breaks blood [stasis and] therefore governs the elimination of malign blood. [Líng yáng jiǎo's] qì is cold; as a result, it clears heat [and] therefore it stops downpour diarrhea. Gǔ venoms are damp-heat toxins, so salty and cold can be used to eliminate this. [Líng yáng jiǎo] wards off malign ghosts and [things that are] inauspicious, [and] permanently prevents nightmares [while] sleeping soundly; [therefore] it has been praised for its magical effect of communicating with the shén.

卷之四

Chapter Four

閩吳航陳念祖修園甫著
男 元豹道彪古愚元犀道照靈石同挍字

Written by Chén Niànzǔ Xiūyuán from Mǐn Wúháng.
Revised by Yuánbào Dàobiāo Gǔyú and Yuánxī Dàozhào Língshí.

中品

Medicinals of the Middle Grade

Lù Róng 鹿茸
Pilose antler of Cervus nippon

氣味甘、溫，無毒。主漏下惡血，寒熱驚癇，益氣，強志，生齒，不老。

The qì and flavor are sweet, warm, and non-toxic. [*Lù róng*] governs spotting and malign blood, cold and heat fright epilepsy; [it] boosts the qì, strengthens the will, grows teeth, and prevents aging.

陳修園曰：鹿為仙獸而多壽，其臥則口鼻對尾閭以通督脈。督脈為通身骨節之主，腎主骨，故又能補腎。腎得其補，則志強而齒固，以志藏於腎，齒為骨餘也。督得其補，則大氣升舉，惡血不漏，以督脈為陽氣之總督也。

Chén Xiūyuán said: The deer is an animal of immortality and lives very long.[313] When it sleeps, the snout faces the coccyx so as to connect with the *dū* vessel. The *dū* vessel is the governor, which connects the body's joints. The kidneys govern the bones; therefore, [*lù róng*] is also able to supplement the kidneys. When the kidneys obtain this supplementation, then the will is strengthened and the teeth are firmed. [This is] because the will is stored in the kidneys, and the teeth are surplus of the bones. When the *dū* vessel obtains [*lù róng's*] supplementation, then the great qì is raised and lifted, and the malign blood [does] not spot, because the *dū* vessel is the governor-general of the yáng qì.

然角中皆血所貫，衝為血海，其大補衝脈可知也。凡驚癇之病，皆挾衝脈而作，陰氣虛不能寧謐於內，則附陽而上升，故上熱而下寒。陽氣虛不能周衛於身，則隨陰而下陷，故下熱而上寒。鹿茸入衝脈，而大補其血，所以能治寒熱驚癇也。至於長而為角，《別錄》謂其主惡瘡，逐惡氣。以一點胚血，發泄已盡，祇有拓毒消散之功也。

---

313. Captive breeds can live up to twenty years, while their free companions usually have shorter lives. This deer has played an important role in ancient marriage ceremonies and in sacrifices. Also, because it lives in herds, it was regarded as an animal of prosperity for the family and the collective, and not so much in regards to the longevity of the individual.

Blood passes through the center of the horn;[314] the *chòng* is the sea of blood, [and] clearly [*lù róng*] greatly supplements the *chòng* vessel. Generally the disease of fright epilepsy is always [related] to the *chòng* vessel. [If] the yīn qì is vacuous and unable to be quiet inside, then the yáng [which is] attached rises upward, and this causes heat in the upper [body] and cold in the lower [body]. If the yáng qì is vacuous and unable to protect the whole body, then [the yáng qì] follows the yīn and sinks downwards, which causes heat in the lower [body] and cold in the upper [body]. *Lù róng* enters the *chòng* vessel and greatly supplements its blood. For this reason, it is able to treat cold and heat fright epilepsy. As for developed antlers that have become a horn, the [*Míng Yī*] *Bié Lù*[315] mentions that [*lù róng*] governs malign sores and expels evil qì. Use a drop of fetal blood to discharge [what is] already exhausted, as [the horn] only has the actions of pushing out toxins [from sores] and dissipating [evil qì].

Biē Jiǎ 鱉甲
Dorsal shell of Amyda sinensis

氣味酸、平，無毒。主心腹癥瘕，堅積寒熱，去痞疾、蝕肉、陰蝕、痔核、惡肉。

The qì and flavor are sour, neutral, and non-toxic. [*Biē jiǎ*] governs concretions and conglomerations of the heart and abdomen, and hard accumulations of cold or heat; [it] expels glomus disease, eroded flesh, genital erosion, hemorrhoids, and malign flesh.

述：鱉甲氣平，稟金氣而入肺。味鹹無毒，得水味而入腎。心腹者，合心下，大腹，小腹，以及脅肋而言也。癥瘕堅硬之積，致發寒熱，為厥陰之肝氣凝聚。鱉甲氣平，可以制肝，味鹹可以軟堅，所以主之也。

Narration: *Biē jiǎ's* qì is neutral and is endowed with metal qì, which enters the lungs. [*Biē jiǎ's*] flavor is salty and non-toxic, [and by] obtaining the water flavor (salty), it enters the kidneys. The heart and abdomen are said to connect below the heart to the greater abdomen, the smaller abdomen, and also the rib-sides. The accumulation of hard concretions and conglomerations causes cold and heat effusion, due to the coagulation of the liver qì of juèyīn. *Biē jiǎ's* qì is neutral, and can be used to control the liver. The flavor is salty and can be used to soften hardness. Therefore, [*biē jiǎ*] governs these [diseases].

314. While this language may appear strange, the idea of the blood passing through the center of a horn conjures up the same images of blood coursing through the *chòng* vessel, which is in the center of the body.
315. This is the short title of *Míng Yī Bié Lù*《名醫別錄》(Specific Recordings by Famous Physicians). This book was written by Táo Hóngjǐng 陶弘景 (456-536).

痞者，肝氣滯也，鹹平能制肝而軟堅，故亦主之。蝕肉、陰蝕、痔核、惡肉，一生於鼻，鼻者肺之竅也。一生於二便，二便者腎之竅也。入肺腎而軟堅，所以消一切惡肉也。

Glomus is [due to] stagnant liver qì. [The] salty [flavor] and neutral [qì] are able to control the liver and soften hardness; therefore, it also governs this. [*Biē jiǎ* also governs] eroded flesh, genital erosion, hemorrhoids, and malign flesh. [Malign flesh] may grow in the nose, and the nose is the orifice of the lungs. [Malign flesh may also] grow in the [openings of the] urine and stools, and the [opening of the] urine and stools are the orifices of the kidneys. [*Biē jiǎ*] enters the lungs and kidneys and softens hardness; therefore, it disperses all types of malign flesh.

Bái Jiāng Cán 白僵蠶
Dried 4th or 5th stage larva of the moth of Bombyx mori

氣味鹹、辛、平，無毒。主治小兒驚癇、夜啼，去三蟲，滅黑䵟，令人面色好，男子陰瘍病。

The qì and flavor are salty, acrid, neutral, and non-toxic. [*Bái jiāng cán*] governs the treatment of children's fright epilepsy and night crying, expels the three worms, eliminates black moles, brings forth a good facial complexion, and [governs] genital itching in men.

凡稟金氣色白之藥，俱不宜炒。

In general, as it is a medicinal endowed with metal qì and a white color, it is completely inappropriate to stir-fry.

述：僵蠶氣平為秋氣，味辛為金味，味鹹為水味，稟金水之精也。治驚癇者，金能平木也。治夜啼者，金屬乾而主天，天運旋轉，晝開夜闔也。

Narration: [*Bái*] *jiāng cán's* qì, is neutral [like the] qì of autumn. The acrid flavor is the metal flavor, and the salty flavor is the water flavor; [therefore, it] inherits the essence of metal and water. [*Bái jiāng cán*] treats fright epilepsy, because metal is able to balance wood. It treats night crying, because metal belongs to dryness and governs heaven. When [the celestial] heavens move and spin, the day opens and the night closes.[316]

---

316. Therefore, night crying ceases when the day begins.

殺三蟲者，蟲為風木所化，金主肅殺也。滅黑䵟、令人面色好者，俾水氣上滋也。治男子陰瘍者，金能制風，鹹能除瘍也。

[*Bái jiāng cán*] kills the three parasites, because worms are the transformation of wind and wood, and metal governs harsh killing. [*Bái jiāng cán*] eliminates black moles and brings forth a good facial complexion, because it enables water qì to enrich the upper [body]. It treats genital itching in men, because metal is able to control wind, and the salty [flavor] is able to eliminate itching.

徐靈胎曰：僵蠶感風而僵，凡風氣之疾，皆能治之，蓋借其氣以相感也。

Xú Língtāi said: [*Bái*] *jiāng cán* affects wind and stiffness; [therefore, it is] able to treat all kinds of wind diseases. Perhaps by means of its qì, [*bái jiāng cán*] has this effect.

或問：因風以僵，何以反能治風？曰：邪之中人也，有氣而無形，穿經透絡，愈久愈深。以氣類相反之藥投之，則拒而不入。必與之同類者，和入諸藥，使為響導，則藥力至於病所，而邪與藥相從，藥性漸發，或從毛孔出，或從二便出，不能復留矣。此即從治之法也。風寒暑濕，莫不皆然。此神而明之之道，不專恃正治奏功矣。

It might be asked: Because stiffness is caused by wind, why [is *bái jiāng cán*] able to treat wind? The answer is: When evil strikes a person, there is qì but no form. It pierces through the channels and penetrates the collaterals. The longer [the disease lasts], the deeper [the evil penetrates]. When a medicinal from a clashing qì[317] category is given, then [the qì] is repulsed, and [the medicinal] is unable to enter. One must give the same category [of medicinals], which harmoniously allows entrance to all the [other] medicinals, which employ it as a guide. Then the strength of the medicinals [will] arrive at the location of the disease, as the evil and the medicinals [will] follow each other. The nature of the medicinal gradually discharges, or follows the pores in the [skin and] hair to issue forth, or follows the two openings [urine and stool] to issue forth, [and the evil is] unable to return and lodge! This then is the method of coacting treatment.[318] [No matter if it is] wind, cold, summerheat, or damp, there is no [evil] for which [this method] is not correct. This is a divine and enlightened way, and does not specifically rely on straight treatment[319] to obtain [the correct] action!

---

317. Clashing in the Wiseman terminology is: The seven relations; e.g., aconite main tuber clashes (i.e., produces side effects) when used with pinellia.

318. The *cóng zhì fǎ* 從治法 (coacting treatment method) is also called paradoxical treatment. For example, it treats heat with hot medicines, when there are only false heat signs, but true cold trapped inside is the cause. See: Wiseman, 1998, p. 428.

319. The *zhèng zhì fǎ* 正治法 (straight treatment method) is treating cold with hot medicines, when the cold is truly cold. See: ibid, p. 583.

Zhà Chán 蚱蟬
Exuviae of Cicada

古人用蟬，今人用蛻，氣性亦相近。氣味寒、鹹。主小兒驚癇、夜啼，癲病寒熱。

People in ancient times used [whole] cicadas, [but] today people use the exuvia, which also has a similar qì and nature. The qì and flavor are salty and cold. [Zhà chán] governs children's fright epilepsy, night crying, and withdrawal disease[320] with cold and heat.

陳修園曰：蚱蟬氣寒稟水氣，味鹹得水味，而要其感涼風清露之氣以生，得金氣最全。其主小兒驚癇者，金能平木也。蚱蟬日出有聲，日入無聲，故止夜啼也。癲病寒熱者，肝膽之風火也，蚱蟬具金水之氣，金能制風，水能制火，所以主之。

Chén Xiūyuán said: *Zhà chán's* qì is cold, and inherits the water qì. [It's] flavor is salty, [and] obtains the water flavor. Yet it must take in the qì of cool wind and clear dew in order to generate, [and thus] obtains the most complete metal qì. [*Zhà chán*] governs children's fright epilepsy, because metal is able to balance wood. *Zhà chán* make sounds at sunrise and are silent at sundown, and are therefore able to stop night crying. Withdrawal disease with cold and heat [is due to] wind and fire of the liver and gallbladder. *Zhà chán* possesses the qì of metal and water. Metal is able to control wind, and water is able to control fire; therefore, it governs this.

張隱庵曰：蟬脫、僵蠶，皆稟金水之精，故《本經》主治大體相同。但蟬飲而不食，溺而不糞。蠶食而不飲，糞而不溺，何以相同？經云：「飲入於胃，上歸於肺。」穀入於胃，乃傳之肺。是飲食雖殊，皆由肺氣之通調，則尿糞雖異，皆稟肺氣以傳化矣。

Zhāng Yǐn'ān said: *Chán tuì* and [*bái*] *jiāng* both inherit the essence of metal and water, therefore their main indications are basically identical in the *Shén Nóng Běn Cǎo Jīng*. However, cicadas drink but do not eat, and urinate but do not defecate; silkworms eat but do not drink, and defecate but do not urinate. Why should they be identical? The classic said: "Fluid enters into the stomach … [where it] rises and returns to the lung."[321] When grains enter into the stomach, then [the qì] is conveyed to the lungs. Although food and drink are [each] unique, they both cause free [flow] and

---

320. See Footnote 206 from Chapter 2.

321. This is a quotation from *Huáng Dì Nèi Jīng Sù Wèn · Jīng Mài Bié Lùn* 《黃帝內經素問·經脈別論》 (Inner Canon of the Yellow Emperor Plain Questions · Further Discussion on the Vessels and Pulses), Chapter 21. 飲入於胃，遊溢精氣，上輸於脾。脾氣散精，上歸於肺，通調水道，下輸膀胱。

regulation of the lung qì; as a result, although the urine and stool differ, both inherit the lung qì in order to convey and transform!

Shí Gāo 石膏
Gypsum

氣味辛、微寒，無毒。主中風寒熱，心下逆氣驚喘，口乾舌焦，不能息，腹中堅痛，除邪鬼，產乳，金瘡。

The qì and flavor are acrid, slightly cold, and non-toxic. [*Shí gāo*] governs wind strike with cold and heat, counterflow qì below the heart, fright panting, dry mouth, parched tongue, inability to breathe, and hardness and pain inside the abdomen; [it also] eliminates evil ghosts, [frees] breast milk, and [heals] incised wounds.

陳修園曰：石膏氣微寒，稟太陽寒水之氣。味辛無毒，得陽明燥金之味。風為陽邪，在太陽則惡寒發熱，然必審其無汗煩燥而喘者，可與麻桂並用。在陽明則發熱而微惡寒，然必審其口乾舌焦大渴而自汗者，可與知母同用。

Chén Xiūyuán said: *Shí gāo's* qì is slightly cold, and inherits the qì of tàiyáng cold water. [*Shí gāo's*] flavor is acrid, non-toxic, [and] obtains the flavor of yángmíng dry metal. Wind is a yáng evil. [When it] is located in the tàiyáng, then [there is] aversion to cold and heat effusion. However, [one] must carefully investigate: [if there is] absence of sweating, vexation, agitation, and panting, then [*shí gāo*] can be used together with *má* [*huáng*] and *guì* [*zhī*].[322] When [the wind] is located in the yángmíng, then [there is] heat effusion and slight aversion to cold. However, [one] must carefully investigate: [if there is] dry mouth, a parched tongue, great thirst, and spontaneous sweating, [then *shí gāo*] can be used together with *zhī mǔ*.[323]

曰心下氣逆，即《傷寒論》氣逆欲嘔之互詞。曰不能息，即《傷寒論》虛羸少氣之互詞。然必審其為解後裏氣虛而內熱者，可與人參、竹葉、半夏、麥冬、甘草、粳米同用。腹中堅痛，陽明燥甚而堅，將至於胃實不大便之症。

When it is said "counterflow qì below the heart," then this is a synonym for "counterflow qì with a desire to retch" from the *Shāng Hán Lùn*.[324] When it is said "inability to breathe," then this is a

322. See: Mitchell, 1999, p. 114.
323. Ibid: p. 317.
324. Shāng Hán Lùn, Line 397. The actual citation should be *tǔ* 吐 (vomit) 氣逆欲吐.

166

synonym for "vacuity emaciation with shortness of breath" from the *Shāng Hán Lùn*.[325] One must investigate: [if there] is internal qì vacuity and interior heat after resolving [cold damage, only then] can [*shí gāo*] be used together with *rén shēn*, *zhú yè*, *bàn xià*, *mài dōng*, *gān cǎo*, and *gēng mǐ*. Abdominal hardness and pain are caused by extreme dryness in the yángmíng that becomes hard. In extreme cases, this leads to the condition of stomach repletion with inability to pass stool.

邪鬼者，陽明邪實，妄言妄見，或無故而生驚，若邪鬼附之 。石膏清陽明之
熱，可以統治之 。陽明之脈從缺盆下乳，石膏能潤陽明之燥，故能通乳 。陽
明主肌肉，石膏外糝，又能愈金瘡之潰爛也 。但石品見火則成石灰，今人畏
其寒而煅用，則大失其本來之性矣 。

Ghost evils are a yángmíng repletion evil [manifesting with] raving, hallucinations, or growing fright without reason, as if the evil ghost was close. *Shí gāo* clears the heat of yángmíng, and can be used to govern this. The vessel of yángmíng follows the supraclavicular fossa[326] and descends to the nipple. *Shí gāo* is able to moisten yángmíng dryness; therefore, [it is] able to free the breast milk. The yángmíng governs the flesh; [therefore, when] *shí gāo* is topically applied,[327] it is able to heal the ulcerations of incised wounds. However, when this mineral sees fire, then it becomes *shí huī* (lime). People nowadays fear its coldness, and use it calcined; as a result, [*shí gāo*] greatly loses its original nature!

---

325. Ibid.

326. Quē Pén (ST 12) Empty Basin.

327. *Shēn* 糝 here means "disperse, spread."

下品
Medicinals of the Lowest Grade

Fù Zǐ 附子
Lateral root of Aconitum carmichaeli

氣味辛、溫，有大毒。主風寒咳逆邪氣，溫中，金瘡，破癥堅積聚、血瘕，寒濕痿躄，拘攣，膝痛不能行步。

The qì and flavor are acrid, warm, and very toxic. [*Fù zǐ*] governs wind-cold, counterflow cough with evil qì, and warms the center. [It treats] incised wounds, breaks concretions, hardenings, accumulations, and gatherings. [In addition it treats women's] blood conglomerations, cold-damp crippling wilt, hypertonicity, and knee pain with inability to walk.

以刀削去皮臍，每個剖作四塊，用滾水微溫泡三日，一日一換，去鹽味，晒半燥，剖十六塊，於銅器炒熟用之。近世以便煮之，非法也。

Use a knife to scrape off the skin and nodes. With each cut, make four pieces; soak for three days in slightly warm boiled water, and change [the water] daily to remove the salty flavor. Sun dry until half dried, cut into sixteen pieces, and stir-fry in bronze ware [until it is] thoroughly cooked [before] utilizing it. In modern times it is simply boiled, [which is] not [adhering to the proper] method.

陳修園曰：《素問》謂以「毒藥攻邪」是回生妙手，後人立補養等法是模棱巧朮，究竟攻其邪而正氣復，是攻之即所以補之也。附子味辛氣溫，火性迅發，無所不到，故為回陽救逆第一品藥。

Chén Xiūyuán said: What the *Sù Wèn* calls "toxic medicinals for attacking evils"[328] is a miraculous method for restoring life. The position of later generations of supplementing and nourishing and other methods are ambiguous [but] skillful techniques, [which] afterall attack the evil and return the right qì. This [is a method of] attack [that] then consequently supplements. *Fù zǐ's* flavor is acrid, its qì is warm, and [its] nature is of fire and rapid effusion; [therefore,] there is no place that cannot be reached by it. Thus [*fù zǐ*] is the number-one medicinal for returning the yáng and rescuing counterflow.

---

328. See: *Huáng Dì Nèi Jīng Sù Wèn · Zàng Qì Fǎ Shí Lùn* 《黃帝內經素問·藏氣法時論》 (Inner Canon of the Yellow Emperor Plain Questions · Discussion on Times and Methods for the Storage of Qì), Chapter 22.

《本經》云：風寒咳逆邪氣，是寒邪之逆於上焦也。寒濕痿躄、拘攣、膝痛不能行步，是寒邪著於下焦筋骨也。癥堅積聚、血瘕，是寒氣凝結，血滯於中也。

The *Shén Nóng Běn Cǎo Jīng* said: wind-cold counterflow cough with evil qì is counterflow cold evil in the upper *jiāo*. Cold damp crippling wilt, hypertonicity, and knee pain with inability to walk are [due to] cold evil adhering to the lower *jiāo*, the sinews, and bones.[329] Concretions, hardenings, accumulations, gatherings, and [women's] blood conglomerations are [due to] cold qì [that has] congealed and bound, as well as blood stagnation in the center.

考《大觀本》「咳逆邪氣」句下，有「溫中，金瘡」四字，以中寒得暖而溫，血肉得暖而合也。大意上而心肺，下而肝腎，中而脾胃，以及血肉筋骨營衛，因寒濕而病者，無有不宜。

Examine the four characters "warms the center, [and] incised wounds" after the sentence "counterflow cough with evil qì" in the *Dà Guān Běn* edition.[330] When cold in the center receives heat, it is warmed, and when blood and flesh receive heat, they are united. The general idea [is that] among the diseases caused by cold-damp [either] in the heart and lungs of the upper [body], in the liver and kidneys of the lower [body], in the spleen and stomach of the center, and also in the blood and flesh, the sinews and bones, and the construction and defense, there is none that [*fù zǐ*] is not appropriate for.

即陽氣不足，寒氣內生，大汗、大瀉、大喘、中風、卒倒等症，亦必仗此大氣大力之品，方可挽回。此《本經》言外意也。

Now, when yáng qì is insufficient, cold qì is internally generated. [This causes] great sweating, great diarrhea, great panting, wind strike, sudden collapse, and other conditions. [One] must also wield this medicinal [with its] great qì and great strength [in] formulas [that] can rescue [the patient] and restore [their life]. This is the meaning behind the words of the *Shén Nóng Běn Cǎo Jīng*.

又曰：附子主寒濕，諸家俱能解到，而仲景用之，則化而不可知之謂神。且夫人之所以生者，陽也，亡陽則死。亡字分二字，一無方切，音忘，逃也，即《春秋傳》「出亡」之義也。一微夫切，音無，無也，《論語》「亡而為有，」孟子問有餘曰「亡矣」之義也。

---

329. This means cold in the liver and kidneys.

330. *Dà Guān Běn*《大觀本》is an edition of the *Shén Nóng Běn Cǎo Jīng*, which was published in the *Sòng* dynasty. *Dà Guān* 大觀 is the name of a reign period (1107-1110).

[Chén Xiūyuán] further said: *Fù zǐ* governs cold and damp. The various schools of thought are all able to understand this. However, when Zhòngjǐng used this, the transformation [of cold and damp] cannot be known and [is] called divine. Moreover, [what gives] people life, is yáng. If yáng collapses, then [there is] death. The character *wáng* 亡 [can be] distinguished into two characters: one is *wú* 無 plus *fāng* 方,[331] pronounced *wàng* 忘,[332] and means *to flee*. The meaning is like [the expression] *chū wáng* 出亡, [meaning *to*] *go into exile*, from the *Chūn Qiū Zhuàn*.[333] The other one is *wēi* 微 plus *fū* 夫, pronounced *wú* 無, and means *no, not to have*. The meaning is like [the passage]: *not to have, but to do as if [one] has*, from the *Lún Yǔ*. Mèngzǐ's reply when asked [about] surplus was: [*better*] *not to have!*[334]

誤藥大汗不止為亡陽，如唐之幸蜀，仲景用四逆湯 、真武湯等法以迎之 。吐利厥冷為亡陽，如周之守府，仲景用通脈四逆湯 、薑附湯以救之 。且太陽之標陽外呈而發熱，附子能使之交於少陰而熱已 。

[If after] inappropriate medicinals [are taken, and the patient] has incessant, great sweating, [this] is yáng collapse, and is like the arrival of the emperor of the *Táng* dynasty in the state of Shǔ.[335] Zhòngjǐng used *Sì Nì Tāng* or *Zhēn Wǔ Tāng*, and similar methods to meet this [head-on.[336] In cases of] vomiting and diarrhea with reversal cold causing yáng collapse; [this is] like the guarded storehouses of the *Zhōu* dynasty.[337] Zhòngjǐng used *Tōng Mài Sì Nì Tāng* or *Jiāng Fù Tāng* in order to rescue this. Moreover, the tip of tàiyáng is yáng, [and this] externally manifests as heat effusion. *Fù zǐ* can cause [tàiyáng] to interact with shàoyīn in order to resolve the heat.

少陰之神機病，附子能使自下而上而脈生，周行通達而厥愈 。合苦甘之芍 、草而補虛，合苦淡之苓 、芍而溫固，玄妙不能盡述 。按其立法，與《 本經 》之說不同，豈仲景之創見歟？然《 本經 》謂「 氣味辛溫有大毒 」七字，仲景即於此悟出附子大功用 。

---

331. This is an old phonetic system called *fǎn qiè* 反切. It uses two Chinese characters, the first indicating the consonant of the given character, and the second, which has the same vowel. So for example, *wú* plus *fāng* is *wàng*.

332. The modern pronunciation is *wáng*.

333. The *Chūn Qiū* 《 春秋 》 (Spring and Autumn Annals) are the historical records of the ancient state of Lǔ 魯國 and are said to have been compiled by Confucius. They cover the time span between 770~475 B.C. There are three major commentaries to this work: *Zuǒ Zhuàn* 《 左傳 》, *Gōng Yáng Zhuàn* 《 公羊傳 》 and *Gǔ Liáng Zhuàn* 《 穀樑傳 》, named after their commentators.

334. See: *Lún Yǔ·Shù Ér* 《 論語· 述而 》 (Analects· Narrations), Chapter 7.

335. The former independent state of Shǔ (modern day Sìchuān) was under imperial sovereignty until it was conquered in the late *Táng*. For the historical background see: Denis Twitchett and John Fairbank (Ed.): *The Cambridge History of China*, Volume 3, Part 1, pp.765-789.

336. The character *yíng* 迎 (Wiseman: receive (guests); meet head-on) implies the receiving someone or something, but under duress. Therefore, one meets the challenge head-on, and faces the problem, but one does not do so lightly.

337. The storehouses of the *Zhōu* dynasty were regarded as especially safe.

If there is a disease of the spirit mechanism of shàoyīn,[338] *fù zǐ* can enable [the blood and qì to flow] from the lower to the upper [part of the body] to engender the pulse, so there is circulation and movement which freely penetrates to resolve the reversal. Combined with the bitterness and sweetness of *sháo [yào]* and *[gān] cǎo*, *[fù zǐ]* supplements vacuity. Combined with the bitterness and lightness of *[fú] líng* and *sháo [yào, fù zǐ]* warms and secures. [I am] unable to exhaust the statement of his[339] profound excellence. Investigating his established methods, they are different from what is said in the *Shén Nóng Běn Cǎo Jīng*. Where is Zhòngjǐng's original opinion from? Now, it is namely from these seven characters in the *Shén Nóng Běn Cǎo Jīng* that say "the qì and flavor is acrid, warm, and very toxic;" thus Zhòngjǐng understood the great use of *fù zǐ*.

溫得東方風木之氣 ，而溫之至則為熱《 內經 》所謂「 少陰之上 」君火主之是也 。辛為西方燥金之味 ，而辛之至則反潤《 內經 》所謂「 辛以潤之 」是也 。凡物性之偏處則毒 ，偏而至於無可加處則大毒 。因「 大毒 」二字 ，知附子之溫為至極 ，辛為至極也 。

Warmth receives the qì of the east, wind, and wood. When warmth is extreme, it turns into heat. This is what the *Nèi Jīng* calls the "highest part of shàoyīn."[340] It is ruled by the sovereign fire. Acrid is the flavor of the west and dry metal. When acidity is extreme, it reverses into moisture. This is what the *Nèi Jīng* calls "moisturizing with acidity."[341] Generally, when the nature of a substance is of a one-sided quality, it is toxic. When its one-sidedness goes so far that no more quality can be added, it is very toxic. By the two characters "very toxic," [we] recognize the warmth as well as the acidity of *fù zǐ* as extreme.

仲景用附子之溫有二法 ：雜於苓 、芍 、甘草中 ，雜於地黃 、澤瀉中 ，如「 冬日可愛 」補虛法也 。佐以薑 、桂之熱 ，佐以麻 、辛之雄 ，如「 夏日可畏 」救陽法也 。

There are two ways in which Zhòngjǐng applied the warmth of *fù zǐ*: First, mixed with *[fú] líng*, *sháo [yào]*, and *gān cǎo*, or mixed with *dì huáng* and *zé xiè*. [Fù zǐ] is like "the loveliness of the sun in

---

338. *Shàoyīn zhī shén jī* 少陰之神機 (the spirit mechanism of shàoyīn) means: the heart and kidneys store the spirit, mind, and essence, and govern the function of the blood vessels (pulse and heartbeat), and the spirit determines life and death.

339. Zhòngjǐng's 仲景.

340. This is tàiyáng and it is governed by heat. See: *Huáng Dì Nèi Jīng·Sù Wèn · Yīn Yáng Lí Hé Lùn* 《 黃帝內經素問· 陰陽離合論 》 (Inner Canon of the Yellow Emperor Plain Questions · Discussion on the Separation and Unity of Yīn and Yáng), Chapter 6, Line 2, and ibid: *Tiān Yuán Jì Dà Lùn* 《 天元紀大論 》 (Great Discussion on the Primary Periods of Heaven), Chapter 66, Line 3.

341. See: *Huáng Dì Nèi Jīng Sù Wèn · Zàng Qì Fǎ Shí Lùn* 《 黃帝內經素問· 藏氣法時論 》 (Inner Canon of the Yellow Emperor Plain Questions · Discussion on Times and Methods for the Storage of Qì), Chapter 22, Line 1.

winter."[342] This is the method for supplementing vacuity. Second, assisted by the heat of [gān] jiāng and guì [zhī], or assisted by the force of má [huáng] and [xì] xīn, [fù zǐ] is like "the loathsomeness of the sun in summer." This is the method for rescuing yáng.

用附子之辛，亦有三法：桂枝附子湯、桂枝附子去桂加白朮湯、甘草附子湯，辛燥以祛除風濕也。附子湯、芍藥甘草附子湯，辛潤以溫補水臟也。若白通湯、通脈四逆湯，加人尿豬膽汁，則取西方秋收之氣，保復元陽，則有大封大固之妙矣。後世虞天民、張景岳、亦極贊其功。然不能從《本經》中細繹其義，以闡發經方之妙，徒逞臆說以極贊之，反為蛇足矣。

[When] using fù zǐ's acridity, Zhòngjǐng also has three methods: Firstly, acridity and dryness for expelling and eliminating wind damp with Guì Zhī Fù Zǐ Tāng, Guì Zhī Fù Zǐ Qù Guì Jiā Bái Zhú Tāng and Gān Cǎo Fù Zǐ Tāng. Secondly, acridity and moistening for warming and supplementing the water viscus with Fù Zǐ Tāng and Sháo Yào Gān Cǎo Fù Zǐ Tāng. Thirdly, when rén niào and zhū dǎn juice are added to Bái Tōng Tāng and Tōng Mài Sì Nì Tāng, then the qì of the west and autumn harvest is obtained, which protects and restores the original yáng. This is excellent for greatly sealing and greatly firming [the yáng]! Physicians of later generations like Yú Tiānmín[343] and Zhāng Jǐngyuè also highly praised the usefulness of [fù zǐ]. However, they were unable to precisely unravel its meaning from the content of the Shén Nóng Běn Cǎo Jīng. And in elucidating the excellence of the classical formulas, they merely indulged in personal views for exceedingly praising [fù zǐ]. On the contrary, these were snake legs![344]

Bàn Xià 半夏
Rhizome of Pinellia ternata

氣味辛、平，有毒。主傷寒寒熱，心下堅，胸脹，咳逆，頭眩，咽喉腫痛，腸鳴，下氣，止汗。

The qì and flavor are acrid, neutral and toxic. [Bàn xià] governs cold and heat in cold damage, hardness below the heart, distention of the chest, counterflow cough, dizziness in the head, throat swelling with pain, and intestinal rumbling. [In addition] it downbears qì and stops sweating.

---

342. *Dōng rì kě ài, xià rì kě wèi.* 冬日可愛，夏日可畏。 (In winter, the sun is lovable. In summer, the sun is detestable.) This is a quotation from the *Chū Qiū Zuǒ Zhuàn*《春秋左傳》(Zuǒ's Commentary to the Spring and Autumn Annals), Chapter 6, Line 2.

343. Yú Tiānmín 虞天民 (1438-1517), also called Yú Tuán 虞摶 was a physician from Zhèjiāng. See: Lǐ, 1985, p. 640.

344. There is a famous Chinese proverb: *Huà shé tiān zú.* 畫蛇添足。 (To paint a snake and add feet.) This is used for ridiculing something superfluous.

陳修園曰：半夏氣平，稟天秋金之燥氣，而入手太陰。味辛有毒，得地西方
酷烈之味，而入手足陽明。辛則能開諸結，平則能降諸逆也。傷寒寒熱、心
下堅者，邪積於半表半裏之間，其主之者，以其辛而能開也。

Chén Xiūyuán said: *Bàn xià's* qì is neutral, inherits the dry qì of heaven and autumn metal, and
enters the hand tàiyīn. [*Bàn xià's*] flavor is acrid, toxic, [and] is of the earth and the west. [*Bàn xià's*]
harsh intense flavor [also] enters the hand and foot yángmíng. Because it is acrid, [*bàn xià*] is able
to open all kinds of binds. Because it is neutral, [*bàn xià*] has the ability to descend all kinds of
counterflow. Cold and heat in cold damage and hardness below the heart are pathogens accumulated between the half exterior and half interior. [*Bàn xià*] governs them, because its acridity is able
to open.

胸脹，咳逆、咽喉腫痛、頭眩上氣者，邪逆於巔頂，胸膈之上，其主之者，
以其平而能降也。腸鳴者，大腸受濕，則腸中切痛而鳴濯濯也。其主之者，
以其辛平能燥濕也。又云止汗者，另著其辛中帶澀之功也。

Distention in the chest, counterflow cough, throat swelling with pain, and dizzy head with ascending qì are evils [that run] counterflow in the vertex, as well as above the chest and diaphragm. Using
[*bàn xià's*] neutrality, which is able to descend, is what governs this. Rumbling in the intestines
[occurs] when the large intestine suffers from dampness, [which also] results in sharp pain and gurgling sounds.[345] [*Bàn xià*] governs this, because its acridity and neutrality are able to dry dampness.
It is further said that [*bàn xià*] stops sweating. This additionally reveals that within the acridity, [*bàn
xià*] brings along the merit of being astringent.

仲景於小柴胡湯用之以治寒熱，瀉心湯用之以治胸滿腸鳴，少陰咽痛亦用
之，《金匱》頭眩亦用之，且嘔者必加此味，大得其開結降逆之旨。用藥悉
遵《本經》，所以為醫中之聖。

Zhòngjǐng uses [*bàn xià*] in his *Xiǎo Chái Hú Tāng* for treating cold and heat, and in his *Xiè Xīn
Tāng*, for treating fullness in the chest and borborygmus. He also uses [*bàn xià*] for shàoyīn pharynx
pain. In the *Jīn Guì*, it is also used [for treating] dizziness, and furthermore, [in cases of] vomiting,
[Zhòngjǐng] definitely adds this flavor. So he greatly achieves its purpose of opening binds and
descending counterflow. [Zhòngjǐng] applies medicinals in conformity with the *Shén Nóng Běn
Cǎo Jīng*. This is the reason why he is a sage in [the field of] medicine.

又曰：今人以半夏功專祛痰，概用白礬煮之，服者往往致吐，且致酸心少
食，製法相沿之陋也。古人祇用湯洗七次，去涎，今人畏其麻口，不敢從
之。

---

345. *Zhuó zhuó* 濯濯 is gurgling, or the sound of water stirring.

[Chén Xiūyuán] further said: Modern people take the function of *bàn xià* especially for expelling phlegm, and they indiscriminately cook it with *bái fán*. [The patients] who take it are often caused to vomit. Furthermore, [*bàn xià*] causes them heartburn with loss of appetite. [The above-mentioned] processing method is an established malpractice. People of antiquity only washed [*bàn xià*] seven times with hot water to remove the mucus. Modern people fear its numbing taste, so they do not dare to follow this [method].

余每年收乾半夏數十斤，洗去粗皮，以生薑汁、甘草水浸一日夜，洗淨，又用河水浸三日，一日一換，濾起蒸熟，晒乾切片，隔一年用之，甚效。蓋此藥是太陰、陽明、少陽之大藥，袪痰卻非專長。故仲景諸方加減，俱云嘔者加半夏，痰多者加茯苓，未聞以痰多加半夏也。

I collect several tens of *jīn*[346] of dried *bàn xià*, wash them, remove the coarse peel, and soak them in fresh *jiāng* juice and *gān cǎo* water for a day and a night. [They are then] washed clean, and again soaked in river water for three days, exchanging [the water] daily. [After] straining [they are] steamed [and then] sun dried and sliced, and divided into [portions] to be used over a year. This is very effective. Now, this is a great medicinal for tàiyīn, yángmíng and shàoyáng. However, expelling phlegm is not [*bàn xià's*] special ability. Therefore, in all of Zhòngjǐng's prescription modifications, it is said: add *bàn xià* for vomiting and add *fú líng* for copious phlegm. It is not conveyed to add *bàn xià* for copious phlegm.

Dà Huáng 大黃
Root of Rheum palmatum

氣味苦、寒，無毒。主下淤血、血閉，寒熱，破癥瘕積聚、留飲宿食，盪滌腸胃，推陳致新，通利水穀，調中化食，安和五臟。

The qì and flavor are bitter, cold and non-toxic. [Dà huáng] governs the precipitation of static blood and blood block with cold and heat. [Dà huáng] breaks concretions, obstructions, accumulations, and gatherings. [It expels] lodged rheum and abiding food, clears up the intestines and stomach, pushes out the old to bring forth the new, unblocks water and grain,[347] harmonizes the center and transforms food, and quiets the five viscera.

---

346. One *jīn* 斤 (a catty) is equal to 597 grams in the *Qīng* dynasty.

347. This means the urinary bladder and bowels.

陳修園曰：大黃色正黃而臭香，得土之正氣正色，故專主脾胃之病。其氣味苦寒，故主下泄。凡血淤而閉，則為寒熱。腹中結塊，有形可徵曰癥，忽聚可散曰瘕。五臟為積，六腑為聚，以及留飲宿食，得大黃攻下，皆能已之。

Chén Xiūyuán said: *Dà huáng's* color is pure yellow and its smell is fragrant, so it receives the right qì and right color of the earth. Therefore, [*dà huáng*] especially governs diseases of the spleen and stomach. It is bitter and cold. Therefore, [*dà huáng*] mainly discharges downwards. Generally, when there is blood stasis or blood block, then there is cold or heat. Lumps in the abdomen have a form, [that] can be examined [because they are palpable] and are called concretions. [Lumps] that suddenly gather and can be dispersed are called obstructions. The [lumps] in the five viscera are accumulations, and the ones in the six bowels are gatherings. The moment lodged rheum and abiding food are attacked and precipitated with *dà huáng*, they are all able to cease.

自「盪滌腸胃」下五句，是申明大黃之效。末一句是總結上四句，又大申大黃之奇效也。意謂人祇知大黃盪滌腸胃，功在推陳，抑知推陳即所以致新乎？

The five sentences from "it clears up the intestines and stomach" onward, are clearly stating *dà huáng's* effect. The final sentence is a summary of the four previous ones, and it is further highly declaring the wonderful effect of *dà huáng*. Its meaning seems to say: people merely know that *dà huáng* clears up the intestines and stomach and that its merit consists in pushing out the old. But are they aware that pushing out the old is what accordingly brings forth the new?

人知大黃通利水穀，功在化食，抑知化食即所以調中乎？且五臟皆稟氣於胃，胃得大黃運化之力而安和，而五臟亦得安和矣，此《本經》所以有黃良之名也。有生用者，有用清酒洗者。

People know that *dà huáng* unblocks water and grain, and functions to transform food, but are they aware that the transformation of food namely is what regulates the center? Furthermore, all the five viscera are endowed with qì by the stomach. When the stomach obtains the strength of transportation and transformation from *dà huáng*, then [the stomach is] peaceful, and the five viscera also obtain peace! This is the reason why [*dà huáng*] has the name *huáng lián* "good yellow" in the *Shén Nóng Běn Cǎo Jīng*. Some use it fresh, some use it washed in clear wine.[348]

---

348. *Qīng jiǔ* 清酒 (clear wine) can be rice wine or old cleared wine, usually not made of grapes.

Táo Rén 桃仁
Seed of Prunus persica

氣味苦、甘、平，無毒。主淤血、血閉、癥瘕邪氣，殺小蟲。雙仁者，大毒。

The qì and flavor are bitter, sweet, neutral, and non-toxic. [*Táo rén*] governs static blood, blood block, concretions, and conglomerations by evil qì, and it kills small crawling animals. *Double kernels are very toxic.*

陳修園曰：桃仁氣平為金氣，味苦為火味，味甘為土味。所以瀉多而補少者，以氣平主降，味苦主泄，甘味之少，不能與之為敵也。

Chén Xiūyuán said: *Táo rén's* neutral qì is that of metal, its bitterness is the flavor of fire, and its sweetness is the flavor of earth. The reason why [*táo rén*] is more draining than supplementing is because the neutral qì governs downbearing and the bitter flavor governs discharging. The mild sweetness is not [enough] to grant opposition [to bitter neutrality].

徐靈胎曰：桃得三月春和之氣以生，而花色鮮明似血，故凡血鬱血結之疾，不能調和暢達者，此能入於其中而和之散之。然其生血之功少，而去淤之功多者，何也？蓋桃核本非血類，故不能有所補益。若淤瘕皆已敗之血，非生氣不能流通。桃之生氣，皆在於仁，而味苦又能開泄，故能逐舊而不傷新也。

Xú Língtāi said: Peaches receive the harmonious spring qì of the third [lunar] month for [their] growth. The color of their blossoms is bright and resembles blood. Therefore, whenever there is the disease of blood depression and bound blood with inability to harmoniously and smoothly pass, this [drug] is able to enter the center [of the blood stasis] in order to harmonize and disperse it. Now, [*táo rén's*] merit of engendering blood is less and its merit of eliminating stasis is more, why is that so? Because *táo hé* was not originally in the blood category. Therefore, it is unable to have a boosting benefit. If the stasis and conglomerations have both already wasted the blood,[349] qì is not engendered and is unable to circulate. The qì engendering [effect] is all in the kernels and their bitterness is further able to open and discharge. Therefore, [*táo hé*] is able to dispel the old without damaging the new.

---

349. *Bài xuě* 敗血 (wasted blood) is static blood that has not been discharged from the body. See: Wiseman, 1998, p. 665.

Xuán Fù Huā 旋覆花
Flowerhead of Inula britannica

氣味鹹、溫，有小毒。主結氣，脅下滿，驚悸，除水，去五臟間寒熱，補中益氣。

The qì and flavor are salty, warm, and slightly toxic. [*Xuán fù huā*] governs bound qì, fullness below the rib-sides, and fright palpitations; [it] eliminates water, expels cold and heat from between the five viscera, supplements the center, and boosts the qì.

陳修園曰：旋覆花氣溫，稟風氣而主散。味鹹，得水味潤下而頓堅。味勝於氣，故以味為主。唯其頓堅，故結氣，脅下滿等症，皆能已之。唯其潤下，故停水，驚悸，及五臟鬱滯而生寒熱等症，皆能已之。

Chén Xiūyuán said: *Xuán fù huā's* qì is warm, [which] inherits the qì of wind, and governs dispersion. [*Xuán fù huā's*] flavor is salty, [which] is the water flavor [that] precipitates with moistness and softens hardness. The flavor dominates that of the qì. Therefore, the flavor is the main [characteristic. *Xuán fù huā*] softens hardness; therefore, bound qì, fullness below the rib-sides, and symptoms of this kind can all be resolved by this. It precipitates by moistening; therefore, detained water, fright palpitations, and also cold and heat produced by depression and stagnation of the five viscera, and symptoms of this kind are all resolved by this.

借鹹降之力，上者下之，水氣行，痰氣消，而中焦自然受補矣。

Through [*xuán fù huā's*] strength of descending with saltiness, that which is ascending is precipitated, water qì is moved, phlegm qì is dispersed, and thus the middle *jiāo* naturally receives supplementation!

《本經》名金沸草。《爾雅》名盜庚。七、八月開花，如金錢菊。相傳葉上露水滴地即生。

In the Shén Nóng Běn Cǎo Jīng, [xuán fù huā] is named "metal boiling herb" and in the Ěr Yǎ 《爾雅》 (Approaching the Refined), it is named "metal robber."[350] *[Xuán fù huā] blooms in the seventh or eighth month [and looks] like a "metal coin chrysanthemum." It has been handed down that the moment dew drops on the ground from its leaves, [one] will live [longer].*[351]

---

350. *Gēng* 庚 is the seventh of the ten celestial stems and equals metal; it can also mean the age of a person.

351. Another translation could be: "it grows, when dew drops onto the ground from the leaves."

Jié Gēng 桔梗
Root of Platycodon grandiflorum

氣味辛 、微溫，有小毒 。主胸脅痛如刀刺，腹滿，腸鳴幽幽，驚恐悸氣 。

The qì and flavor are acrid, slightly warm, and slightly toxic. [*Jié gēng*] governs stabbing pain in the chest and rib-sides, fullness in the abdomen, deep and long-lasting intestinal rumbling, and fright, fear, and palpitation qì.

張隱庵曰：桔梗治少陽之脅滿，上焦之胸痹，中焦之腸鳴，下焦之腹滿 。又驚則氣上，恐則氣下，悸則動中，是桔梗為氣分之藥，上中下皆可治也 。

Zhāng Yǐn'ān said: *Jié gēng* treats fullness in the rib-sides of shàoyáng, chest impediment in the upper *jiāo*, intestinal rumbling in the middle *jiāo*, and abdominal fullness in the lower *jiāo*. Furthermore, when there is fright, then the qì ascends; when there is fear, then the qì descends; and when there are palpitations, then the center is stirred. This [means that] *jié gēng* is a medicinal for the qì aspect. The upper, the middle, and the lower [*jiāos*] all can be treated.

張元素不參經義，謂桔梗乃舟楫之藥，載諸藥而不沉 。今人熟念在口，終身不忘，以元素杜撰之言為是，則《 本經 》幾可廢矣！醫門豪傑之士，能明神農之《 本經 》、軒岐之《 靈 》《 素 》、仲祖之《 論 》《 略 》，則千百方書，皆為糟粕 。設未能也，必為方書所囿，而蒙蔽一生矣 。可畏哉！

Zhāng Yuánsù did not counsel on the meaning of the classics and thought *jié gēng* to be a boat medicinal, which carries all medicinals without sinking. The people of today carefully study [Zhāng Yuánsù's words] by reading them out loud, so they will not forget them [throughout] their life. If Yuánsù's invented words were right, the *Shén Nóng Běn Cǎo Jīng* [would] become almost useless! If this "heroic scholar of medicine" had been able to clearly understand Shén Nóng's *Běn Cǎo Jīng*, the *Líng* [*Shū*], and *Sù* [*Wèn*] of Xuān and Qí,[352] ancestor Zhòng's [*Shāng Hán*] *Lùn* and [*Jīn Guì Yào*] *Lüè*, then numerous formula books would all be useless rubbish. Supposing that he was unable to [comprehend the classics], it is surely due to the limitations of the remedy books, and [Zhāng Yuánsù] was deceived all his life! What a pity!

---

352. Xuān 軒 and Qí 岐 are Huáng Dì 黄帝 and Qí Bó 岐伯.

神
農
本
草
經
讀
・
卷
四

Tíng Lì Zǐ 葶藶子
Seeds of Lepidium apetalum

味辛寒 。主癥瘕、積聚、結氣，水飲所結之疾。飲食寒熱，破堅逐邪，亦
皆水氣之疾。通利水道。肺氣降則水道自通。

The qì and flavor are acrid and cold. [*Tíng lì zǐ*] governs concretions and obstructions, accumulations and gatherings, and bound qì. *These are retained water-rheum conglomeration diseases.* [It also governs] cold or heat due to [inappropriate] drink or food, breaks hardness, and expels evil. *These are also all [pathogenic] water qì diseases.* [It also] unblocks the waterways. *When the lung qì descends, the waterways are opened spontaneously.*

徐靈胎曰：葶藶滑潤而香，專瀉肺氣，肺為水源，故能瀉肺，即能瀉水，凡
積聚寒熱從水氣來者，此藥主之 。

Xú Língtāi said: *Tíng lì zǐ* is slippery, moist, fragrant, and special [for] draining the lung qì. The lungs are the source of water. Therefore, [*tíng lì zǐ*] is able to drain the lungs and accordingly drain water. In general, accumulations and gatherings of cold or heat are all derived from [pathogenic] water qì, and this medicinal governs them.

大黃之瀉，從中焦始 。葶藶之瀉，從上焦始 。故《傷寒論 》中承氣湯用大
黃，而陷胸湯用葶藶也 。

The draining of *dà huáng* begins from the middle *jiāo* and the draining of *tíng lì zǐ* begins from the upper *jiāo*. Therefore, *dà huáng* is used in the *Chéng Qì Tāng* [formulas] from the *Shāng Hán Lùn*, and *tíng lì zǐ* is used in *Xiàn Xiōng Tāng*.[353]

---

353. None of the chest bind decoctions contain *tíng lì zǐ* 葶藶子, but *Dà Xiàn Xiōng Wán* 大陷胸丸 (Major Chest Bind Pills) do.

Lián Qiáo 連翹
Fruit of Forsythia suspensa

氣味苦、平。主寒熱，鼠瘻，瘰癧，癰腫，惡瘡，癭瘤，結熱，蠱毒。

The qì and flavor are bitter and neutral. [*Lián qiáo*] governs cold and heat, mouse fistulae, lymphadenitis, welling-abscess swelling, malign sores, goiters and tumors of the neck, bound heat, and *gǔ* toxins.

Xià Kū Cǎo 夏枯草
Flower spike of Prunella vulgaris

氣味苦、辛，寒。主寒熱，瘰癧，鼠瘻，頭瘡，破癥，散癭，結氣，腳腫，濕痹，輕身。

The qì and flavor are bitter, acrid, and cold. [*Xià kū cǎo*] governs cold and heat, scrofula, mouse fistulae, and head sores. [It also] breaks concretions; disperses goiters, bound qì, swollen legs, and damp impediment; and lightens the body.

Dài Zhě Shí 代赭石
Hematite

氣味苦、寒，無毒。主鬼疰，賊風，蠱毒，殺精物惡鬼，腹中毒，邪氣，女子赤沃漏下。

The qì and flavor are bitter, cold, and non-toxic. [*Dài zhě shí*] governs demonic infixation, bandit wind,[354] and *gǔ* toxins; kills demons and evil spirits, toxins inside the abdomen, and evil qì; and [it governs] women's red spotting.[355]

---

354. *Zèi fēng* 賊風 (bandit wind) means harmful pathogenic wind, and incorrect, untimely qì of any of the four seasons.

355. *Chì wò* 赤沃 (red irrigation) is an old name for the dripping of red-colored sticky discharge.

述：代赭石氣寒入腎，味苦無毒入心。腎為坎水，代赭氣寒益腎，則腎水中一陽上升。心為離火，代赭味苦益心，則心火中一陰下降。

Commentary: *Dài zhě shí's* qì is cold and enters the kidneys. The flavor is bitter, non-toxic, and enters the heart. The kidneys are *kǎn*[356] water, and the qì of *dài zhě shí* is cold, [which] boosts the kidneys, [resulting in] the ascent of the yáng of kidney water. The heart is *lí*[357] fire, and the flavor of *dài zhě shí* is bitter, [which] boosts the heart, [resulting in] the descent of the yīn of heart fire.

水升火降，陰陽互藏其宅，而天地位矣。故鬼疰，賊風，精魅惡鬼，以及蠱毒，腹中邪毒，皆可主之。腎主二便，心主血，血熱則赤沃漏下。

When water ascends and fire descends, yīn and yáng are stored in each other's residence, and heaven and earth dwell![358] Therefore, demonic infixation, bandit wind, spirits, demons, and malign ghosts, as well as *gǔ* toxins, and evil toxins in the abdomen, can all be governed by [*dài zhě shí*]. The kidneys govern the two excretions and the heart governs blood. When the blood is hot, there is red spotting.

苦寒清心，心腎相交，所以主女子赤沃漏下。仲景旋覆花代赭湯，用之極少。後人昧其理而重用之，且賴之以鎮納諸氣，皆荒經之過也！

Bitterness and coldness clear the heart and cause the heart and kidneys to mutually interact. Therefore, [*dài zhě shí*] governs women's red spotting. Zhòngjǐng used *Xuán Fù Huā Dài Zhě Tāng* very rarely. [However], people of later generations ignored [*dài zhě shí's*] intrinsic texture and used it heavily. Moreover, they relied on [*dài zhě shí*] to suppress and restrain all the qì. This is entirely out-of-the-way and goes beyond the proper limits of the classics!

---

356. *Kǎn* 坎 is the trigram for water ☵.

357. *Lí* 離 is the trigram for fire ☲.

358. *Wèi* 位 (seat) means to dwell, to place oneself in. This is again making use of the metaphorical picture of a state for the body. When the state is kept in the right order, there is peace. When the organs take their *seats*, there is physical harmony. It also means yáng has to be within yīn and vice versa.

本草附錄
Appendix to the Materia Medica

《別錄》、《唐本草》、《拾遺》、《藥性》、海藏、《蜀本》、《開寶》
、《圖經》、《日華》、《補遺》。

[The appendix is made of excerpts from the following books:] *Bié Lù* 《別錄》(Supplementary Records),[359] *Táng Běn Cǎo* 《唐本草》(Materia Medica of the *Táng*),[360] *Shí Yí* 《拾遺》(Picking up Lost Property),[361] *Yào Xìng* 《藥性》(On the Nature of Medicines),[362] *Hǎi Zàng* 海藏 (Hǎi Zàng),[363] *Shǔ Běn Cǎo* 《蜀本》(Materia Medica of the State Shǔ),[364] *Kāi Bǎo* 《開寶》(Kāi Bǎo),[365] *Tú Jīng* 《圖經》(Illustrated Materia Medica),[366] *Rì Huà* 《日華》(Materia Medica of Rì Huàzǐ),[367] and *Bǔ Yí* 《補遺》(Addendum).[368]

359. This is the short title of the *Míng Yī Bié Lù* 《名醫別錄》(Supplementary Records of Famous Physicians). This book was written by Táo Hóngjǐng 陶弘景 (456~536).

360. Another title of this book is *Xīn Xiū Běn Cǎo* 《新修本草》(Newly Revised Materia Medica). It was compiled by *Sū Jìng* 蘇敬 (599-674) et al in 659 and is based on the Bié Lù 《別錄》(Supplementary Records).

361. This is the *Běn Cǎo Shí Yí* 《本草拾遺》(Picking up Lost Property of the Materia Medica) by Chén Cángqì 陳藏器, compiled in 739.

362. The full title of this book is *Yào Xìng Běn Cǎo* 《藥性本草》(Materia Medica on the Nature of Medicines) and it was written by Zhēn Quán 甄權 (541-643). The original book is lost, but pieces of it have been assembled under the title *Yào Xìng Lùn* 《藥性論》(Treatise on the Nature of Medicines).

363. This is actually not a book title, but another name of Wáng Hàogǔ 王好古 (1200-1264), who is the author of the *Tāng Yè Běn Cǎo* 《湯液本草》(Materia Medica of Decoctions), so most likely, this is the book referenced here.

364. This book was compiled between 935 and 960 by Hán Bǎoyì 韓保異 et al.

365. *Kāi Bǎo Chóng Dìng Běn Cǎo* 《開寶重定本草》(Kāi Bǎo Revised Materia Medica).

366. This is an abbreviation for the *Tú Jīng Běn Cǎo* 《圖經本草》(Illustrated Materia Medica). It was compiled in 1061 by Sū Sòng 蘇頌 (1020-1101) et al. The original is lost.

367. The full title of this book is *Rì Huà Zǐ Zhū Jiā Běn Cǎo* 《日華子諸家本草》(Materia Medica of Various Schools by Rì Huàzǐ) or *Dà Míng Běn Cǎo* 《大明本草》(Dà Míng's Materia Medica). Dà Míng 大明 is the original name of Rì Huàzǐ 日華子, who lived in the tenth century. The book is said to have had more than six hundred entries, but is now lost. See Footnote 31 of the preface.

368. This is a book by the famous Zhū Zhènhēng 朱震亨 (1281-1358). The full title of the book is *Běn Cǎo Yǎn Yì Bǔ Yí* 《本草衍義補遺》(Addendum to the Amplified Meanings of the Materia Medica). The original is also lost.

Hé Shǒu Wū 何首烏
Root of Polygoni multiflori

氣味苦、溫，無毒。主瘰癧，消癰腫，療頭面風瘡，治五痔，止心痛，益血氣，黑髭髮，悅顏色。久服長筋骨，益精髓，延年不老。亦治婦人產後及帶下諸疾。《開寶》

The qì and flavor are bitter, warm, and non-toxic. [*Hé shǒu wū*] governs scrofula, disperses welling-abscess swelling, [and] cures wind sores[369] of the head and face. [It also] treats the five hemorrhoids, stops heart pain, boosts blood and qì, blackens the moustache and hair, and promotes a pleasant facial complexion. When taken over a long period of time, it grows the sinews and bones, boosts essence and marrow, prolongs life, and prevents aging. It also cures all kinds of postnatal and vaginal discharge diseases in women. (*Kāi Bǎo Chóng Dìng Běn Cǎo*)[370]

陳修園曰：後世增入藥品，余多置之而弗論，唯何首烏於久瘧久痢多取用之。蓋瘧少陽之邪也，久而不愈，少陽之氣慣為瘧邪所侮，俯首不敢與爭，任其出入往來，絕無忌憚，縱舊邪已退，而新邪復乘虛入之，則為瘧。縱新邪未入，而營衛不調之氣，自襲於少陽之界，亦為瘧。

Chén Xiūyuán said: I often ignore medicinals added by later generations and do not discuss them. It is only *hé shǒu wū* that I utilize often in cases of long-lasting malaria and long-lasting dysentery. Now, malaria is an evil of the shàoyáng. If it lasts long without recovery, the shàoyáng becomes accustomed to the malarial evil's insult, bows its head and does not dare to fight with [the evil], allowing [it to] intermittently come and go. [The evil] is entirely fearless, and even if the old evil has already retreated, a new one will avail itself of the vacuity and enter [the shàoyáng], resulting in malaria. Even if the new evil has not yet entered, when the qì of the construction and defense are not harmonious, [the pathogen] will spontaneously raid the boundaries of shàoyáng, also resulting in malaria.

首烏妙在直入少陽之經，其氣甚雄，雄則足以折瘧邪之勢。其味甚澀，澀則足以堵瘧邪之路。邪若未淨者，佐以柴、苓、橘、半。邪若已淨者，佐以參、朮、耆、歸。一、二劑效矣。設初瘧而即用之，則閉門逐寇，其害有不可勝言者矣。

The excellence of *hé shǒu wū* lies in its [ability to] directly enter the shàoyáng channel and in the vigorousness of its qì. Because it is vigorous, [*hé shǒu wū*] sufficiently breaks the strength of the

---

369. *Fēng chuāng* 風瘡 (wind sores) are a disease of the eyelids with redness, blisters, erosions, soreness, itching, and ulceration. See: Wiseman, 1998, p. 691.

370. Hereafter, simply listed as the *Kāi Bǎo*.

malaria evil. The flavor of [hé shŏu wū] is very astringent. Because it is astringent, then [hé shŏu wū] sufficiently stops up the pathway of the malarial evil. If the evil has not yet been wiped out, assist [hé shŏu wū] with chái [hú, fú] líng, jú [pí], and bàn [xià]. If the evil has already been cleared, assist [hé shŏu wū] with [rén] shēn, [bái] zhú, [huáng] qí and [dāng] guī. One or two packets [of medicinals will be] sufficient! Supposing that [these medicinals] were immediately used at the onset of malaria, then the door would be closed for [properly] expelling the bandit, and the harm would be inexpressible!

久痢亦用之者，以土氣久陷，當於少陽求其生發之氣也，亦以首烏之味最苦而澀，苦以堅其腎，澀以固其脫。宜溫者，與薑、附同用。宜涼者，與芩、連同用。亦捷法也。此外，如疽瘡，五痔之病，則取其蔓延而通經絡。瘰癧之病，則取其入少陽之經。

[I] also use [hé shŏu wū] for enduring dysentery, because when the earth qì is sunken for a long [period of time], one should seek out the emergent qì of shàoyáng. The flavor of hé shŏu wū is extremely bitter and astringent; the bitterness firms the [patient's] kidneys and the astringency secures desertion. For warming, it is appropriate to use [hé shŏu wū] together with jiāng and fù zĭ. For cooling, it is appropriate to use [hé shŏu wū] together with [huáng] qín and [huáng] lián. These are also quick methods. Apart from this, for diseases like flat-abscesses and the five hemorrhoids, [I] take [hé shŏu wū's] spreading [nature] to free the channels and collaterals. For the disease of scrofula, [I] make use of [hé shŏu wū's ability to] enter the shàoyáng channel.

精滑，泄瀉，崩漏之病，則取其澀以固脫。若謂首烏滋陰補腎，能烏須髮，益氣血，悅顏色，長筋骨，益精髓，延年，皆耳食之誤也。凡物之能滋潤者，必其脂液之多也。物之能補養者，必氣味和也。試問：澀滯如首烏，何以能滋？苦劣如首烏，何以能補？今之醫輩竟奉為補藥上品者，蓋惑於李時珍《綱目》「不寒不燥，功居地黃之上」之說也。余二十年來，目擊受害者比比。以醫為蒼生之司命，不敢避好辯之名也。

For diseases like seminal leakage, diarrhea, flooding and spotting, [I] employ [hé shŏu wū's] astringent [quality] to secure the desertion. Saying that hé shŏu wū nourishes the yīn and supplements the kidneys, is able to blacken the beard and hair, boosts qì and blood, promotes a pleasant facial complexion, grows sinews and bones, boosts essence and marrow, and prolongs life, are all mistakes due to rumors. Generally, for moisturizing, a substance must have plenty of fat and humors. For supplementing and nourishing, a substance must have harmonious qì and flavor. May I ask: How can a stagnating astringent [medicinal] like hé shŏu wū be able to moisten? How can a slightly bitter [medicinal] like hé shŏu wū be able to supplement? Those among today's generation of physicians who indeed regard [hé shŏu wū] as a supplementing herb of highest grade, were probably mislead by what is said in Lĭ Shízhēn's Gāng Mù: "... it is neither cold nor dry, its merit is in a higher position than that of dì huáng ...." For twenty years I have witnessed that persons who have suffered damage from [this erroneous belief] can be found everywhere. I believe physicians are responsible for the lives of ordinary people, and as such I do not dare avoid becoming famous for being fond of disputes.

Yán Hú Suǒ 延胡索
Rhizome of Corydalis yanhuosuo

氣味辛、溫，無毒。主破血，婦人月經不調，腹中結塊，崩中淋露，產後諸血症，血暈，暴血衝上，因損下血。煮酒或酒磨服。《開寶》

The qì and flavor are acrid, warm, and non-toxic. [*Yán hú suǒ*] governs breaking blood, women's menstrual irregularities, lumps in the abdomen, flooding and strangury dew, all kinds of postpartum blood patterns, blood fainting,[371] sudden surging of blood, and bleeding caused by injuries. *To be taken cooked with wine or ground with wine.* (*Kāi Bǎo*)

Ròu Dòu Kòu 肉豆蔻
Seed of Myristica fragrans

氣味辛、溫，無毒。主溫中，消食，止泄，治精冷，心腹脹痛，霍亂，中惡，鬼氣，冷痃，嘔沫冷氣，小兒乳霍。《開寶》

The qì and flavor are acrid, warm, and non-toxic.[372] [*Ròu dòu kòu*] warms the center, disperses food, stops diarrhea, [and] treats seminal cold.[373] [It also treats] distention and pain in the [region below] the heart and in the abdomen, sudden turmoil,[374] malignity stroke,[375] demonic qì, cold infixation, cold qì with vomiting of foam and children's vomiting, and sudden [letting down] of mother's milk. (*Kāi Bǎo*)

---

371. *Xuè yūn* 血暈 (blood dizziness, fainting) refers to circulation problems due to blood loss during childbirth.

372. In fact, they are toxic when a dosage higher than five grams is taken. For children, they are even more dangerous and can be lethal.

373. *Jīng lěng* 精冷 (seminal cold) is cold, thin, and scant semen attributed to kidney qì or yáng insufficiency. See: Wiseman, 1998, p. 523.

374. In Western medicine, this is known as cholera.

375. *Zhòng è* 中惡 (malignity stroke) is stroke by demons with sudden counterflow cold, goose pimples etc., and even collapse. See: ibid, p. 384.

Bǔ Gǔ Zhī 補骨脂
Fruit of Psoralea corylifolia

氣味辛、溫，無毒。主五勞七傷，風虛冷，骨髓傷敗，腎冷精流，及婦人血氣，墮胎。《開寶》

The qì and flavor are acrid, warm, and non-toxic. [*Bǔ gǔ zhī*] governs the five taxations and the seven damages, wind vacuity cold, damage or loss of bone marrow, seminal flowing due to kidney cold, as well as women's blood and qì [disharmony], and abortion. (*Kāi Bǎo*)

陳修園曰：墮胎者，言其人素有墮胎之病，以此藥治之，非謂以此藥墮之也。上文主字，直貫至此。蓋胎借脾氣以長，借腎氣以舉，此藥溫補脾腎，所以大有固胎之功。數百年來，誤以黃芩為安胎之品，遂疑溫藥礙胎，見《開寶》有「墮胎」二字，遽以「墮」字不作病情解，另作藥功解，與上文不相連貫。李瀕湖、汪訒庵、葉天士輩因之，貽害千古。或問《本經》牛膝本文，亦有「墮胎」二字，豈非以「墮」字作藥功解乎？曰彼頂「逐血氣」句來，唯其善逐，所以善墮。古書錯綜變化，難與執一不通？同者道。

Chén Xiūyuán said: [Here] abortion [signifies that] this patient constitutionally has this disease, and this medicinal cures it. It does not mean that this medicinal induces abortion. The main characters of the text above are directly hinting at this [disease]. Now, the fetus avails itself of spleen qì for growth and it makes use of the kidney qì for being born. This medicinal supplements the spleen and kidneys with warmth. Therefore, [*bǔ gǔ zhī*] has a great fetus securing effect. Over the last few centuries, [bitter cold] *huáng qín* has been mistaken as a fetus calming herb, and forthwith it had been suspected that warming herbs are fetus deterring. Looking at the two characters "abortion of fetus" in the *Kāi Bǎo* [*Chóng Dìng Běn Cǎo*], immediately the character "abortion" is not understood as a patient's condition, but rather as a pharmaceutical effect. This is not coherent with the text above. The generation of Lǐ Bīnhú,[376] Wāng Rèn'ān,[377] and Yè Tiānshì[378] followed this, and harm had been handed down for a long, long time. Someone may ask: "In the *Shén Nóng Běn Cǎo Jīng's* original text on *niú xī*, the the two characters 'fetus abortion' also appear. How come the character 'abortion' is not understood as a pharmaceutical effect?" The answer is at: "The top of the line: '*it expels blood and qì*,' and because [*niú xī*] is good at expelling, it is good at aborting. Ancient books are intricate and variable, so it is difficult to maintain a single, unobstructed way [of thinking]."

---

376. Lǐ Bīnhú 李瀕湖: Also known as Lǐ Shízhēn 李時珍 (1518-1593), author of the *Běn Cǎo Gāng Mù* 《本草綱目》.

377. Wāng Rèn'ān 汪訒庵: Also known as Wāng Áng 汪昂 (1615-1699), author of the *Běn Cǎo Bèi Yào* 《本草備要》.

378. Yè Tiānshì 葉天士: Also known as Yè Guì 葉桂 (1666-1745), author of the *Wēn Rè Lùn* 《溫熱論》.

神
農
本
草
經
讀
・
卷
附

Bái Dòu Kòu 白豆蔻
Round fruit of Amomum kravanh

氣味辛，溫，無毒。主積冷氣，止吐逆，反胃，消穀下氣。《開寶》

The qì and flavor are acrid, warm, and non-toxic. [*Bái dòu kòu*] governs accumulated cold qì, stops vomiting counterflow and stomach reflux, digests food, and downbears qì. (*Kāi Bǎo*)

Suō Shā Rén 縮砂仁
Fruit of Amomum villosum

氣味辛、溫、澀，無毒。主虛勞冷瀉，宿食不消，赤白泄痢，腹中虛痛，下氣。《開寶》

The qì and flavor are acrid, warm, astringent, and non-toxic. [*Suō shā rén*] governs cold diarrhea due to vacuity taxation, non-dispersion of abiding food, red and white dysentery,[379] and vacuity pain in the abdomen; [it also] downbears qì. (*Kāi Bǎo*)

Yù Jīn 鬱金
Tuber of Curcuma aromatica

氣味苦、寒，無毒。主血積，下氣，生肌，止血，破惡血，血淋，尿血，金瘡。《唐本草》

The qì and flavor are bitter, cold, and non-toxic. [*Yù jīn*] governs blood accumulation, downbears qì, engenders flesh, stops bleeding, [and] breaks malign blood. [It also treats] blood strangury, urination of blood, and [governs] incised wounds. (*Táng Běn Cǎo*)

---

379. *Chì bái xiè lì* 赤白泄痢 (red and white dysentery) is blood and pus in the stool. See: Wiseman, 1998, pp. 495 and 675.

陳修園曰：時醫徇名有二誤：一曰生脈散，因其有「生脈」二字，每用之以救脈脫，入咽少頃，脈未生而人已死矣。一曰鬱金，因其命名為「鬱」，往往取治於氣鬱之症，數服之後，氣鬱未解，而血脫立至矣。醫道不明，到處皆然，而江、浙、閩、粵尤其甚者。

Chén Xiūyuán said: there are two mistakes occurring when contemporary physicians take words too literally[380]: the first occurs with *Shēng Mài Săn*: because of the two characters "pulse engendering," they always use it for saving pulse desertion. A short while after [the powder] has entered the throat, the pulse is not engendered, and the patient is already dead! The second [mistake] happens with *yù jīn*: because it is named "depressed,"[381] [*yù jīn*] is often taken for the treatment of qì depression patterns. After several dosages, the qì is [still] depressed and not resolved, but the blood desertion will immediately become extreme! There are [people], who fail to understand the Dào of medicine everywhere. However, [the situation] in Jiāng 江, Zhè 浙, Mǐn 閩, and Yuè 粵,[382] is particularly severe.

Shén Qū 神麴
Medicated leaven

氣味辛、甘、溫，無毒。主化水穀宿食，癥結積聚，健脾暖胃。《藥性》

The qì and flavor are acrid, sweet, warm, and non-toxic. [*Shén qū*] governs the transformation of water, grains and abiding food, concretions, binds, accumulations, and gatherings [in the bowels. *Shén qū* also] strengthens the spleen and warms the stomach. (*Yào Xìng Běn Căo*)

陳修園曰：凡麴糱皆主化穀，穀積服此便消。或鼻中如聞酒香，《藥性》所言主治，亦不外此。

Chén Xiūyuán said: In general, all kinds of brewer's yeast[383] govern the transformation of food. When [patients, who have] food accumulation take it, the stool disperses. Sometimes [*shén qū*] smells like alcohol, and the main indications listed in the *Yào Xìng Běn Căo* are also not beyond the scope of this.

---

380. The meaning of *xùn míng* 徇名 is "to give one's life to become famous," [which] means to take words too literally. *Xùn* 徇 "to die for a cause" is interchangeable with "to be buried with the dead."
381. *Yù jīn* 鬱金 literally means "depressed gold."
382. These are old names for the modern provinces of Jiāngsū, Zhèjiāng, Fùjiàn, and Guǎngdōng.
383. *Qū niè* 麴糱 means brewer's yeast.

癥結積聚者，水穀之積久而成也 。健脾暖胃者，化水穀之效也 。除化水穀之外，並無他長 。今人以之常服，且云祛百病，怪甚！

Concretions, binds, accumulations, and gatherings [in the bowels] develop out of long-lasting accumulations of water and grains. [*Shén qū's*] function of strengthening the spleen and warming the stomach is the effect on the transformation of water and grains. Apart from eliminating and transforming water and grains, it has no other strong points. The people of today regard [*shén qū*] as a [medicinal] for frequent intake and further claim it would expel one hundred diseases. This is very bewildering!

考造麴之法：六月六日，是六神聚會之日，用白麴百斤，青蒿 、蒼耳 、野蓼各自然汁三升，杏仁研泥 、赤小豆為末各三升，以配青龍 、白虎 、朱雀 、玄武 、勾陳 、螣蛇六神，通和作餅，麻葉或楮葉包罨，如造醬黃法，待生黃衣，晒乾收之 。陳久者良 。

Examine the manufacturing method of [*shén*] *qū*: [On] the sixth day of the sixth [lunar] month, is the gathering day of the six gods,[384] and [one should] use one hundred *jìn*[385] of plain flour,[386] three *shēng*[387] each of the natural juice of *qīng hāo*, *cāng ěr*, and *yě liǎo*, and three *shēng* each of *xìng rén* [which has been] ground into a paste, and powdered *chì xiǎo dòu*, in order to match them with the six gods *Qīng Lóng* 青龍 (Black Dragon), *Bái Hǔ* 白虎 (White Tiger), *Zhū Què* 朱雀 (Vermilion Bird), *Xuán Wǔ* 玄武 (Dark Tortoise), *Gōu Chén* 勾陳 (Hooked Old), and *Téng Shé* 螣蛇 (Winged Snake).[388] Blend them thoroughly and form cakes [out of the mass]; wrap and cover [the cakes] with hemp leaves or paper-mulberry leaves with the same method as if making fermented soybean paste. Wait until a yellow coating grows [on top of the cakes], sun dry, and collect them. The old ones are good.

---

384. *Liù shén* 六神 (the six gods) could be either six Daoist deities, the six organs heart, liver, kidneys, spleen, and gallbladder, or the six star constellations.

385. One hundred often simply means "a lot."

386. This can also mean bran.

387. One *shēng* is equal to 1.0355 liter in the *Qīng* dynasty.

388. These are the above mentioned star constellations of the east, west, south, north, and the North Star as well as a folklore god. The sequence of matches is slightly different in Miào Xīyōng's 繆希雍 (1546-1627) book *Pào Zhì Dà Fǎ · Mǐ Gǔ Bù* 《 炮炙大法· 米穀部 》 (Great Methods for Processing Medicines · Section on Rice and Grains). Miào was a physician from Jiāngsū, and a predecessor of Chén Xiūyuán. This book was published in 1622 and Miào's sequence is as follows: plain flour equates with *Bái Hǔ* 白虎, *cāng ěr* 蒼耳 equates with *Gōu Chén* 勾陳, *yě liǎo* 野蓼 equates with *Téng Shé* 螣蛇, *qīng hāo* 青蒿 equates with *Qīng Lóng* 青龍, *xìng rén* 杏仁 equates with *Xuán Wǔ* 玄武, and *chì xiǎo dòu* 赤小豆 equates with *Zhū Què* 朱雀.

藥用六種，以配六神聚會之日，罨發黃衣作麵，故名六神麵。今人除去「六」字，衹名神麵，任意加至數十味，無非剋破之藥，大傷元氣。且有百草神麵，害人更甚！

This medicinal has six ingredients, [which] matches with the gathering day of the six deities, and it is covered until it effuses a yellow coating to become yeast. Therefore, it is called *liù shén qū*.[389] The people of today removed the character "six" and simply call it *shén qū*. [In addition] they randomly add several tens of medicinals to it, [so it becomes] nothing but a ruined medicinal, which greatly damages the original qì. Moreover, there is a *bǎi cǎo shén qū* 百草神麵,[390] which is even more harmful to people!

近日通行福建神麵，其方於六神本方中，去赤小豆，惡其易蛀，加五苓散料、平胃散料及麥芽、穀芽、使君子、榧子、大黃、黃芩、大腹皮、砂仁、白蔻、丁香、木香、藿香、香附、良薑、芍藥、防風、秦艽、羌活、獨活、川芎、蘇葉、荊芥、防己、黨參、茯苓、萊菔子、苡米、木通、茶葉、乾薑、乾葛、枳椇、山楂、檳榔、青皮、木瓜、薄荷、蟬蛻、桃仁、紅花、三棱、莪朮、鬱金、菖蒲、柴胡、菊花等。

From the formula of the recently fashionable *shén qū* in Fújiàn, the *chì xiǎo dòu* is removed from the original formula, because [*chì xiǎo dòu*] is easily eaten by insects. And grains of *Wǔ Líng Sǎn* and *Píng Wèi Sǎn*[391] are added, as well as *mài yá, gǔ yá, shǐ jūn zǐ, fěi zǐ, dà huáng, huáng qín, dà fù pí, shā rén, bái kòu, dīng xiāng, mù xiāng, huò xiāng, xiāng fù,* high-quality *jiāng, sháo yào, fáng fēng, qín jiāo, qiāng huó, dú huó, chuān xiōng, sū yè, jīng jiè, fáng jǐ, dǎng shēn, fú líng, lái fú zǐ, yǐ mǐ, mù tōng,* tea leaves, *gān jiāng, gān gě, zhǐ jǔ, shān zhā, bīng láng, qīng pí, mù guā, bò hé, chán tuì, táo rén, hóng huā, sān léng, é zhú, yù jīn, chāng pú, chái hú, jú huā* etc.

為末，製為方塊，以草罨發黃衣晒乾。此方雜亂無序，誤人匪淺。而竟盛行一時者，皆誤信招牌上夸張等語。而慣以肥甘自奉之輩，單服此剋化之品，未嘗不通快一時，而損傷元氣，人自不覺。

[This is] powdered and processed into cubes, covered with herbs, and sun-dried once the yellow coating has developed. This formula is chaotic and the harm it causes to people is not light. Indeed, it was in fashion for a while, all because [people] erroneously believed the boasting words on the shop signs. Contemporary [people] who are used to supplying themselves with luxuriant food [and who] only take this digestive drug, are not necessarily overjoyed, and [are] unaware that their original qì was injured.

---

389. *Liù shén qū* 六神麵 (six gods leaven).

390. *Deities Yeast with One Hundred Herbs*: It is still available today.

391. *Stomach-Calming Powder*.

若以入方，則古人之方，立法不苟，豈堪此雜亂之藥，礙此礙彼乎？且以藥末合五穀，罯造發黃而為麴，祇取其速於釀化，除消導之外，並無他長，何以統治百病？且表散之品，因罯發而失其辛香之氣。攻堅之品，以罯發而失其雄入之權。

If they made a prescription, the established methods for the formulas of the people of antiquity were not thoughtless. How could they have endured this mess of medicinals [which] block this and block that? Furthermore, when medicinal powder is combined with the five grains, covered until it becomes yellow and turns into leaven, one only applies it [because it is] quick to ferment. Apart from eliminating, dispersing, and transmitting, [leaven] has no further advantage. How [is it] used to govern the one hundred diseases? In addition: exterior diffusing drugs lose their acrid and fragrant qì by being fermented. Hardness-attacking drugs lose their authority to vigorously enter by being fermented.

補養之藥，氣味中和，以罯發而變為臭腐穢濁之物，傷脾妨胃，更不待言，明者自知。余臨證二十年，而泉州一帶，先救誤服神麴之害者，十居其七。如感冒病，宜審經以發散，若服神麴，則裏氣以攻伐而虛，表邪隨虛而入裏矣。

Supplementing and nourishing medicinals have neutral qì and flavor. By being fermented, they turn into a thing of fetid decay and foul turbidity, which damages the spleen and harms the stomach. It is needless to say more about this, because the clever ones know it by themselves. I have clinical [experience] for twenty years now. In the region of Quánzhōu,[392] I have previously saved victims numbering seven out of ten residents from the wrongful use of *shén qū*. For instance, [with] the common cold, it is appropriate to examine the channels for effusing and dispersing. If [the patient] takes *shén qū*, the interior qì is attacked and becomes vacuous, [and] the external evil follows the vacuity and enters the interior!

傷食新病，宜助胃以剋化。傷食頗久，宜承氣以攻下。若服神麴，則釀成甜酸穢腐之味，滯於中焦，漫無出路，則為惡心脹痛矣。吐瀉是陰陽之不交，泄瀉是水穀不分，赤白痢是濕熱下注，噎隔是賁門乾槁，翻胃是命門火衰，痰飲是水氣泛溢，與神麴更無乾涉。若誤服之，輕則致重，重則致死，可不慎哉！

In recently acquired food damage, it is appropriate to assist the stomach in digestion. In rather long-lasting food damage, it is appropriate to coordinate the qì for offensive precipitation. If [the patient] takes *shén qū*, then the ferment forms into a sweet and sour foul and rotten flavor, which stagnates in the middle *jiāo* and spreads all over [the abdomen] without an exit. This results in nausea and painful distention! Vomiting and diarrhea occur when yīn and yáng fail to communicate. Dys-

392. Quánzhōu 泉州 is a prefecture-level city in Fújiàn.

entery occurs, when water and grains are not separated. Red and white dysentery is the result of the down-pour of damp-heat. Dysphagia-occlusion[393] is [due to] dryness of the cardiac opening. Stomach reflux occurs, when the fire of the Life Gate is feeble. [When] phlegm-rheum floats and [there is] overflowing water qì, then [one] should not further interfere with *shén qū*. If [*shén qū*] is wrongly taken, it causes mild [cases] to become serious, and in serious cases it leads to death. How can [people] not be cautious [in using it]!?

唯「范志」字號藥品精，製法妙，餘與吳先生名條光同年，因知其詳。可恨市中多假其字號，宜細辨之。

Only the medicinal drug of the "Fàn Zhì" brand[394] is refined. Its manufacturing method is excellent. Mister Wú named Tiáoguāng[395] and I are of the same age. This is the reason why I know the details [of his medicinal]. It is detestable that in the markets his brand is often faked. One should distinguish them precisely.

Huò Xiāng 藿香
Whole plant Agastache rugosa

氣味辛、甘、溫，無毒。主風水毒腫，去惡氣，止霍亂，心腹痛。《別錄》

The qì and flavor are acrid, sweet, warm, and non-toxic. [*Huò xiāng*] governs toxic wind and water swelling,[396] expels malign qì, and stops sudden turmoil and pain [in the region below] the heart and abdomen. (*Míng Yī Bié Lù*)

---

393. *Yē gé* 噎隔 (dysphagia-occlusion) is a blockage on swallowing and or immediate vomiting after eating. See: Wiseman, pp. 163.

394. The *Fàn Zhì* 范志 brand is *lǎo fàn zhì wàn yìng shén qū* 老范志萬應神麴 (Old Fan Zhi´s Ten Thousand Compliances Medicated Leaven) is an invention of doctor Wú Yìfēi 吳亦飛 (eighteenth century) from Quánzhōu 泉州. It started being produced with a secret method in 1733 and soon after became locally famous. It is named after the statesman Fàn Zhòngyān 范仲淹 (989-1052).

395. Wú Tiáoguāng 吳條光 (late eighteenth to early nineteenth century) seems to be the grandson of Wú Yìfēi 吳亦飛.

396. *Fēng shuǐ* 風水 (wind and water) here means external wind contraction with water swelling. See: Wiseman, 1998, p. 694.

Qián Hú 前胡
Root of Peucedanum praeruptorum

氣味苦、微寒，無毒。主痰滿，胸脅中痞，心腹結氣，風頭痛，去痰，下氣，治傷寒寒熱，推陳致新，明目益精。《別錄》

The qì and flavor are bitter, slightly cold, and non-toxic. [*Qián hú*] governs phlegm fullness, glomus in the chest and rib-sides, bound qì in the heart and abdomen, as well as wind headache. It expels phlegm, downbears qì, treats cold and heat in cold damage, pushes out the old to bring forth the new, brightens the eyes, and boosts essence. (*Míng Yī Bié Lù*)

Hóng Huā 紅花
Flower of Carthamus tinctorius

氣味辛、溫，無毒。主產後血暈口噤，腹內惡血不盡，絞痛，胎死腹中。並酒煮服。亦主蠱毒。《開寶》

The qì and flavor are acrid, warm, and non-toxic. [*Hóng huā*] governs postpartum blood fainting with inability to speak, endless malign blood in the abdomen, gripping pain, and death of the fetus in utero. *Take it cooked in wine.* It also governs *gǔ* venoms. (*Kāi Bǎo*)

Xiāng Fù 香附
Rhizome of Cyperus rotundus

氣味甘、微寒，無毒。除胸中熱，充皮毛。久服令人益氣，長須眉。《別錄》

The qì and flavor are sweet, slightly cold, and non-toxic. [*Xiāng fù*] eliminates heat from within the chest and replenishes the skin and hair. When taken over a long period of time, people have their qì boosted, and the beard and eyebrows grow. (*Míng Yī Bié Lù*)

Jīn Yīng Zǐ 金櫻子
Fruit of Rosa laevigata

氣味酸、澀，平，無毒。主脾泄下痢，止小便利，澀精氣。久服令人耐寒輕身。

The qì and flavor are sour, astringent, neutral, and non-toxic. [*Jīn yīng zǐ*] governs spleen diarrhea and dysentery, stops disinhibited urination, and astringes essence and qì. When taken over a long period of time, it makes people resistant to cold and lightens the body.[397]

Fú Shén 茯神
Sclerotium (i.e., white, hardened core in the center) of Poria cocos

氣味甘、平，無毒。主辟不祥，療風眩風虛，五勞口乾，止驚悸，多恚怒，善忘，開心益智，安魂魄，養精神。《別錄》

The qì and flavor are sweet, neutral, and non-toxic. [*Fú shén*] governs the warding off of the inauspicious, cures wind dizziness, wind vacuity, and the five taxations with dryness of the mouth. [It] stops fright palpitations and excessive rage and anger; remedies forgetfulness, makes [one] happy, boosts the intelligence, quiets the ethereal and corporeal souls, and nourishes [the] essence and spirit. (*Míng Yī Bié Lù*)

張隱庵曰：離松根而生者為茯苓，抱松根而生者為茯神，總以茯苓為勝。茯苓皮、茯神木，後人收用，各有主治，然皆糟粕之藥，並無精華之氣，不足重也。

Zhāng Yǐn'ān said: What grows distant from the roots of pine trees is *fú líng*, and [that] which grows embracing the pine roots is *fú shén*. [*Fú shén*] is always surpassed by *fú líng*. *Fú líng* has the bark and *fú shén* has the wood [for growing]. The people of later generations had indications for each of their applications. However, [*fú shén*] is an entirely useless medicinal and has absolutely no essential qì. It is not worth emphasizing.

---

397. Editor's note: Chén does not give a source for this quote, so we can only guess as to where the original source came from. However, the earliest text we could find that has the same sentence structure is the *Běn Cǎo Pǐn Huì Jīng Yào* 《本草品匯精要》 (Essential Collection of the Materia Medica) by Liú Wéntài 劉文泰 in 1505.

Dīng Xiāng 丁香
Flower bud of Syzygium aromaticum

氣味辛 、溫，無毒 。主溫脾胃，止霍亂，壅脹，風毒諸種，齒疳䘌，能發諸
香 。《開寶》

The qì and flavor are acrid, warm, and non-toxic. [*Dīng xiāng*] governs warming of the spleen and stomach, stops sudden turmoil, congestion, and distention, [as well as] all kinds of wind toxins, swelling and caries,[398] and is able to emit various fragrances. (*Kāi Bǎo*)

Shǔ Jiāo 蜀椒
Seed capsules of Zanthoxylum bungeanum

氣味辛 、溫，有毒 。主邪氣咳逆，溫中，逐骨節皮膚死肌，寒濕痹痛，下
氣 。久服頭不白，輕身增年 。

The qì and flavor are acrid, warm, and toxic. [*Shǔ jiāo*] governs the evil qì of counterflow cough, warms the center, expels joint and skin numbness, [treats] cold-damp impediment pain, and down-bears the qì. When taken over a long period of time, [the hair on] the head does not turn white, the body is lightened, and the lifespan expanded.

去閉口去目。椒目同巴豆、菖蒲、松脂、黃蠟為挺，納耳中，治聾。

Remove the closed fruits and the seeds.[399] [Shǔ] jiāo seeds are similar to bā dòu, chāng pú, sōng zhí, and huáng là at pulling out. So, when put into the ears, they [can] treat deafness.

---

398. *Nì* 䘌 (gadfly), in this case, it means caries.

399. The closed fruits and seeds are regarded as toxic; only the fruit pericarpium is used. See: Bensky 2004, p. 692.

Chén Xiāng 沉香
Wood of Aquilaria sinensis

氣味辛 、微溫，無毒 。療風水毒腫，去惡風 。《別錄》

The qì and flavor are acrid, slightly warm, and non-toxic. [*Chén xiāng*] treats wind water toxic swelling and removes malign wind. (*Míng Yī Bié Lù*)

Wū Yào 烏藥
Root of Lindera strychnifolia

氣味辛 、溫，無毒 。主中惡，心腹痛，蠱毒，痊忤鬼氣，宿食不消，天行疫瘴，膀胱 、腎間冷氣 。攻衝背膂，婦人血氣，小兒腹中諸蟲 。《拾遺》

The qì and flavor are acrid, warm, and non-toxic. [*Wū yào*] governs malignity stroke, pain in the heart and abdomen, *gǔ* venoms, infixation of disobedient demonic qì, abiding food which is not digested, seasonal epidemic malaria, and cold qì between [the] urinary bladder and kidneys. [It also treats that] which attacks and dashes against the spine, women's [disharmony of] blood and qì, and all kinds of children's worms in the abdomen. (*Běn Cǎo Shí Yí*)

Hǔ Pò 琥珀
Succinum

氣味甘 、平，無毒 。主安五臟，定魂魄，殺精魅邪氣，消淤血，通五淋 。《別錄》

The qì and flavor are sweet, neutral, and non-toxic. [*Hǔ pò*] governs the quieting of the five viscera, settles the ethereal and corporal souls, kills the evil qì of ghosts and demons, disperses static blood, and frees the five stranguries. (*Míng Yī Bié Lù*)

Zhú Rù 竹茹
Shavings of the stripped core Phyllostachys stalks

氣味甘、微寒，無毒。主嘔啘，溫氣，寒熱，吐血，崩中。《別錄》

The qì and flavor are sweet, slightly cold, and non-toxic. [*Zhú rù*] governs vomiting and retching,[400] warm qì, cold and heat, vomiting of blood, and flooding. (*Míng Yī Bié Lù*)

張隱庵曰：此以竹之脈絡，而通人之脈絡也。人身脈絡不和，則吐逆而為熱矣。脈絡不和，則或寒或熱矣。充膚熱肉、澹滲皮毛之血，不循行於脈絡，則上吐血而下崩中矣。竹茹通脈絡，皆能治之。

Zhāng Yǐn'ān said: This uses the veins of the bamboo [in order to] enter the human blood vessels. If a human's blood vessels are not in harmony, this [will] result in vomiting counterflow which turns into heat! If the blood vessels are not in harmony, then there is either cold or heat! The blood replenishes the skin, heats the flesh, and quietly seeps into the skin and hair, but [if the blood] does not move inside the blood vessels in an orderly fashion, then this results in vomiting of blood in the upper and flooding in the lower [body]! *Zhú rù* frees the blood vessels; [therefore it] always is able to treat this.

Zhú Lì 竹瀝
Sap of Phyllostachys

氣味甘、大寒，無毒。療暴中風，風痹，胸中大熱，止煩悶，消渴，勞復。《別錄》

The qì and flavor are sweet, very cold, and non-toxic. [*Zhú lì*] treats fulminant wind strike, wind impediment, and great heat inside the chest; [it] stops anguish, dispersion-thirst, and taxation relapse.[401] (*Míng Yī Bié Lù*)

---

400. *Yuē* 啘 (to retch; to hiccup).

401. *Láo fù* 勞復 (taxation relapse) is relapse due to taxation, when blood and qì have not yet returned to normal in convalescence. See: Wiseman 1998, p. 604.

Qīng Jú Pí 青橘皮
Unripe peel of Citrus reticulata

氣味苦、辛、溫，無毒。主氣滯，下食，破積結及膈氣。《圖經》

The qì and flavor are bitter, acrid, warm, and non-toxic. [*Qīng jú pí*] governs qì stagnation, descends food, and breaks accumulations and binds, as well as diaphragm qì.[402] (*Tú Jīng Běn Cǎo*)

Mù Guā 木瓜
Fruit of Chaenomeles sinensis

氣味酸、溫，無毒。主濕痹腳氣，霍亂大吐下，轉筋不止。《別錄》

The qì and flavor are sour, warm, and non-toxic. [*Mù guā*] governs damp impediment and leg qì,[403] severe vomiting and diarrhea in sudden turmoil, and unstoppable muscle cramps. (*Míng Yī Bié Lù*)

Pí Pá Yè 枇杷葉
Leaf of Eriobotrya japonica

氣味苦、平，無毒。主卒啘不止，下氣。刷去毛。《別錄》

The qì and flavor are bitter, neutral, and non-toxic. [*Pí pá yè*] governs sudden unstoppable retching and downbears qì. *Brush to remove the hair.* (*Míng Yī Bié Lù*)

---

402. *Gé qì* 膈氣 (diaphragm qì) seems to be retching counterflow with food stagnation.

403. *Jiǎo qì* 腳氣 (leg qì) is characterized by numbness, pain, limpness etc. in the calves due to accumulated damp evil and wind toxin. In Western medicine, this is referred to as either beriberi or fungal infection. See: Wiseman 1998, p. 342.

Lóng Yǎn Ròu 龍眼肉
Flesh of the fruit of Euphoria longan

氣味甘、平，無毒。主五臟邪氣，安志，厭食，除蠱毒，去三蟲。久服強魂聰明，輕身不老，通神明。《別錄》

The qì and flavor are sweet, neutral, and non-toxic. [*Lóng yǎn ròu*] governs evil qì of the five viscera, quiets the mind, [governs] aversion to food, eliminates *gǔ* venoms, and expels the three parasites. When taken over a long period of time, it strengthens the ethereal soul, sharpens sight and hearing, lightens the body, prevents aging, and improves the mental abilities. (*Míng Yī Bié Lù*)

Shān Zhā Zǐ 山楂子
Fruit of Crataegus pinnatifida

氣味酸、冷，無毒。煮汁服，止水痢。沐頭洗身，治瘡癢。

The qì and flavor are sour, cold, and non-toxic. When taken cooked as a juice, [*shān zhā zǐ*] stops watery dysentery. When used for bathing and washing the head and body, it cures sores and itching.

Xiǎo Mài 小麥
Seed of Triticum aestivum

氣味甘、寒，無毒。主除客熱，止煩渴咽燥，利小便，養肝氣，止漏血唾血，令女人易孕。《別錄》

The qì and flavor are sweet, cold, and non-toxic. [*Xiǎo mài*] governs the elimination of seasonal heat, stops vexation thirst with dryness of the throat, disinhibits urine, nourishes the liver qì, stops spotting and spitting of blood,[404] and causes women to become easily pregnant. (*Míng Yī Bié Lù*)

---

404. *Tuò xuè* 唾血 (spitting of blood) is either coughing of blood or expulsion of blood with saliva due to the spleen failing to manage the blood. See: Wiseman 1998, p. 551.

Mǎ Liào Dòu 馬料豆
Seed of Glycine soja

氣味甘、平，無毒。生研塗癰腫，煮汁殺鬼毒，止痛。久服令人身重。

The qì and flavor are sweet, neutral, and non-toxic. Raw and finely ground, [*mǎ liào dòu* can be] applied to welling-abscess swelling. Cooked as juice, it [can] kill demonic poison and stop pain. When taken over a long period of time, [*mǎ liào dòu*] makes people's bodies heavy.

Lǜ Dòu 綠豆
Seed of Phaseolus radiatus

氣味甘、寒，無毒。主丹毒，煩熱，風疹，藥石發動熱氣奔豚。生研絞汁服，亦煮食，消腫下氣，壓熱。解砒石[405]之毒，用[之勿]去皮，令人小壅。《開寶》

The qì and flavor are sweet, cold, and non-toxic. [*Lǜ dòu*] governs cinnabar toxin,[406] wind measles, and running piglet [caused by erroneously applied] herbs and minerals that effuse stirring heat qì. [This can be] taken fresh and finely ground to wring [out] the juice, [or] also cooked as food. [*Lǜ dòu*] disperses swelling, downbears the qì, and suppresses heat. It resolves arsenic toxin. When used [without][407] removing the skin, it causes slight obstruction. (*Kāi Bǎo*)

Biǎn Dòu 扁豆
Seed of Dolichos lablab

氣味甘、微溫，無毒。主和中下氣。《別錄》

The qì and flavor are sweet, slightly warm, and non-toxic. [*Biǎn dòu*] governs harmonizing the center and downbears qì. (*Míng Yī Bié Lù*)

---

405. Other versions of the text have *fán shí* 礬石 (alum).

406. *Dān dú* 丹毒 (cinnabar toxin) is localized sudden redness of the skin. See: ibid: p. 62

407. The text versions also differ here.

Gǔ Yá 穀芽
Sprouted fruit of Setaria italica[408]

氣味苦、溫，無毒。主寒中，下氣，除熱。《別錄》

The qì and flavor are bitter, warm, and non-toxic. [*Gǔ yá*] governs cold strike, downbears qì, and eliminates heat. (*Míng Yī Bié Lù*)

陳修園曰：凡物逢春萌芽而漸生長，今取乾穀透發其芽，更能達木氣以制化脾土，故能消導米穀積滯。推之麥芽、黍芽、大豆黃卷，性皆相近。而麥春長夏成，尤得木火之氣，凡怫鬱致成膨脹等症，用之最妙。人但知其消穀，不知其疏肝，是猶稱驥以力也。

Chén Xiūyuán said: Generally, plants sprout every spring and gradually grow. When the dry grains are taken and their sprouts are set off, they are increasingly able to reach the wood qì for the control and transformation of spleen earth. Therefore, [*gǔ yá*] is able to dissipate and dredge food accumulation and stagnation. Sprouted *mài yá*,[409] *shǔ yá*,[410] and *dà dòu huáng juàn*[411] are all of a similar nature. However, *mài* grows in spring and ripens in summer, so it especially receives the qì of wood and fire. So generally, it is most excellent to use [*mài*] against swelling and distention caused by worry and depression and other symptoms of this kind. People only know about [*mài's* ability of] dissipating food, but they do not know that it courses the liver, [and therefore] it is also referred to as [having] "the power of a thoroughbred horse."

Dòu Chǐ 豆豉
Preparation of Glycine max

氣味苦、寒，無毒。主傷寒頭痛寒熱，瘴氣惡毒，煩燥滿悶，虛勞喘吸，兩腳疼冷。《別錄》

The qì and flavor are bitter, cold, and non-toxic. [*Dòu chǐ*] governs cold damage headache with cold or heat, miasmic toxin, vexation, agitation, fullness and melancholy, vacuity taxation with gasping, and cold pain in the legs. (*Míng Yī Bié Lù*)

---

408. This plant is also listed in some sources under the botanical name Oryza sativa or rice sprout.

409. Barley or wheat sprouts.

410. Millet sprouts.

411. Sprouted soybean.

Yí Táng 飴糖
Malt sugar

氣味甘、大溫，無毒。主補虛乏，止渴，去血。《別錄》

The qì and flavor are sweet, very warm, and non-toxic. [*Yí táng*] governs supplementing vacuity and lack [of any kind], stops thirst, and removes [malign or static] blood. (*Míng Yī Bié Lù*)

Bò Hé 薄荷
Leaves of Mentha arvensis

氣味辛、溫，無毒。主賊風傷寒，發汗，惡氣心腹脹滿，霍亂，宿食不消，下氣。煮汁服，亦堪生食。《唐本草》

The qì and flavor are acrid, warm, and non-toxic. [*Bò he*] governs cold damage due to bandit wind, the promotion of sweat, distention and fullness in the heart and abdomen due to malign qì, sudden turmoil, and undigested abiding food; [it also] downbears qì. *Taken cooked as a juice, [but can] also be eaten raw.* (*Táng Běn Cǎo*)

Xiāng Rú 香薷
Leaves of Elsholtzia ciliata

氣味辛、微溫，無毒。主霍亂腹痛吐下，散水腫。《別錄》

The qì and flavor are acrid, slightly warm, and non-toxic. [*Xiāng rú*] governs abdominal pain as well as vomiting and diarrhea in sudden turmoil; [it also] disperses water swelling. (*Míng Yī Bié Lù*)

Bái Jiè Zǐ 白芥子
Seed of Sinapis alba

氣味辛、溫，無毒。發汗，主胸膈痰冷，上氣，面目黃赤。醋研，敷射工毒。《別錄》

The qì and flavor are acrid, warm, and non-toxic. [*Bái jiè zǐ*] promotes sweating and governs phlegm and coldness in the chest and diaphragm, qì ascent, and yellowing as well as redness of the face and eyes. *Grind with vinegar and apply on "archer"*[412] *venom.* (*Míng Yī Bié Lù*)

Wǔ Líng Zhī 五靈脂
Feces of Trogopterus xanthipes

氣味甘、溫，無毒。主療心腹冷氣，小兒五疳，辟疫，治腸風，通利血脈，女子月閉。酒研。

The qì and flavor are sweet, warm, and non-toxic. [*Wǔ líng zhī*] governs the treatment of cold qì of the heart and abdomen, and the five *gān*[413] diseases in children, warding off of epidemics, treating intestinal wind, unblocking the blood vessels, and [treating] women's menstrual obstructions. *Grind with alcohol.*

---

412. *Shè gōng* 射工 (archer) is either a legendary insect or an insect found in mountain streams in Jiàngnán. It is said to "shoot" its venom at people, which can be deadly. The term can also hint at venomous insects in general.

413. *Wǔ gān* 五疳 (the five *gān* diseases) are a childhood disease characterized by dry hair, heat effusion, abdominal distention, emaciation, yellow face, and loss of vitality. It affects the five viscera and is usually caused by malnutrition and or parasites. See: Wiseman 1998, p. 236.

Hǔ Gǔ 虎骨
Bone of Panthera tigris[414]

氣味辛、微熱，無毒。主邪惡，殺鬼疰毒，止驚悸，治惡瘡、鼠瘻。頭骨尤良。《別錄》

The qì and flavor are acrid, slightly hot, and non-toxic. [*Hǔ gǔ*] governs evil malignity, kills demonic infixation toxin, stops fright palpitations, and cures malign sores and mouse fistulae. *The skull is especially good.* (*Míng Yī Bié Lù*)

Xiǎo Huí Xiāng 小茴香
Fruit of Foeniculum vulgare

氣味辛、溫，無毒。主小兒氣脹，霍亂嘔逆，腹冷，不下食，兩筋[415]痞滿。《拾遺》

The qì and flavor are acrid, warm, and non-toxic. [*Xiǎo huí xiāng*] governs children's qì distention,[416] sudden turmoil with retching counterflow, abdominal coldness, inability to get food down, glomus, and fullness in both ribsides. (*Běn Cǎo Shí Yí*)

Tǔ Fú Líng 土茯苓
Rhizome of Smilax glabra

氣味甘、淡、平，無毒。主治食之當穀不飢，調中止泄，健行不睡。藏器

The qì and flavor are sweet, bland, neutral, and non-toxic. The indications for [*tǔ fú líng*] are: [when used] as a food, it prevents hunger, harmonizes the center, stops dysentery, and [governs the] ability to walk around without sleeping.[417] (*Cáng Qì*)

---

414. Any part of the tiger is listed under Appendix 1 of CITES.

415. This is likely to be a printing error. Instead of *jīn* 筋 (tendon) it should be written *xié* 脅 (ribside).

416. *Qì zhàng* 氣脹 (qì distention) is either distention from congestion of the qì pathways caused by affect-mind binding depression (liver) with abdominal distention and emaciation of the limbs, or abdominal distention with fullness that is empty (drum distention). See: Wiseman 1998, p. 479.

417. *Jiàn xíng bù shuì* 健行不睡 can also be translated as: "prevents sleepiness while hiking" or "it strengthens motion without sleepiness."

治拘攣骨痛，惡瘡癰腫，解汞銀朱毒。時珍

[*Tǔ fú líng*] cures hypertonicity and pain in the bones, malign sores, [and] welling-abscess swelling; [it also] resolves mercury and vermillion toxins. ([Lǐ] Shízhēn)

Bì Xiè 萆薢
Rhizome of Dioscorea hypoglauca

氣味苦、平，無毒。主腰脊痛，強骨節，風寒濕周痹，惡瘡不瘳，熱氣。《本經》

The qì and flavor are bitter, neutral, and non-toxic. [*Bì xiè*] governs pain and tension in the lumbar spine, strengthens the bones and joints, [and treats] generalized wind-cold-damp impediment, malign sores that do not recover, and heat qì. (*Běn Jīng*)[418]

傷中，恚怒，陰痿，失溺，老人五緩，關節老血。《別錄》

[*Bì xiè* governs] damage to the center, rage and anger, impotence, urinary incontinence, the five chronic conditions in elderly people,[419] and old blood in the joints. (*Míng Yī Bié Lù*)

Bīng Láng 檳榔
Fruit of Areca catechu

氣味苦、辛、澀、溫，無毒。主消穀逐水，除痰癖，殺三蟲，伏尸，療寸白。《別錄》

The qì and flavor are bitter, acrid, astringent, warm, and non-toxic. [*Bīng lang*] governs dispersing food and expelling water, eliminates phlegm aggregation,[420] kills the three parasites, [governs] "hid-

---

418. Actually, this herb should belong to the herbs of middle grade in the *Shén Nóng Běn Cǎo Jīng*.

419. This could be the five stranguries. It could also be chronic diseases in any of the five phases/viscera.

420. *Tán pǐ* 痰癖 (phlegm aggregation) is enduring water-rheum transforming into phlegm, which flows into the ribsides, causing periodic pain. See: Wiseman 1998, p. 433.

den corpse"[421] and treats inch white [worms].[422] (*Míng Yī Bié Lù*)

Qiān Niú Zǐ 牽牛子
Seed of Pharbitis nil

氣味苦、寒，有毒。主下氣，療腳滿，水脹，除風毒，利小便。《別錄》

The qì and flavor are bitter, cold, and toxic. [*Qiān niú zǐ*] governs the downbearing of qì, treats fullness in the legs [and] water distention, eliminates wind toxin, and disinhibits urine. (*Míng Yī Bié Lù*)

陳修園曰：大毒大破之藥，不堪以療內病。惟楊梅瘡，或毒發周身，或結於一處，甚則陰器剝，鼻柱壞，囟潰不合，其病多從陰器而入，亦必使之從陰器而出也。法用牽牛研取頭末，以土茯苓自然汁泛丸，又以燒褌散為衣。每服一錢，生槐蕊四錢，以土茯苓湯送下，一日三服。服半月效。

Chén Xiūyuán said: [*Qiān niú zǐ*] is a very toxic and destructive medicinal and may not be used for treating internal diseases. [It can] only [be used internally against] red bayberry sores,[423] or when the toxins erupt on the whole body, or when [the toxins] are bound in one location. In severe cases, then the genitals peel off, the stem of the nose rots, and the fontanels burst apart. This disease often enters via the genitals, so it also has to be enabled to exit via the genitals. The method of employment is: grind *qiān niú* [*zǐ*] and take the top of the powder, [mix it with] the natural juice of *tǔ fú líng* and make pills [with honey and water]. Further coat [the pills] with *Shāo Kūn Sǎn* (Burnt Trousers Powder).[424] Take one *qián* as one dosage with four *qián* of fresh *huái ruǐ*[425] and swallow it together with *Tǔ Fú Líng Tāng*.[426] Take three doses a day. After half a month, there will be an effect.

---

421. See Footnote 42 above.

422. *Cùn bái chóng* 寸白蟲 (inch white worms) is the spleen worm disease, which is the same as tapeworm infestation. See: Wiseman 1998, p. 298.

423. This is syphilis.

424. This is using the ashes of a burnt pair of male trousers for female patients and female burnt trousers for a male patient.

425. Stamen or pistil of Sophora japonica.

426. *Smilax Decoction* or *Smooth Greenbrier Decoction*.

Rěn Dōng 忍冬
Lonicera japonica

氣味甘、溫，無毒。主寒熱，身腫。久服輕身，長年益壽。《別錄》

The qì and flavor are sweet, warm, and non-toxic. [*Rěn dōng*] governs cold and heat, and swelling of the body. When taken over a long period of time, it lightens the body, prolongs life, and boosts longevity. (*Míng Yī Bié Lù*)

陳修園曰：氣溫得春氣而入肝，味甘得土味而入胃。何以知入胃不入脾？以此物質輕味薄，偏走陽分，胃為陽土也。其主寒熱者，忍冬延蔓善走，花開黃白二色，黃入營分，白入衛分，營衛調而寒熱之病愈矣。

Chén Xiūyuán said: The qì of [*rěn dōng*] is warm, obtains the qì of spring, and enters the liver. The flavor is sweet, [which] obtains the earth flavor, and enters the stomach. How [can one] know that [*rěn dōng*] enters the stomach and not the spleen? Because it is a light substance with a thin flavor; thus, [*rěn dōng*] is inclined to go into the yáng aspect. The stomach is the yáng aspect of the earth. It governs cold and heat, because the tendrils of *rěn dōng* are good at entering [the liver and stomach]. It blossoms in two colors, yellow and white. Yellow enters the construction aspect and white enters the defense aspect. When construction and defense are harmonized, diseases of cold and heat are cured!

其主身腫者，以風木之氣傷於中土，內則病脹，外則病腫，昔人統名為蠱，取卦象山風之義。忍冬甘入胃，胃為艮土，艮為山。溫入肝，肝為風木，巽為風。內能使土木合德，外能使營衛和諧，所以善治之也。

[*Rěn dōng*] governs swelling of the body: when the qì of wind and wood damages the center-earth, this results in the internal disease of distention and the external disease of swelling. Former people gave [the qì of wind and wood that damages the center-earth] the collective name *gǔ* venom. The significance [here] is that it takes the shape of the mountain and wind trigrams.[427] The sweetness of *rěn dōng* enters the stomach. And the stomach is *gèn* earth, *gèn* is mountain. The warmth of [*rěn dōng*] enters the liver. And the liver is wind and wood, *xùn is wind*. Internally, [*rěn dōng*] can enable the earth and wood to be in united virtue. Externally, it can enable construction and defense to be in peaceful harmony.[428] Therefore, [*rěn dōng*] is good at curing those [diseases].

---

427. The trigram for *shān* 山 (mountain) is called *gèn* 艮 and looks like this ☶. The trigram for *fēng* 風 (wind) is called *xùn* 巽 and looks like this ☴.

428. *Hé dé* 合德 (united virtue) is attributed to *gèn* 艮 and *hé xié* 和諧 (peaceful harmony) is attributed to *xùn* 巽. Chén Xiūyuán parallels the eight trigrams with the five elements and their diseases here, in order to give his statements more authority.

神農本草經讀・卷附

久服長年益壽者，夸其安內調外之功也 。至於瘡毒，腫毒等證，時醫重其功，而《別錄》反未言及者，以外科諸效，特疏風祛濕，調和營衛之餘事耳 。

Saying that it prolongs life and boosts longevity when taken over a long period of time is praising [rěn dōng's] merit of quieting the interior and harmonizing the exterior. With regards to sore toxins, swelling toxins and other patterns of this kind, contemporary physicians emphasize [rěn dōng's] effect. However, the *Míng Yī Bié Lù* on the contrary does not speak extensively of this, because all the effects of external medicinals, especially clearing wind and expelling damp, are [already] the surplus of harmonizing construction and defense, and that is all!

Mǎ Dōu Líng 馬兜鈴
Fruit of Aristolochia debilis[429]

氣味苦 、寒，無毒 。主肺熱咳嗽，痰結喘促，血痔瘻瘡 。《開寶 》

The qì and flavor are bitter, cold, and non-toxic. [*Mǎ dōu líng*] governs heat in the lungs with cough, hasty panting induced by bound phlegm, bleeding hemorrhoids, and fistulae. (*Kāi Bǎo*)

陳修園曰：氣寒得水氣入腎，味苦得火味入心，雖云無毒，而偏寒之性，多服必令吐利不止也 。《內經 》云：肺喜溫而「 惡寒 」。若《開寶 》所云「 肺熱咳嗽 」，為絕少之症，且所主咳嗽痰結喘促之症，與血痔瘻瘡外症，同一施治，其為涼瀉攻堅之性無疑 。今人惑於錢乙補肺阿膠散一方，取用以治虛嗽，百服百死 。

Chén Xiūyuán said: The qì [of *mǎ dōu líng*] is cold, obtains the qì of water, and enters the kidneys. [*Mǎ dōu líng's*] flavor is bitter, obtains the fire flavor, [and] enters the heart. Although it is said that, [*mǎ dōu líng*] is non-toxic, it has an extremely cold nature. When taken in excess, [*mǎ dōu líng*] definitely causes unstoppable vomiting and diarrhea. The *Nèi Jīng* said: The lungs like warmth and "have an aversion to cold." If the *Kāi Bǎo* speaks of "lung heat cough," this is an extremely rare pattern. Further, that which governs the [internal] pattern of cough with bound phlegm and hasty panting, as well as the external pattern of bleeding hemorrhoids and fistulae, is the application of the identical cure. [This] is no doubt [because of *mǎ dōu líng's*] nature of draining with coolness and attacking with hardness. The people of today confuse [*mǎ dōu líng*] with Qián Yǐ's[430] formula of *Bǔ Fèi Ē Jiāo Sǎn*,[431] and use it for treating vacuity cough. Of one hundred takings, there are one hundred deaths.

---

429. Today, this substance is obsolete because of its unacceptable toxicity. See: Bensky 2004, p. 1044.

430. Qián Yǐ 錢乙 (1032-1113) was a famous pediatrician from Shāndōng.

431. *Bǔ Fèi Ē Jiāo Sǎn* 補肺阿膠散 (Lung Supplementing Ass Hide Glue Powder).

Gōu Téng 鈎藤
Twigs of Uncaria rhynchophulla

氣味微寒，無毒。主小兒寒熱，十二驚癇。《別錄》

The qì and flavor are slightly cold and non-toxic. [*Gōu téng*] governs children's cold and heat and the twelve kinds of fright epilepsy. (*Míng Yī Bié Lù*)

Rén Rǔ 人乳
Human breast milk

氣味甘、鹹，平，無毒。主補五臟，令人肥白悅澤。《別錄》

The qì and flavor are sweet, salty, neutral, and non-toxic. [*Rén rǔ*] governs supplementing the five viscera and makes people fat, white, happy, and lustrous. (*Míng Yī Bié Lù*)

Xiǎo Biàn 小便
Human urine

氣味鹹、寒，無毒。主療寒熱，頭痛，溫氣。*童男者尤良*。《別錄》

The qì and flavor are salty, cold, and non-toxic. [*Xiǎo biàn*] governs the treatment of cold and heat, headaches, and warm [pathogenic] qì. *Boy's urine is especially good.* (*Míng Yī Bié Lù*)

按：虻蟲、水蛭及芫花、大戟、甘遂等不常用之藥，集隘不能具載。柯韻伯抵當湯、十棗湯方論極妙，宜熟讀之。

Note: the collected works on the rarely used drugs *méng chóng*,[432] *shuǐ zhì*,[433] *yuán huā*,[434] *dà jǐ*,[435]

---

432. Horsefly.

433. Leech.

434. Genkwa flower.

435. Knoxia root.

and *gān suí*[436] etc. are confined and cannot be recorded in detail. Kē Yùnbó's[437] formula theories on *Dǐ Dàng Tāng*[438] and *Shí Zǎo Tāng*[439] [both from the *Shāng Hán Lùn*] are extremely excellent and worth [further] careful study.

---

436. Kan-sui root.

437. Kē Yùnbó 柯韻伯 was a physician from Zhèjiāng. He lived at the beginning of the Qīng dynasty and was a specialist in the *Shāng Hán Lùn* 《傷寒論》 (Discussion on Cold Damage). See Footnote 19 of the preface.

438. *Dead-On Decoction.*

439. *Ten Jujubes Decoction.*

English Titles

Bensky, Dan et al.: *Chinese Herbal Medicine. Materia Medica, 3rd Edition.* Seattle: Eastland Press, 2004.

Loewe, Michael (Ed.): *Early Chinese Texts: A Bibliographical Guide.* Berkeley: Institute of East Asian Studies, 1993.

Mair, Victor H (Ed.): *The Columbia Anthology of Traditional Chinese Literature.* Columbia University Press 1994.

Mitchell, Craig et al: *Shāng Hán Lùn* 《傷寒論》(On Cold Damage). Brookline: Paradigm Publications, 1999.

Pothmann, Raymund (Ed.): *33 Fallbeispiele zur Akupunktur aus der VR China. (Thirty-three actupuncture cases from the People's Republic of China).* Stuttgart, 1996.

Twitchett, Denis and Fairbank, John (Ed.): *The Cambridge History of China,* Volume 3. Cambridge: Cambridge University Press, 1979.

Wiseman, Nigel and Ye, Feng. *A Practical Dictionary of Chinese Medicine.* Brookline: Paradigm Publications, 1998.

Chinese Titles

Zhōng Guǒ Yī Rén Wù Cí Diǎn Zhǔ Biān Lǐ Jīng Wěi, Shànghǎi Cí Shū Chū Bǎn Shè. 《中國醫人物詞典》主編李經緯上海辞書出版社 Lǐ Jīng Wěi (Ed.) (Dictionary of Chinese Medical Physicians) Shanghai Dictionary Publishing House, 1985.

Zhōng Guo Yī Xuě Dà Cí Diǎn 《中國醫學大辭典》(Great Dictionary of Chinese Medicine), 1988.

Historical References

Bái Xiāng Shān Shī Jù	《白香山詩句》	Verse of the "White Fragrant Mountain"
Bèi Jí Qiān Jīn Yào Fāng	《備急千金要方》	Essential Prescriptions Worth a Thousand in Gold For Every Emergency
Běn Cǎo Bèi Yào	《本草備要》	Complete Essentials of Materia Medica
Běn Cǎo Chóng Yuán	《本草崇原》	Honored Originals of the Materia Medica
Běn Cǎo Gāng Mù	《本草綱目》	Compendium of the Materia Medica

Běn Cǎo Jīng Jiě	《本草經解》	Explaining the Materia Medica Classic
Běn Cǎo Shí Yí	《本草拾遺》	Picking up Lost Property of the Materia Medica
Běn Cǎo Yǎn Yì Bǔ Yí	《本草衍義補遺》	Addendum to the Amplified Meanings of the Materia Medica
Cháo Shì Zhū Bìng Yuán Hòu Zǒng Lùn	《巢氏諸病源候總論》	Treatise on the Origins and Symptoms of Disease by Master Cháo
Chūn Qiū Fán Lù	《春秋繁露》	Spring and Autumn Annals
Chū Qiū Zuǒ Zhuàn	《春秋左傳》	Zuǒ's Commentary to the Spring and Autumn Annals
Dà Míng Běn Cǎo	《大明本草》	Dà Míng's Materia Medica
Dà Xué	《大學》	The Great Learning
Huáng Dì Nèi Jīng Sù Wèn	《黃帝內經素問》	Inner Canon of the Yellow Emperor, Plain Questions
Jīn Gùi Yào Lüè Lùn Zhù	《金匱要略論注》	Commentary on the Discussion of the Formulas of the Golden Cabinet
Kāi Bǎo Chóng Dìng Běn Cǎo	《開寶重定本草》	Kāi Bǎo Revised Materia Medica
Léi Gōng Pào Zhì Lùn	《雷公炮炙論》	Master Léi's Discussion on Processing of Medicinals
Lèi Jīng	《類經》	Categorized Classic
Lín Zhèng Zhǐ Nán Yī Àn	《臨證指南醫案》	Guide to Clinical Practice in Cases
Lǚ Shān Táng Lèi Biàn	《侶山堂類辨》	The Differentiation of Categories from the Lǚ Shān Hall
Lún Yǔ	《論語》	The Analects
Mèng Zǐ	《孟子》	Mencius
Míng Yī Bié Lù	《名醫別錄》	Supplementary Records of Famous Physicians
Nán Jīng	《難經》	Classic of Difficult Issues
	Also known as *Huáng Dì Bā Shí Yī Nán Jīng* 《黃帝八十一難經》 (Huáng Dǐ's Classic on Eighty One Difficult Issues)	
Pào Zhì Dà Fǎ, Mǐ Gǔ Bù	《炮炙大法·米穀部》	Great Methods for Processing Medicines, Section on Rice and Grains
Pí Wèi Lùn	《脾胃論》	Treatise on the Spleen and Stomach
Rì Huà Zǐ Zhū Jiā Běn Cǎo	《日華子諸家本草》	Materia Medica of Various Schools by Rì Huàzǐ
Shāng Hán Bái Wèn	《傷寒百問》	One Hundred Questions on Cold Damage
Shāng Hán Lùn	《傷寒論》	Discussion on Cold Damage

213

Shén Nóng Běn Cǎo Jīng	《神農本草經》	Divine Farmer's Classic of Materia Medica
Shí Xìng Běn Cǎo	《食性本草》	Materia Medica on the Nature of Food
Tāng Yè Běn Cǎo	《湯液本草》	Materia Medica of Decoctions
Tú Jīng Běn Cǎo	《圖經本草》	Illustrated Materia Medica
Wài Tái Mì Yào	《外臺秘要》	Essential Secrets from Outside the Metropolis
Xīn Xiū Běn Cǎo	《新修本草》	Newly Revised Materia Medica
Yào Xìng Běn Cǎo	《藥性本草》	Materia Medica on the Nature of Medicines
Yào Xìng Lùn	《藥性論》	Treatise on the Nature of Medicines
Yī Mén Fǎ Lǜ	《醫門法律》	Regulations of Medicine
Yì Jīng	《易經》	Book of Changes
Zhēn Zhū Náng Yào Xìng Fù	《珍珠囊藥性賦》	Poetic Essay on the Nature of Medicinals of the Bag of Pearls
Zhōu Yì Hán Shū Yuē Cún	《周易函書約存》	Stored Letters on the Book of Changes

Chén's Collected Works (revisions marked as R)

Huó Rén Bǎi Wèn	《活人百問》	One Hundred Questions on How to Save Lives	R
Jīn Guì Dú	《金匱讀》	Reading the Formulas from the Golden Cabinet	
Jīn Guì Yào Lüè Qiǎn Zhù	《金匱要略淺注》	Superficial Commentary on the Formulas from the Golden Cabinet	
Jǐng Yuè Xīn Fāng Biān	《景岳新方砭》	A Critique of Jǐngyuè's New Prescriptions	
Kē Zhù Shāng Hán Lùn	《柯注傷寒論》	Kē Qín's Commentary to the Discussion on Cold Damage	R
Shāng Hán Lùn Dú	《傷寒論讀》	Reading the Discussion on Cold Damage	
Shāng Hán Lùn Qiǎn Zhù	《傷寒論淺注》	Shallow Commentary to the Discussion on Cold Damage	
Shāng Hán Yī Jué Chuàn Jiě	《傷寒醫訣串解》	The Medical Method of the Discussion on Cold Damage Collected and Explained	
Shāng Hán Yī Yuē Lù	《傷寒醫約錄》	Record on the Medical Outlines of the [Discussion on] Cold Damage	
Shāng Hán Zhēn Fāng Gē Kuò	《傷寒真方歌括》	True Prescriptions from the Discussion on Cold Damage with Poems	
Yī Jué	《醫訣》	Methods of Medicine	

| *Yī Xué Cóng Zhòng Lù* | 《 醫學從眾錄 》 | A Record of Medicine by Others | |
| *Yī Yī Ǒu Lù* | 《 醫醫偶錄 》 | Medical Records in Pairs | |

神
農
本
草
經
讀

Internet Resources

Lǐ Jiāngjūn 李將軍	See: http://vr.theatre.ntu.edu.tw/fineart/painter-ch/lisixun/lisixun.htm
Máo Shī 《 毛詩 》 (Book of Odes by the Two Máo)	See http://www.ct.taipei.gov.tw/zh-tw/C/Sage/Confucian/2/2/67.htm
Musk deer	See: http://www.cites.org/gallery/species/mammal/mammals.html
Rì Huàzǐ 日華子	See http://yibian.hopto.org/book/?bno=219
Shāng Hán Bái Wèn 《 傷寒百問 》	See http://so.med.wanfangdata.com.cn/ViewHTML/PeriodicalPaper_zhyszz201103010.aspx
Shī Jīng 《 詩經 》 (Book of Odes)	See http://ctext.org/book-of-poetry/odes-of-zhou-and-the-south
Shí zhī 石脂	See http://webmineral.com/data/Halloysite.shtml
Tiger	See: http://cites.org/eng/res/all/12/E12-05R15.pdf
Yè Tiānshì 葉天士	See http://www.chinesemedicinedoc.com/misc-chinese-medicine-articles/ye-tian-shi-the-eight-extraordinary-channels/
Zhāng Jièbīn 張介賓	See http://ejournal.nricm.edu.tw/nricm2/pages/show.php?qry_dtnbr=23&qry_dsnbr=498
Zhāng Jiégǔ 張潔古	See http://ejournal.nricm.edu.tw/nricm2/pages/show.php?qry_dtnbr=23&qry_dsnbr=489
Zhuāng Zǐ 莊子	See http://ctext.org/zhuangzi/enjoyment-in-untroubled-ease

Mentioned People

Bái Jūyì 白居易 (772-846)	A *Táng* poet, who lived on Xiāng Shān 香山, a mountain in Luòyáng.
Bào Pùzǐ 抱朴子 (284-363 or 283-343)	Also known as Gě Hóng 葛洪. Bào was a famous physician, Daoist, alchemist, natural scientist, and chemist from Jiāngsū.
Chén Cángqì 陳藏器	Compiler of the *Běn Cǎo Shí Yí* 《 本草拾遺 》 (Picking up Lost Property of the Materia Medica) in 739.
Chén Chéng 陳承 (12th century)	A physician from Sìchuān, whose expertise was in using cooling herbs.

Chén Shìliáng 陳士良 (tenth century)	Author of the *Shí Xìng Běn Cǎo* 《 食性本草 》 (Materia Medica on the Nature of Food) is a physician of the Later *Táng* from the city of Kāifēng.
Chén Yuánbào 陳元豹	Chén Xiūyuán's 陳修園 eldest son.
Chén Yuánxī 陳元犀	Chén Xiūyuán's 陳修園 second son.
Huà Tuó 華佗 (~145-208)	Also known as Huà Yuánhuà 華元化, the famous physician who first applied surgical techniques.
Kē Qín 柯琴	A *Qīng* physician, named Yùn Bó 韵伯, who was born in Zhèjiāng. His life dates are unknown, but from a preface written by his own hand to his commentary, it is known, that his commentary the *Shāng Hán Lùn Zhù* 《 傷寒論注 》 (Commentary to The Discussion on Cold Damage) was written in 1669.
Léi Gōng 雷公	The legendary physician of Chinese antiquity.
Léi Xiào 雷斅 (5th century)	A scholar of medicinals who lived during the time of the *Sòng* of the Southern dynasties (420-479). Author of the three volume *Léi Gōng Páo Zhì Lùn* 《 雷公炮制論 》 (Master Léi's Discussion on Processing of Medicinals), in which he gave a written account of the methods of blast-frying, honey-frying, stir-frying, calcining, drying in the sun, and distilling for seventy different kinds of medicinals.
Lǐ Gǎo 李杲 (1180-1251)	Also known as Lǐ Dōngyuán 李東垣. Lǐ was the author of the *Pí Wèi Lùn* 《 脾胃論 》 (Treatise on the Spleen and Stomach).
Lǐ Jiāngjūn 李將軍	Whose real name is Lǐ Sīxùn 李思訓 (651-716), was a landscape artist of the *Táng*, famous for his elaborated "Green landscapes," which were partially gilded.
Lǐ Shìcái 李士材 (1588-1655)	Also known as Lǐ Zhōngzǐ 李中梓 is a physician from Jiāngsū.
Lǐ Shízhēn 李時珍 (1518-1593)	Also known as Lǐ Bīnhú 李瀕湖, is the author of the *Běn Cǎo Gāng Mù* 《 本草綱目 》 (Compendium of the Materia Medica) (1578).
Lú Biǎn 盧扁 (407-310 B.C.)	Also known as the ancient physician Biǎn Què 扁鹊, because he was from the city of Lú. He is said to have invented pulse diagnosis.
Mèngzǐ 孟子 (372~289 B.C.)	The great philosopher.
Miào Xīyōng 缪希雍 (1546—1627)	Author of the *Pào Zhì Dà Fǎ·Mǐ Gǔ Bù* 《 炮炙大法·米穀部 》 (Great Methods for Processing Medicines·Section on Rice and Grains), as well as a physician from Jiāngsū.
Qián Yǐ 錢乙 (1032-1113)	A famous pediatrician from Shāndōng.

神農本草經讀

Rì Huàzǐ 日華子	Rì is most likely the same person as Dà Míng 大明 (of the tenth century). There is a book with the title *Rì Huàzǐ Zhū Jiā Běn Cǎo* 《日華子諸家本草》 (Materia Medica of Various Schools by Rì Huàzǐ), which was compiled in the state of *Wú* 吳 during the Five Dynasties and Ten States period (907-979).
Sū Jìng 蘇敬 (599-674)	Compiler of the *Xīn Xiū Běn Cǎo* 《新修本草》 (Newly Revised Materia Medica).
Sū Sòng 蘇頌 (1020-1101)	Compiler of the *Tú Jīng Běn Cǎo* 《圖經本草》 (Illustrated Materia Medica) in 1061.
Sūn Sīmiǎo 孫思邈 (581-682)	Author of the *Bèi Jí Qiān Jīn Yào Fāng* 《備急千金要方》 (Essential Prescriptions Worth a Thousand in Gold For Every Emergency).
Táo Hóngjǐng 陶弘景 (456~536)	A famous Daoist, and an outstanding physician. He called himself Huà Yáng Yǐnjū 華陽隐居 the hermit of Huà Yáng. He is also referred to as Táo Yǐnjū 陶隱居.
Wáng Hàogǔ 王好古 (1200-1264)	A famous representative of the spleen-fortifying school and successor of Lǐ Gǎo 李杲 (1180-1251).
Wáng Rèn'ān 汪訒庵 (1615-1699)	Also known as Wáng Áng 汪昂 of Ānhuī. Wáng was a physician who came from a poor family and had more than thirty years of textual study and clinical practice. He wrote the *Běn Cǎo Bèi Yào* 《本草備要》 (Complete Essentials of Materia Medica).
Wáng Tāo 王濤 (670-755)	Author of the *Wài Tái Mì Yào* 《外臺秘要》 (Essential Secrets from Outside the Metropolis).
Xú Lingtāi 徐靈胎 (1693-1771)	He was from Jiāngsū.
Xú Bīn 徐彬	A *Qīng* dynasty physician who compiled the *Jīn Gùi Yào Lüè Lùn Zhù* 《金匱要略論注》 (Commentary on the Discussion of the Formulas of the Golden Cabinet) in 1671.
Xú Zhīcái 徐之才 (492~572 to 505~572)	A physician who learned his skills via oral tradition from his father and grandfather.
Xú Zhōngkě 徐忠可 (seventeenth century)	Also known as Xú Bīn 徐彬. Xú was a physician who wrote an important commentary to the *Jīn Gùi Yào Lüè* 《金匱要略》 (Essential Prescriptions of the Golden Cabinet) with the title *Jīn Gùi Yào Lüè Lùn Zhù* 《金匱要略論注》 (Treatise on the Essential Prescriptions of the Golden Cabinet) published in 1671.
Xuē Lìzhāi 薛立齋 (1487~1559)	Also named Xuē Jǐ 薛己. Xuē was a physician from Jiāngsū.

Yè Tiānshì 葉天士 (1666-1745)	Also known as Yè Guì 葉桂 of Jiāngsū. Yè was influential in the development of warm disease theory. He is the author of the *Wēn Rè Lùn* 《 溫熱論 》 (Discussion on Warm Disease) and his disciples made the *Lín Zhèng Zhǐ Nán Yī Àn* 《 臨證指南醫案 》 (Guide to Clinical Practice in Cases) out of his notes.
Yú Tiānmín 虞天民 (1438-1517)	Also known as Yú Tuán 虞摶, was a physician from Zhèjiāng.
Yù Jiāyán 喻嘉言 (1585-1664)	Also known as the physician Yù Chāng 喻昌 from Jiāngxī.
Zhāng Chángshā 張長沙	This is another name for Zhāng Zhòngjǐng 張仲景.
Zhāng Jièbīn 張介賓 (1563-1640)	Also known as Zhāng Jǐngyuè 張景岳, author of the *Xīn Fāng Bā Zhèn* 《 新方八陣 》 (New Prescriptions Divided into the Eight Classifications), the *Jǐng Yuè Quán Shū* 《 景岳全書 》 (Collected Treatise's of Zhāng Jǐngyuè), and the *Lèi Jīng* 《 類經 》 (Classic of Categories).
Zhāng Jiégǔ 張潔古 (1151-1234)	Also known as Zhāng Yuánsù 張元素. Zhāng was a scholar physician of the Western *Yuán* dynasty.
Zhāng Yǐn'ān 張隱庵 (1644-1722)	Also known as Zhāng Zhìcōng 張志聰 was a scholar physician of Zhèjiāng, who specialized in six levels theory.
Zhāng Zǐhé 張子和 (1151-1231 or 1156-1228)	Originator of the *gōng xià pài* 攻下派 (purgative school).
Zhēn Quán 甄權 (541-643)	Author of the *Yào Xìng Běn Cǎo* 《 藥性本草 》 (Materia Medica on the Nature of Medicines).
Zhū Dānxī 朱丹溪 (1281-1358)	Also named Zhū Zhènhēng 朱震亨, is the founder of the yīn-nourishing school.
Zhū Gōng 朱肱 (1050-1125)	Author of the book *Huó Rén Shū* 《 活人书 》 (Book on How to Save People's Lives), which is also known as the *Shāng Hán Bái Wèn* 《 傷寒百問 》 (One Hundred Questions on Cold Damage).
Zhū Xī 朱熹 (1130-1200)	*Sì Shū Zhāng Jù Jí Zhù, Gào Zi Zhāng Jù Shàng* 《 四書章句集注·孟子集注 》 告子章句上 (Collection of Commentaries to Writings from The Four Books, Collection of Comments to Mèngzǐ, first chapter of Gàozǐ's writings).
Zhū Zhènhēng 朱震亨 (1281-1358)	Author of the *Běn Cǎo Yǎn Yì Bǔ Yí* 《 本草衍義補遺 》 (Addendum to the Amplified Meanings of the Materia Medica).
Zhuāng Zǐ 莊子 (369-286 B.C.)	Also known as Zhuāng Zhōu 莊周, is the most influential philosopher in Daoism.

General Index

concretions and con-glomerations of the heart and abdomen	162	-- or loss of bone marrow	186
confusion of a suck-ling child	77	-- to the center	25-26, 29, 34, 46, 69, 88-89, 105, 112, 129, 205
congealed phlegm	107	damp-heat	33, 40, 97, 99-100, 109, 126, 144, 159, 192
conglomerations	28, 93, 99, 101-102, 108-109, 130, 143, 168-169, 176	damp-heat diarrhea	150
construction and defense	62, 116, 169, 183, 207-208	damp impediment	23, 36, 47, 60-61, 66, 69, 92, 108, 151-152, 180, 195, 198, 205
copious phlegm	174	damp jaundice	123-124
cough	21, 74, 79, 83-84, 103, 119, 124-125, 136, 139, 144-145, 155, 208	damp qì	24, 98, 146
		dān tián	76
		dead flesh	23, 145-146, 156-157
		death of the fetus in utero	58, 195
counterflow		deafness	193
-- cold of the four limbs	154	demons	59, 101, 180-181, 185, 196
-- cough	56, 72, 75-76, 99, 101-102, 153-154, 168-169, 172-173, 195	depression	22, 79, 102, 122, 176-177, 188, 201, 204
		desiccated water	123
-- cough evil qì in the heart and abdomen	96	diarrhea	19, 39-40, 97-99, 118, 128, 149-150, 154, 169-170, 184-185, 187, 191, 194, 198, 202, 208
-- cough qì ascent	36, 49-50, 58, 114		
-- qì	82, 156		
-- qì ascent	114, 119, 124-125, 136, 144-145, 154-155		
		diarrhea afflux	95
-- qì below the heart	166	diarrhea with pus and blood	101-102
-- qì of the chest and rib-sides	72	difficult lactation	42-43, 47-48, 95, 138
-- retching	77	dispersion-thirst	85, 97, 126, 136-137, 139, 144, 197
crippling wilt	136, 168-169	distention	68, 84, 146, 173, 185, 191, 195, 201-204, 206-207
D			
damage			
-- and tearing at the canthus of the eye	39		
-- due to hunger	27, 34-35	distention of the chest	172

神農本草經讀

dizziness	41, 134, 172-173, 185, 194
dizzy	79, 173
dizzy vision	66
downpour diarrhea	158-159
dreams	86-87, 106
dribbling urinary block	95
dripping after urination	143
dry mouth	166
dry tongue	72, 111
dryness of the throat	199
dū vessel	161
dysentery	39, 59, 97, 114-115, 126, 148, 183-184, 187, 191-192, 194, 199, 204
dysphagia-occlusion	68, 192
E	
edema	79
enduring decaying sores	21
enuresis	111, 133
epidemic disorders	64
epidemics	86-87, 203
epilepsy	22, 36, 62-63, 66-67, 101-102, 106-108, 131-132, 145, 161-163, 165, 209
eroded flesh	162-163

essence	13, 18, 26, 29, 33, 35, 37-39, 46-49, 51, 53-54, 59, 61, 64, 69, 74, 80-82, 86-88, 91, 94-96, 98, 101, 106, 108-109, 111-112, 122, 124, 130, 140, 147, 152, 156, 158, 163, 165, 171, 183-184, 193-194
essence vacuity	28, 50
evil	
-- ghosts	94-95, 110, 157-158, 166
-- qì	18-19, 24-26, 31, 37, 39, 44-45, 56, 64-67, 85-87, 89, 91, 97, 107-108, 131-132, 135-138, 140-141, 144-145, 147, 151, 162, 168-169, 176, 180, 195-196, 199
-- qì in the heart and abdomen	93, 96, 130
-- toxins	67-68, 181
expiration of the stomach vessel	34
expiring pulse	88
expiry	35, 53, 66-67, 91, 105, 121-122, 139
external evil	18, 191
extreme shivering	103
eye pain	40
F	
facial complexion	81-82, 163-164, 183-184
falling sinews	54
fear of cold on the upper back	71
fear palpitations	72

神農本草經讀

神農本草經讀

神農本草經讀

神農本草經讀

神農本草經讀

Medicinals

bā jǐ tiān	巴戟天	Root of Morinda officinalis	morinda root	41, 44-46
bā dòu	巴豆	Seed of Croton tiglium	croton seed	195
bái dòu kòu	白豆蔻	Round fruit of Amomum kravanh	round cardamom	187
bái jiāng cán	白僵蠶	Dried 4th or 5th stage larva of the moth of Bombyx mori	body of sick silkworm	163-164
bái jiāo	白膠	Glue produced from Cervus nippon	deer antler glue	105-106
bái jiè zǐ	白芥子	Seed of Sinapis alba	white mustard seed	203
bái shí yīng	白石英	White quartz	quartz, white fluorite	97
bái tóu wēng	白頭翁	Root of Pulsatilla chinensis	pulsatilla root	40
bái zhǐ	白芷	Root of Angelica dahurica	Dahurian Angelica root	143
bái zhú	白朮	Rhizome of Atractylodes macrocephala	white atractylodes rhizome	23-24, 74, 79-80, 117, 172
bǎi hé	百合	Bulb of Lilium brownii	lily bulb	79
bǎi láo shuǐ	百勞水	medically prepared water	flowing water that has been stirred intensely with a spoon for "one thousand" times to produce bubbles	71
bǎi shí	柏實	Seed of Platycladus orientalis	arborvitae seed	92
bàn xià	半夏	Rhizome of Pinellia ternata	pinellia rhizome	13, 19, 84, 139-140, 167, 172-174
bèi mǔ	貝母	Bulb of Fritillaria cirrhosa	fritillaria cirrhosa bulb	83-84, 138-139
bì xiè	萆薢	Rhizome of Dioscorea hypoglauca	fish-poison yam rhizome/ seven-lobed yam rhizome	205
biǎn dòu	扁豆	Seed of Dolichos lablab	hyacinth bean	200

biē jiǎ	鱉甲	Dorsal shell of Amyda sinensis	Chinese soft-shelled turtle shell (dorsal aspect)	162-163
bīng láng	檳榔	Fruit of Areca catechu	betel nut	79, 190, 205
bò hé	薄荷	Leaves of Mentha arvensis	mentha	190, 202
bǔ gǔ zhī	補骨脂	Fruit of Psoralea corylifolia	psoralea fruit	186
cāng ěr	蒼耳	Fruit of Xanthium sibiricum	Siberian cockelbur	189
cāng zhú	蒼朮	Rhizome of Atractylodes lancea	atractylodes rhizome	13, 23
chán tuì	蟬蛻	Exuviae of Cicada	cicada molting	165, 190
chāng pú	菖蒲	Rhizome of Acorus gramineus	sweetflag rhizome	58-59, 190, 195
chái hú	柴胡	Root of Bupleurum chinense	bupleurum	19, 37-39, 117, 173, 190
chē qián zǐ	車前子	Seed of Plantago asiatica	plantago seeds	60, 79
chén jiǔ	陳酒		aged wine	71
chén xiāng	沉香	Wood of Aquilaria sinensis	aquilaria wood	196
chì jiàn	赤箭	Rhizome of Gastrodia elata	gastrodia rhizome	59
chì shí zhī	赤石脂	Red Halloysite	red hallyosite	97-98
chì xiǎo dòu	赤小豆	Fruit of Phaseolus calcaratus	adzuki bean	79, 189-190
chuān xiōng	川芎	Root of Ligusticum wallichii	chuanxiong root	120-121, 190
cōng bái	蔥白	Stalk of Allium fistulosum	white scallion	118
dà fù pí	大腹皮	Pericarpium of Areca catechu	areca husk	79, 190
dà huáng	大黃	Root of Rheum palmatum	rhubarb root and rhizome	13, 174-175, 179, 190
dà zǎo	大棗	Mature fruit of Ziziphus jujuba	jujube	93, 116
dài zhě shí	代赭石	Hematite	hematite	19, 180-181
dān shēn	丹參	Root of Salvia miltiorrhiza	salvia root	60, 129-131
dāng guī	當歸	Root of Angelica sinensis	Chinese angelica root	22, 78-79, 119-120
dǎng shēn	黨參	Root of Codonopsis pilosula	codonopsis root	190
dì huáng	地黃	Root of Rehmannia glutinosa	rehmannia root	14, 29-32, 120, 171, 184
dīng xiāng	丁香	Flower bud of Syzygium aromaticum	clove	190, 195

dòu chǐ	豆豉	Preparation of Glycine max	prepared soybean	201
dú huó	獨活	Root and rhizome of Angelica pubescens	pubescent angelica root	62-63, 190
dù zhòng	杜仲	Bark of Eucommia ulmoidis	eucommia bark	87-88
ē jiāo	阿膠	Gelatinous glue produced from Equus asinus	ass hide glue	26, 31, 103-104, 208
é zhú	莪朮	Rhizome of Curcuma zedoaria	curcuma	190
fà bì	髮髲	Crinis Carbonisatus Hominis	charred human hair	100-101
fáng fēng	防風	Root of Ledebouriella divaricata	ledebouriella root	13, 41-42, 45-46, 65, 190
fáng jǐ	防己	Root of Aristolochia fangchi/ Root of Stephaniae tetrandrae	stephania root/or southern fangji root	65, 132-134, 142, 190
fěi zǐ	榧子	Seeds of Torreya grandis	torreya seeds	190
fú líng	茯苓	Dried fungus of Poria cocos	poria cocos	19, 72, 74, 79-80, 116, 129, 133, 190, 194, 204-206
fú shén	茯神	Sclerotium (i.e., white, hardened core in the center) of Poria cocos	root poria	194
fù zǐ	附子	Lateral root of Aconitum carmichaeli	aconite root	13-14, 31, 77, 79, 168-172, 184
gān cǎo	甘草	Root of Glycyrrhiza uralensis	licorice	19-20, 24-25, 80, 83-84, 100, 115, 167, 171-172, 174
gān gě	乾葛	Dried root of Pueraria lobata	dried kudzu root	190
gān jiāng	乾薑	Dried root of Zingiber officinale	dried ginger	14, 19, 50, 114-115, 190
gān jú huā	甘菊花	Flower of Chrysanthemum morafolii	chrysanthemum flower	66
gé gēn	葛根	Root of Pueraria lobata	pueraria root	126-127
gě gǔ	葛穀	Seeds of Pueraria lobata	pueraria bean seeds	126
gǒu jǐ	狗脊	Rhizome of Cibotium barometz	cibotium rhizome	134

gǒu qǐ	枸杞	Bark of the root of Lycium chinensis	lyceum bark	14, 85-86
gōu téng	鉤藤	Twigs of Uncaria rhyncho-phulla	uncaria vine	13, 209
gǔ yá	穀芽	Sprouted fruit of Setaria italica	grain sprouts	190, 201
guā lóu gēn	栝蔞根	Root of Trichosanthes kirilowii	trichosanthes root	139-140
guī bǎn	龜板	Shell of Chinemys reevesii	freshwater turtle plastron	108-109, 111
guì	桂	Bark of Cinnamonum cassia	cinnamon bark	5, 9, 13, 76, 79, 82, 102, 115, 133, 138-140, 152, 166, 173, 178, 186, 214, 218
guì pí	桂皮	Bark of Cinnamonum cassia	cinnamon bark	75
guì zhī	桂枝	Twigs of Cinnamonum cassia	cinnamon twig	19, 74-75, 77-78, 80-81, 116, 137, 172
hǎi jīn shā	海金砂	Spores of Lygodium japoni-cum	Japanese climbing fern	79
hé shǒu wū	何首烏	Root of Polygoni multiflori	processed fleeceflower root	183-184
hēi zhī má	黑芝麻	Black seeds of Sesamum indicum	black sesame seeds	69
hóng huā	紅花	Flower of Carthamus tinctorius	safflower	190, 193
hòu guì	厚桂	Thick bark of Cinnamonum cassia	thick cinnamon	75
hòu pò	厚朴	Bark of Magnolia officinalis	magnolia bark	19, 79, 145-146, 149
hǔ gǔ	虎骨	Bone of Panthera tigris	tiger bone	204
hǔ pò	琥珀	Succinum	amber, fossilized resin	196
huá shí	滑石	Talcum	talcum	95-96
huái ruǐ	槐蕊	Stamen or pistil of Sophora japonica	sophora stamen or pistil	206
huái shí	槐實	Fruit of Sophora japonica	sophora fruit	91
huáng bǎi	黃柏	Bark of Phellodendron amurense	phellodendron bark	128, 149-150

huáng jīng	黃精	Rhizome of Polygonatum sibricum	Solomon's seal rhizome	13
huáng lián	黃連	Rhizome of Coptis chinensis	coptis rhizome	13, 19, 31, 39-40, 128, 143, 175
huáng qí	黃耆	Root of Astragalus membranaceus	astragalus root	14, 21-23, 133
huáng qín	黃芩	Root of Scutellaria baicalensis	scutellaria	13, 19, 128-129, 186, 190
huò xiāng	藿香	Whole plant Agastache rugosa	patchouli	190, 192
jī tóu shí	雞頭實	Seeds of Euryale ferox	euryale seeds	69
jiāo bái zhú	焦白朮	Scorch-fried rhizome of Atractylodes macrocephala	scorch-fried white atractylodes rhizome	79
jié gēng	桔梗	Root of Platycodon grandiflorum	platycodon root	178
jīn yīng zǐ	金櫻子	Fruit of Rosa laevigata	Cherokee rosehip	194
jīng jiè	荊芥	Foliage, stem, or flower buds of Schizonepeta tenuifolia	schizonepeta stem or bud	123-124, 190
jú hóng	橘紅	Pericarpium of Citrus erythrocarpa	red tangerine peel	83
jú huā	菊花	Flower of Chrysanthemum morafolii	chrysanthemmum flower	66, 190
jú pí	橘皮	Peel of Citrus reticulata	tangerine peel	82-84, 198
jūn gēn	菌根	Bark of Cinnamonum cassia	the root of incense wood	75
jūn guì	菌桂	Bark of Cinnamonum cassia	cinnamon bark	75, 81-82
kǔ shēn	苦參	Root of Sophora flavescens	sophora root	60, 143
kuǎn dōng huā	款冬花	Flower of Tussilago farfara	tussilago flower	144-145
lái fú zǐ	萊菔子	Seed of Raphanus Sativus	radish seeds	190
lián qiáo	連翹	Fruit of Forsythia suspensa	forsythia fruit	180
líng yáng jiǎo	羚羊角	Horn of the male Saiga tatarica	antelope horn	158-159
lóng dǎn	龍膽	Root and rhizome of Gentiana scabra	Chinese gentian root	66-67
lóng gǔ	龍骨	Os draconis	dragon bone	101-102
lóng yǎn ròu	龍眼肉	Flesh of the fruit of Euphoria longan	flesh of the longan fruit	199
lú rú	蘆茹	Root of Rubia cordifolia	rubia root	70-71

神
農
本
草
經
讀

lù róng	鹿茸	Pilose antler of Cervus nippon	deer velvet	105-106, 161-162
lù dòu	綠豆	Seed of Phaseolus radiatus	mung bean	200
luó bó zǐ	蘿卜子	Seed of Raphanus Sativus	radish seeds	79
má huáng	麻黃	Stalk of Ephedra sinica	ephedra stem	124-125
mǎ dōu líng	馬兜鈴	Fruit of Aristolochia debilis	aristolochia fruit	208
mǎ liào dòu	馬料豆	Seed of Glycine soja	black bean	200
mài mén dōng	麥門冬	Tuber of Ophiopogon japonicus	ophiopogon tuber	14, 33-35
mài yá	麥芽	Shoots of Hordeum vulgare	malt or barley sprouts	190, 201
mǔ dān pí	牡丹皮	Bark of the root of Paeonia suffruticosa	moutan root bark	131-132
mǔ guì	牡桂	Bark of Cinnamonum cassia	cinnamon bark	75-77, 82
mǔ lì	牡蠣	Shell of Ostrea rivularis	oyster shell	102, 110-111
mù guā	木瓜	Fruit of Chaenomeles sinensis	chaenomeles fruit	190, 198
mù tōng	木通	Stalk of Akebia quinata	akabia caulis	65, 79, 141-142, 190
mù xiāng	木香	Root of Aucklandia lappa	aucklandia root	86-87, 190
niú huáng	牛黃	Bezoar of Bos taurus domesticus	cow bezoar	106
niú xī	牛膝	Root of Achyranthes bidentata	achyranthes root	43, 79, 186
ǒu shí, jīng	藕實，莖	Node of Nelumbo nucifera	node of the lotus rhizome	68
péng shā	硼砂	Hydrated Sodium Tetraborate	borax	83
pí pá yè	枇杷葉	Leaf of Eriobotrya japonica	loquat leaf	198
pò xiāo	朴硝	Impure mirabilite	mirabilite	93-94
qiān niú zǐ	牽牛子	Seed of Pharbitis nil	morning glory seeds	206
qián hú	前胡	Root of Peucedanum praeruptorum	peucedanum root	193
qiàn cǎo gēn	茜草根	Root of Rubia cordifolia	rubia root	70-71
qiāng huó	羌活	Root of Notopterygii	notopterygium root	13, 62-63, 190
qín jiāo	秦艽	Root of Gentiana macrophylla	macrophylla root	65, 135, 190
qīng hāo	青蒿	Leaves of Artemisia annua	sweet wormwood	189

qīng jú pí	青橘皮	Unripe peel of Citrus reticulata	unripe tangerine peel	198
qīng pí	青皮	Pericarpium of Citri immaturis	immature orange peel	190
qīng yán	青鹽	Halite		83-84
rén rǔ	人乳	Human breast milk	human milk	209
rén shēn	人參	Root of Panax ginseng	ginseng root	18-20, 26, 60, 83-84, 154, 167
rěn dōng	忍冬	Lonicera japonica	honeysuckle	207-208
ròu cōng róng	肉蓯蓉	Fleshy stalk of Cistanche salsa	cistanche	27-28
ròu dòu kòu	肉豆蔻	Seed of Myristica fragrans	nutmeg seeds	185
ròu guì	肉桂	Trunk and branch bark of Cinnamonum cassia	cassia	75, 77-79
sān léng	三棱	Rhizome of Sparganium stoloniferum	bur-reed	190
sāng gēn bái pí	桑根白皮	Bark of the root of Morus alba	mulberry root bark	88-90
sāng piāo xiāo	桑螵蛸	Cocoon-like egg capsules of Paratenodera sinensis	mantis egg-case	112
sāng shàng jì shēng	桑上寄生	Branches and foliage of Viscum coloratum	taxillus	90
shā rén	砂仁	Seed pods of Amomum villosum	grains of paradise	187, 190
shā shēn	沙參	Root of Adenophora tetraphylla	adenophora root	55, 60
shā yuàn jí lí	沙苑蒺藜	Seed of Astragalus complanatus	complanate astragalus seed	26
shān zhā zǐ	山楂子	Fruit of Crataegus pinnatifida	crataegus fruit	199
shān zhū yú	山茱萸	Fruit of Cornus officinalis	cornus fruit	151-152
shāng lù	商陸	Root of Phytolacca acinosa	poke root	79
sháo yào	芍藥	Root of Paeonia rubra	red peony root	79, 129, 137, 140-141, 172, 190
shè xiāng	麝香	Dried secretion from the musk pod of Moschus moschiferus	musk	106-107
shén qū	神麴	Medicated leaven	medicated leaven	188-192

shēng jiāng	生薑	Fresh root of Zingiber officinale	fresh ginger	19, 116-117
shēng má	升麻	Rhizome of Cimifuga foetida	cimicifuga	
shí gāo	石膏	Gypsum	gypsum	19, 166-167
shí hú	石斛	Whole plant of Dendrobium nobile	dendrobium	46-47
shí mì	石蜜	Crystalized honey of Apis cerana	rock honey	107-108
shǐ jūn zǐ	使君子	Fruit of Quisqualis indica	Rangoon creeper fruit with seeds	190
shú dì huáng	熟地黃	Prepared root of Rehmannia glutinosa	rehmannia root	14, 30-32
shú dì tàn	熟地炭	Charred prepared root of Rehmannia glutinosa	charred rehmannia root	79
shǔ jiāo	蜀椒	Seed capsules of Zanthoxylum bungeanum	Sichuan pepper	195
shǔ yù	薯蕷	Root of Dioscorea opposita	dioscorea rhizome	25
shuǐ píng	水萍	Whole plant of Spirodela polyrhiza	duckweed	144
sū yè	蘇葉	Foliage of Perilla frutescens	perilla leaves	190
suān zǎo rén	酸棗仁	Seed of Ziziphus spinosa	spiny ziziphus seeds	14
suō shā rén	縮砂仁	Fruit of Amomum villosum	amomum fruit	187
táo rén	桃仁	Seed of Prunus persica	peach kernel	176, 190
tiān má	天麻	Rhizome of Gastrodia elata	gastrodia rhizome	13, 59-60
tiān mén dōng	天門冬	Tuber of Asparagus cochinchinensis	asparagus tuber	32-33
tíng lì zǐ	葶藶子	Seeds of Lepidium apetalum	tingli seeds	179
tōng cǎo	通草	Stalk of Akebia quinata	akabia caulis	142
tóng biàn	童便	Infantis Urina	child's urine	71
tǔ fú líng	土茯苓	Rhizome of Smilax glabra	smilax	204-206
tù sī zǐ	菟絲子	Seed of Cuscuta chinensis	cuscuta seeds	26, 53
wēi ruí	葳蕤	Rhizome of Polygonatum odoratum	scented Solomon´s seal rhizome	26, 54-55
wū gǔ bái sī máo jī	烏骨白絲毛雞	Gallus gallus domesticus Brisson	black-boned silky fowl	71
wū méi	烏梅	Unripe fruit of Prunus mume	mume fruit	40, 83-84, 152, 156-157

神農本草經讀

241

wū yào	烏藥	Root of Lindera strychnifolia	lindera root	65, 196
wū zéi yú gǔ	烏鰂魚骨	Calcified shell of Sepiella maindroni	cuttlefish shell	70-71
wú zhū yú	吳茱萸	Unripe fruit of Evodia rutaecarpa	evodia fruit	19, 117, 153-154
wǔ líng zhī	五靈脂	Feces of Trogopterus xanthipes	flying squirrel feces	203
wǔ wèi zǐ	五味子	Fruit of Schisandra chinensis	schisandra fruit	49-50
xī jiǎo	犀角	Horn of Rhinoceros	rhinoceros horn	157-158
xì xīn	細辛	Complete plant including root of Asarum heteropoides	asarum root and rhizome	36-37
xià kū cǎo	夏枯草	Flower spike of Prunella vulgaris	prunella	180
xiāo shí	硝石	Niter	saltpeter	94
xiǎo biàn	小便	Human urine	urine	209
xiǎo huí xiāng	小茴香	Fruit of Foeniculum vulgare	fennel fruit	204
xiǎo mài	小麥	Seed of Triticum aestivum	wheat	199
xiāng fù	香附	Rhizome of Cyperus rotundus	cyperus rhizome	190, 193
xiāng rú	香薷	Leaves of Elsholtzia ciliata	mosla	202
xìng rén	杏仁	Dried seed of Prunus armeniaca	apricot kernel	154-155, 189
xù duàn	續斷	Root of Dipsacus asper	dipsacus root	42-43
xuán / yuán shēn	玄 / 元參	Root of Scrophularia ningpoensis	scrophularia root	129
xuán fù huā	旋覆花	Flowerhead of Inula britannica	inula flower	177, 181
yán hú suǒ	延胡索	Rhizome of Corydalis yanhuosuo	corydalis rhizome	185
yí táng	飴糖	Malt sugar	malt sugar	202
yì mǔ cǎo zǐ	益母草子	Seeds of Leonurus artemisia	Chinese motherwort seeds	69-70
yì yǐ rén	薏苡仁	Seed kernel of Coix lachryma-jobi	coix seeds	50-51
yīn chén hāo	茵陳蒿	Shoots and leaves of Artemisia capillaris	Artemisia capillaris shoots and leaves	65-66

神農本草經讀

Formulas

Bā Wèi Wǎn	八味丸	152
Bái Hǔ Jiā Rén Shēn Tāng	白虎加人參湯	19
Bái Hǔ Tāng	白虎湯	111
Bái Tōng Tāng	白通湯	31, 118, 172
Bái Zhú Tāng	白朮湯	74, 117, 172
Bàn Xià Xiè Xīn Tāng	半夏瀉心湯	19
Bǔ Fèi Ē Jiāo Sǎn	補肺阿膠散	208
Chái Hú Guì Zhī Tāng	柴胡桂枝湯	19
Dà Chéng Qì Tāng	大承氣湯	31, 149
Dà Xiàn Xiōng Wán	大陷胸丸	179
Dāng Guī Liù Huáng Tāng	當歸六黃湯	22
Dǐ Dàng Tāng	抵當湯	210
Fáng Jǐ Fú Líng Tāng	防己茯苓湯	133
Fáng Jǐ Huáng Qí Tāng	防己黃耆湯	133
Fáng Jǐ Jiā Fú Líng Máng Xiāo Tāng	防己加茯苓芒硝湯	133
Fēng Yǐn Tāng	風引湯	102
Fú Líng Guì Zhī Tāng	茯苓桂枝湯	116
Fú Líng Sì Nì Tāng	茯苓四逆湯	19
Fù Zǐ Tāng	附子湯	31, 172
Gān Cǎo Fù Zǐ Tāng	甘草附子湯	172
Gān Cǎo Gān Jiāng Tāng	甘草乾薑湯	115
Gān Jiāng Huáng Qín Huáng Lián Rén Shēn Tāng	乾薑黃芩黃連人參湯	19
Gé Gēn Tāng	葛根湯	127
Guì Líng Gān Zhú Tāng	桂苓甘朮湯	78
Guì Líng Wán	桂苓丸	77
Guì Zhī Fù Zǐ Qù Guì Jiā Bái Zhú Tāng	桂枝附子去桂加白朮湯	172
Guì Zhī Fù Zǐ Tāng	桂枝附子湯	172
Guì Zhī Qù Guì Jiā Fú Líng Bái Zhú Tāng	桂枝去桂加茯苓白朮湯	74
Guì Zhī Rén Shēn Tāng	桂枝人參湯	19
Guì Zhī Sháo Yào Zhī Mǔ Tāng	桂枝芍藥知母湯	137
Guì Zhī Tāng	桂枝湯	19, 77, 116
Hòu Pò Shēng Jiāng Bàn Xià Rén Shēn Tāng	厚朴生薑半夏人參湯	19
Huáng Lián Ē Jiāo Jī Zǐ Tāng	黃連雞子黃湯	31

神農本草經讀

Zhū Líng Tāng	豬苓湯	31, 74
Zhú Pí Dà Wán	竹皮大丸	77
Zhú Yè Shí Gāo Tāng	竹葉石膏湯	19

Pinyin

Ā Jǐng	阿井	Ā wells	103
bǎi cǎo shén qū	百草神麴	Deities Yeast with One Hundred Herbs	190
Bái Hǔ	白虎	White Tiger	111, 189
bái lài	白癩	white leprosy	147
bài xuě	敗血	wasted blood	176
bēng duò	崩墮	flooding and miscarriage, can also mean abortion of the fetus.	104
bēng lòu	崩漏	flooding	88
bēng zhōng	崩中	flooding	88, 197
bì	啓	open, or to open	3
bì	痹	impediment	23
bì	髲	wig or human hair.	100
bì	躄	cripple, lame	136
bí chì	鼻赤	red nose	147
bō	剝	prosperity	42
bǔ	補	supplement	5
bǔ tiān	補天	a Daoist method to preserve health.	50
cháng chóng	長蟲	longworm (tapeworm)	32
cháng pì	腸澼	intestinal afflux	39, 97
chè zhǒu	掣肘	to hold somebody by the elbow	48
chì bái xiè lì	赤白泄痢	red and white dysentery	
chì chóng	赤蟲	redworm (roundworm)	32
chì wò	赤沃	red irrigation	180
chōng hé zhī qì	衝和之氣	qì of harmonious flow	114
chōng mài	衝脈	penetrating vessel	97
chǎn yú nán fāng zhī bā dā	產於南方之叭噠	almonds produced in the south	155
cóng zhì fǎ	從治法	coacting treatment method	164
cùn bái chóng	寸白蟲	inch white worms	206

dà fēng	大風	pestilential wind	41
dà fēng lài jí	大風癩疾	great wind leprosy	21
dān dú	丹毒	cinnabar toxin	200
dān tián	丹田	cinnabar field	76
dāng dào	當道	to be in power	60
dāo guī	刀圭	an ancient tool for measuring tiny amounts of medicine	3
dì suǐ	地髓	an alternate name for *dì huáng* 地黃.	30
diān	癲	convulsions or epileptic spasms	102
dōng rì kě ài, xià rì kě wèi	冬日可愛，夏日可畏。	In winter, the sun is lovable. In summer, the sun is detestable.	172
è ròu	惡肉	malign flesh	156, 162-163
è xuè	惡血	malign blood	158
fā chén	發陳	creating from the old	65
fà	髮	human hair	101
fēng chuāng	風瘡	wind sores	183
fēng lún	風輪	wind wheel	44
fēng shuǐ	風水	wind and water	192
fóu yǐ	苤苢	plantago major	60-61
fú shī	伏尸	hidden corpse	32, 205
fú zhǒng	浮腫	puffy swelling	118
fù	復	decline	42, 45
gān	疳	*gān* disease	128
gān lán shuǐ fǎ	甘瀾水法	the method of worked water	71
gé qì	膈氣	diaphragm qì	198
gōng	攻	attack	5
gōng chén	功臣	one, who has made a significant contribution to a specific task.	9
gōng xià pài	攻下派	purgative school	3, 218
Gōu Chén	勾陳	Hooked Old	189
gǔ zhù	蠱疰	summer influx or infixation	73
gǔ	蠱	a legendary venomous worm.	59-67
gù	固	firm	5
guān gé	關格	block and repulsion	100
guī	圭	jade tablet	94
hé	和	harmonize	5

hēi shuǐ shén guāng	黑水神光	black water spirit light	129
hóu bì	喉痹	throat impediment	75, 138, 144
hú	斛	an ancient measure for grain and is equal to fifty liters.	47
hù	芐	an alternate name for *dì huáng* 地黃.	30
huà lóng diǎn jīng yù fēi	畫龍點睛欲飛	to [paint] a dot [as] eye [of a painted dragon, to make it] want to fly.	102
huà shé tiān zú	畫蛇添足。	to paint a snake and add feet.	172
huǒ qí	火齊	a degree of heat, the time, and the temperature in which the medicine is prepared.	3
huǒ yáng	火瘍	fire-ulcers	128
Jǐ Shuǐ	濟水	the name of a river in ancient China.	103
jiǎ mù	甲木	first of the ten heavenly stems	67
jiàn xíng bù shuì	健行不睡	prevents sleepiness while hiking or it strengthens motion without sleepiness.	204
jiǎo qì	腳氣	leg qì	198
jīn lún	金輪	metal wheel	44
jīn	筋	tendon	204
jīng lěng	精冷	seminal cold	185
jiōng	扃	door	3
jiǔ pào zhā bí	酒皰齇鼻	alcohol blisters and pimples on the nose	147
jiǔ tiān	九天	the Ninth Heaven is the highest of all heavens, but can as well mean the center of heaven and the eight directions.	87
kòng lún	空輪	emptiness wheel	44
kūn	坤	earth/ stillness	45, 61
láo fù	勞復	taxation relapse	197
láo nüè	勞瘧	taxation malaria	103
lǎo yù néng jiě	老嫗能解	easy to comprehend.	4
lìn lù	淋露	filter, distillation or soak, drip	86
lìn lù hán rè	淋露寒熱	soaking dew cold and heat	86
lǐng jiāng	領薑	dry ginger	118
liù jí	六極	six extremes	88
liù shén	六神	the six gods	189
liù shén qū	六神麴	six gods leaven	190
liù yín	六淫	six excesses	107
lóng dǎn	龍膽	dragon bile	66-67

shēn	穆	disperse, spread	107, 167
shén qì	神氣	spirit qì	76
shèn gōng	腎宮	kidney palace	118
shèn zuò qiáng [zhī guān]	腎作強[之官]	the kidney holds the office of labor	112
shòu kǎo	壽考	longevity	27
shǔ lòu	鼠瘻	mouse fistulae	21, 110, 123, 180, 204
shuǐ lún	水輪	water wheel	44
sǐ jī	死肌	numb or insensible flesh/ necrosis	23, 36, 145, 156
sì lún	四輪	four wheels	44
tán pǐ	痰癖	phlegm aggregation	205
tàn	炭	charcoal	20
Téng Shé	螣蛇	Winged Snake	189
tiān dōng	天冬	heaven winter	
tiān guǐ	天癸	heavenly tenth	140
tǔ	吐	vomit	18-19, 166
tù chǎo	土炒	earth-frying	120
tuó yuè	橐籥	a bellows is a tool with a bag of air, which upon pressing two handles together, emits a stream of air, and is used to make the fire of a forge hotter.	20
tuò xuè	唾血	spitting of blood	199
wěi	骫	originally meant buckled bone.	3
wèi	位	(seat) means to dwell, to place oneself in.	181
wēn nüè	溫瘧	warm malaria	106, 119, 124
wǔ gān	五疳	five gān diseases	203
wǔ jīn	五金	five metals	128
wǔ láo	五勞	five taxations	27
wǔ lín	五淋	five stranguries	100
wǔ lóng	五癃	five stranguries	100
wǔ yùn	五運	the five movements	59
wǔ zhì	五痔	five kinds of hemorrhoids	21, 91
xī	觹	a kind of tool made of bones, a bodkin for undoing knots.	3
xǐ xǐ	洗洗	tidal trembling	119
xián	鹹	all, or whole	33, 157, 165, 209

xiǎo ér jīng [fēng]	小兒驚[風]	infantile convulsions	100
xiào lián	孝廉	filial and upright	8
xié	脅	ribside	204
xīn zhī huà zài miàn	心之華在面	the bloom of the heart is in the face	147
xīn zhǔ hàn	心主汗	heart governs sweat	124-125
xū sǔn	虛損	vacuity detriment	77
Xuán Wǔ	玄武	Dark Tortoise	189
xuě hǎi	血海	sea of blood	97
xuè yú huī	血餘灰	ashed surplus of the blood	100
xuè yūn	血暈	blood dizziness, fainting	185
xùn míng	徇名	to give one´s life to become famous	188
yào jī	藥雞	medicinal chicken	71
yē gé	噎隔	dysphagia-occlusion	192
yì xiàng	易象	shape of changes	42
yīn	因	causal	5,171
yīn mái sì bù	陰霾四布	a yin dust-storm in all directions	79
yīn shí	陰蝕	genital erosion	97, 162-163
yīn xià yǎng shī	陰下癢濕	itchy damp below the genitals	87
yīn	蔭	to shade, to shelter, to protect.	47
yíng	迎	receive (guests); meet head-on	170
yù	豫	comfort	45
yuán zhēn	元真	true origin	77
yuē	啘	to retch; to hiccup	197
zèi fēng	賊風	bandit wind	180-181
zhēn yuán	真元	true origin	77
zhèn	震	thunder	45, 61
zhèn yǔ	鴆羽	feathers of the legendary bird zhèn	157
zhèng zhì fǎ	正治法	straight treatment method	164
zhì	櫛	comb	8
zhōng	尰	swollen	24
zhòng è	中惡	malignity stroke	185
zhòng fēng chì zòng	中風瘈瘲	wind strike with tugging and slackening	131
zhòng shuǐ	重水	heavy water	104
Zhū Què	朱雀	Vermilion Bird	189
zhū shū	朱書	cinnabar book	11

251

神農本草經讀

zhù	疰	influx or infixation	101, 157
zhuāng huǒ	壯火	strong fire	151
zhuó zhuó	濯濯	gurgling, or the sound of water stirring	173
zōng jīn	宗筋	ancestral sinews	138
zōng yǎn	宗眼	ancestral eyes	83

People

Bái Jūyì	白居易	4, 215
Bào Pùzǐ	抱朴子	57-58, 60, 215
Biǎn Què	扁鵲	79, 216
Chén Chéng	陳承	37, 216
Chén Shìliáng	陳士良	142, 216
Féng Chǔdǎn	馮楚瞻	27
Gě Hóng	葛洪	57, 215
Guō Rǔcōng	郭汝聰	7, 9
Huà Tuó	華佗	15, 54, 216
Huà Yáng Yǐn Jū	華陽隐居	10
Huà Yuánhuà	華元化	15, 54, 216
Huáng Dì	黃帝	2, 9, 13, 19, 31, 38, 44, 57, 65, 68, 71, 86, 100, 103, 120, 125, 133, 138, 151, 153, 165, 168, 171, 178
Kē Qín	柯琴	5, 214, 216
Léi Gōng	雷公	8, 14, 83, 213, 216
Léi Xiào	雷斅	8, 83, 216
Lǐ Bīnhú	李瀕湖	8, 186, 216
Lǐ Dōngyuán	李東垣	8, 10, 42, 133-134, 216
Lǐ Gǎo	李杲	3, 8, 134, 216-217
Lǐ Shízhēn	李時珍	3, 8, 12, 15, 18, 54, 60, 99, 127, 134, 184, 186, 216
Lǐ Shìcái	李士材	15, 19, 139, 216
Lǐ Zhōngzǐ	李中梓	15, 216
Liú Wéntài	劉文泰	194
Lú Biǎn	盧扁	79, 216
Miào Xīyōng	缪希雝	189, 216
Qí Bó	岐伯	2, 178

神農本草經讀

Books

Bái Xiāng Shān Shī Jù	《白香山詩句》	Verse of the "White Fragrant Mountain"	4, 212
Bèi Jí Qiān Jīn Yào Fāng	《備急千金要方》	Essential Prescriptions Worth a Thousand in Gold for Every Emergency	7, 217
Běn Cǎo Bèi Yào	《本草備要》	Complete Essentials of Materia Medica	8, 12, 186, 212, 217
Běn Cǎo Chóng Yuán	《本草崇原》	Honored Originals of the Materia Medica	12, 35, 89, 212
Běn Cǎo Pǐn Huì Jīng Yào	《本草品匯精要》	Essential Collection of the Materia Medica	194
Běn Cǎo Gāng Mù	《本草綱目》	Compendium of the Materia Medica	3-4, 12, 15, 18, 99, 186, 212, 216
Běn Cǎo Jīng Dú	《本草經讀》	Reading the [Divine Farmer's] Classic of Materia Medica	3-4, 8-9
Běn Cǎo Jīng Jiě	《本草經解》	Explaining the Materia Medica Classic	12, 213
Běn Cǎo Jīng Sān Zhù	《本草經三注》	The Divine Farmer's Classic of Materia Medica Commented [on] by [the] Three	9
Běn Cǎo Shí Yí	《本草拾遺》	Picking up Lost Property of the Materia Medica	182, 215
Běn Cǎo Yǎn Yì Bǔ Yí	《本草衍義補遺》	Addendum to the Amplified Meanings of the Materia Medica	182, 213, 218
Cháo Shì Zhū Bìng Yuán Hòu Zǒng Lùn	《巢氏諸病源候總論》	Treatise on the Origins and Symptoms of Disease by Master Cháo	32, 213
Chū Qiū Zuǒ Zhuàn	《春秋左傳》	Zuǒ´s Commentary to the Spring and Autumn Annals	172, 213
Dà Míng Běn Cǎo	《大明本草》	Dà Míng´s Materia Medica	182, 213
Dà Xué	《大學》	The Great Learning	11
Ěr Yǎ	《爾雅》	Approaching the Refined	30, 177
Huáng Dì Bā Shí Yī Nán Jīng	《黃帝八十一難經》	Huáng Dì´s Classic on Eighty-One Difficult Issue	15, 213
Huó Rén Bǎi Wèn	《活人百問》	One Hundred Questions on How to Save Lives	5, 214
Huó Rén Shū	《活人书》	Book on How to Save People's Lives	5, 218
Jīn Guì Dú	《金匱讀》	Reading the Formulas from the Golden Cabinet	5, 214
Jīn Guì Yào Lüè	《金匱要略》	Essential Prescriptions of the Golden Cabinet	7, 40, 45, 50, 77-78, 80, 122, 213, 217
Jīn Guì [Yào Lüè] Qiǎn Zhù	《金匱[要略]淺注》	Superficial Commentary on Formulas from the Golden Cabinet	5

Jīn Gùi Yào Lüè Lùn Zhù	《金匱要略論注》	Treatise on the Essential Prescriptions of the Golden Cabinet	77, 122, 213, 217
Jǐng Yuè Quán Shū	《景岳全書》	Complete Works of Jǐngyuè	5, 218
Jǐng Yuè Xīn Fāng Biān	《景岳新方砭》	A Critique of Jǐngyuè's New Prescriptions	5, 214
Kāi Bǎo Chóng Dìng Běn Cǎo	《開寶重定本草》	Kāi Bǎo Revised Materia Medica	11, 149, 182-183, 213
Kē Zhù Shāng Hán Lùn	《柯注傷寒論》	Commentary to the Discussion On Cold Damage	5, 214
Léi Gōng Páo Zhì Lùn	《雷公炮制論》	Master Léi's Discussion on Processing of Medicinals	8, 216
Lěng Zhāi Yè Huà	《冷齋夜話》		4
Lín Zhèng Zhǐ Nán Yī Àn	《臨證指南醫案》	Guide to Clinical Practice in Cases	9, 81, 213, 218
Lǚ Shān Táng	《侶山堂》		13, 213
Lǚ Shān Táng Lèi Biàn	《侶山堂類辨》	The Differentiation of Categories from the Lǚ Shān Hall	13, 213
Lún Yǔ	《論語》	The Analects	11, 170, 213
Máo Shī	《毛詩》	Book of Odes by the Two Máo	60, 215
Mèng Zǐ	《孟子》	Mencius	11, 213
Míng Yī Bié Lù	《名醫別錄》	Specific Recordings by Famous Physicians	11, 162, 182, 192-194, 196-209, 213
Nán Jīng	《難經》	Classic of Difficult Issues	15, 213
Pào Zhì Dà Fǎ	《炮炙大法》	Great Methods for Processing Medicines	189, 213, 216
Pí Wèi Lùn	《脾胃論》	Treatise on the Spleen and Stomach	3, 213, 216
Rì Huàzǐ Zhū Jiā Běn Cǎo	《日華子諸家本草》	Materia Medica of Various Schools by Rì Huàzǐ	8, 217
Shāng Hán Lùn	《傷寒論》	Discussion on Cold Damage	5, 7, 19, 40, 127, 138-139, 148, 154, 156, 166-167, 179, 210, 212-214, 216
Shāng Hán Lùn Dú	《傷寒論讀》	Reading the Discussion On Cold Damage	5, 214
Shāng Hán Lùn [Qiǎn] Zhù	《傷寒論[淺]注》	[Shallow] Commentary to the Discussion On Cold Damage	5
Shāng Hán Yī Jué Chuàn Jiě	《傷寒醫訣串解》	The Medical Method of the Discussion on Cold Damage Collected and Explained	5, 214
Shāng Hán Yī Yuē Lù	《傷寒醫約錄》	Record on the Medical Outlines of the Discussion on Cold Damage	5, 214
[Shāng Hán] Zhēn Fāng Gē Kuò	《[傷寒]真方歌括》	True Prescriptions from On Cold Damage with Poems	5

Shén Nóng Běn Cǎo Jīng	《神農本草經》	Divine Farmer's Classic of Materia Medica	1, 3-4, 7-8, 20, 30, 34, 40, 44-45, 50, 60, 70, 86, 99, 105, 109, 117, 128-129, 134, 137, 142, 145-146, 149, 152-154, 165, 169, 171-173, 175, 177-178, 186, 205, 214
Shén Xiān Fú Shí Jīng	《神仙服食經》	Dietary Classic of the Immortals	61
Shī [Jīng]	《詩[經]》	Book of Odes	61
Shí Xìng Běn Cǎo	《食性本草》	Materia Medica on the Nature of Food	142, 214, 216
Tāng Yè Běn Cǎo	《湯液本草》	Materia Medica of Decoctions	182, 214
Tú Jīng Běn Cǎo	《圖經本草》	Illustrated Materia Medica	182, 198, 214, 217
Wài Tái Mì Yào	《外臺秘要》	Essential Secrets from Outside the Metropolis	7, 214, 217
Wēn Rè Lùn	《溫熱論》	Discussion on Warm Diseases	9, 186, 218
Xīn Fāng Bā Zhèn	《新方八陣》	New Prescriptions Divided into the Eight Classifications	5, 218
Xīn Xiū Běn Cǎo	《新修本草》	Newly Revised Materia Medica	182, 214, 217
Xún Zǐ	《荀子》	Xúnzǐ	56
Yào Xìng Běn Cǎo	《藥性本草》	Materia Medica on the Nature of Medicines	182, 188, 214, 218
Yào Xìng Lùn	《藥性論》	Treatise on the Nature of Medicines	182, 214
Yī Jué	《醫訣》	Methods of Medicine	5, 214-215
Yī Lín Zhǐ Nán	《醫林指南》	Medical Guide Book	81
Yī Mén Fǎ Lù	《醫門法律》	Regulations of Medicine	78, 214
Yī Xué Cóng Zhòng Lù	《醫學從眾錄》	A Record of Medicine by Others	5, 215
Yī Yī Ǒu Lù	《醫醫偶錄》	Medical Records in Pairs	5, 215
Yī Yuē	《醫約》	Outlines of Medicine	5, 214
Yì Jīng	《易經》	Book of Changes	42, 61, 158, 214
Zhēn Zhū Náng Yào Xìng Fù	《珍珠囊藥性賦》	Poetic Essay on the Nature of Medicinals of the Bag of Pearls	12, 214
Zhōng Yōng	《中庸》	The Doctrine of the Mean	11
Zhuāng Zǐ	《莊子》	Zhuāng zǐ	215, 218

The Chinese Medicine Database

www.cm-db.com

The Chinese Medicine Database has been organized around one central principle -- translation of Classical Asian texts, and dissemination of that information.

There are thousands of Asian medicine texts that have never been translated. We have compiled a small list on our website of the ones that we have found, but we believe that there are tens of thousands of documents that span from the *Hàn* Dynasty to pre-Republican times. Most of these documents will never be read by people in the West, simply because of lack of translation.

We have created a vehicle, that allows interested practitioners, students, institutions, and scholars to help support and fund the translation of these documents, and then mine and synthesize the data that is gained from these texts.

The Database contains:

Monographs on:
690 Single Herbs
1510 Formulas
Mayway's Patents
ITM's Formulations
Golden Flowers Formulations
Classical Pearls Formulations by Heiner Fruehauf
OBGYN Modifications to Formulas
Single Points: the 361 Regular Points
Timeline of the History of Chinese Medicine

Beer Hall Lecture Series
Watch videos from our monthly Beer Hall lecture series with guest speakers such as: Arnaud Versluys, Subhuti Dharmananda, Jason Robertson, Craig Mitchell, Michael Max, Lorraine Wilcox, and Ed Neal.

Play STORT
Play our free online game STORT where you can learn Chinese while having a bit of fun (www.cm-db.com/stort).

15,000 Western Diagnoses with ICD-9 Codes

A Chinese-English dictionary:
Containing over 103,843 terms, including the Eastland and the WHO term sets.

A Western Book search containing:
Fenner's Complete Formulary
by B. Fenner

The 1918 Dispensatory of the United States of America
    Edited by Joseph P. Remington, Horatio C. Woods and others
The Eclectic Materia Medica, Pharmacology and Therapeutics
    by Harvey Wickes Felter, M.D.

Translations:

Shāng Hán Lái Sū Jí	傷寒來蘇集	Renewal of Treatise on Cold Damage
Qí Jīng Bā Mài Kǎo	奇經八脈考	Explanation of the Eight Vessels of the Marvellous Meridians
Shāng Hán Míng Lǐ Lùn	傷寒明理論	Treatise on Enlightening the Principles of Cold Damage
Wú Jū Tōng Yī Àn	吳鞠通医案	Case Studies of Wú Jūtōng
The Nàn Jīng	難經	The Classic of Difficulties
The Zàng Fǔ Biāo Běn Hán Rè Xū Shí Yòng Yào Shì	臟腑標本寒熱虛實用藥式	Viscera and Bowels, Tip and Root, Cold and Heat, Vacuity and Repletion Model for Using Medicinals
Wēn Rè Lún	溫熱論	Treatise on Warm Heat Disease
Shāng Hán Shé Jiàn	傷寒舌鑒	Tongue Mirror of Cold Damage
Xǔ Shì Yī Àn	許氏醫案	Case Histories of Master Xǔ
Fǔ Xìng Jué Zāng Fǔ Yòng Yào Fǎ Yào	輔行決臟腑用藥法要	Secret Instructions for Assisting the Body: Essential Methods for the Application of Drugs to the Viscera & Bowels
Biāo Yōu Fù	標幽賦	Indicating the Obscure
Liú Juān Zǐ Guǐ Yí Fāng	劉涓子鬼遺方	Liu Juanzi's Formulas Inherited from Ghosts
Shèn Jí Chú Yán	慎疾芻言	Precautions in Illness: My Humble Thoughts
Yào Zhèng Jì Yí	藥症忌宜	Medicinals & Patterns Contraindications & Appropriate [Choices]
Fù Kē Wèn Dá	婦科問答	Questions and Answers in Gynecology
Nèi Jīng Zhī Yào	內經知要	Essential Knowledge from the Nèijīng
Běn Cǎo Bèi Yào	本草備要	The Essential Completion of Traditional Materia Medica
Bǎi Zhèng Fù (Jù Yīng)	百症賦《聚英》	Ode of the Hundred Diseases from The Great Compendium of Acupuncture-Moxibustion

Benefits:

Subscribers to the Database receive a 10% discount on our published books when they are in pre-release.

We translate texts as often, and in quantities that reflect our user base. The larger amount of subscribers that we have, the more translation that we can accomplish.

2008 Bèi Jí Qiān Jīn Yào Fāng 備急千金要方:
Essential Prescriptions Worth a Thousand Gold Pieces For Emergencies. vol. 2-4
by Sūn Sīmiǎo 孫思邈
Translated by Sabine Wilms.
ISBN 978-0-9799552-0-4
Out of Print

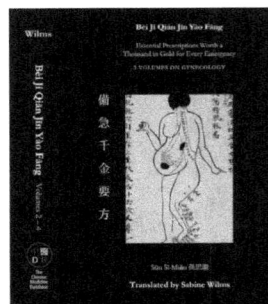

2010 Zhēn Jiǔ Dà Chéng 針灸大成:
The Great Compendium of Acupuncture & Moxibustion vol. I
by Yáng Jìzhōu 楊繼洲
Translated by Sabine Wilms.
ISBN 978-0-9799552-2-8

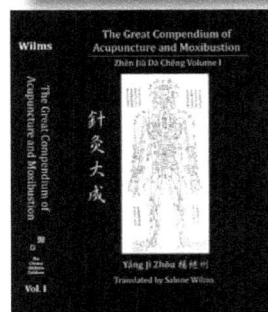

2010 Zhēn Jiǔ Dà Chéng 針灸大成:
The Great Compendium of Acupuncture & Moxibustion vol. V
by Yáng Jìzhōu 楊繼洲
Translated by Lorraine Wilcox.
ISBN 978-0-9799552-4-2

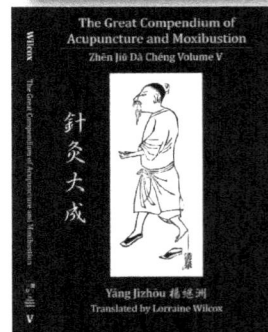

2010 Jīn Guì Fāng Gē Kuò 金匱方歌括:
Formulas from the Golden Cabinet with Songs vol. I - III
by Chén Xiūyuán 陳修園
Translated by Sabine Wilms.
ISBN 978-0-9799552-5-9

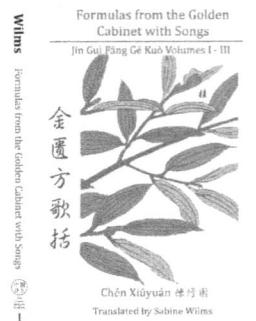

2011 Zhēn Jiǔ Dà Chéng 針灸大成:
The Great Compendium of Acupuncture & Moxibustion vol. VIII
by Yáng Jìzhōu 楊繼洲
Translated by Yue Lu.
ISBN 978-0-9799552-7-3

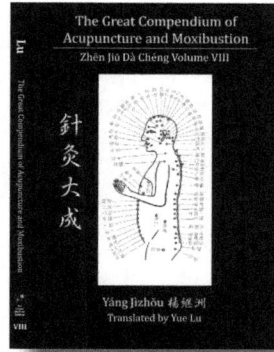

2011 Zhēn Jiǔ Dà Chéng 針灸大成:
The Great Compendium of Acupuncture & Moxibustion vol. IX
by Yáng Jìzhōu 楊繼洲
Translated by Lorraine Wilcox.
ISBN 978-0-9799552-6-6

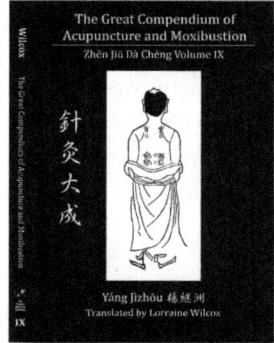

2012 Raising the Dead and Returning Life: Emergency Medicine of the Qīng
Dynasty
by Bào Xiāng'áo 鮑相璈
Translated by Lorraine Wilcox.
ISBN 978-0-9799552-3-5

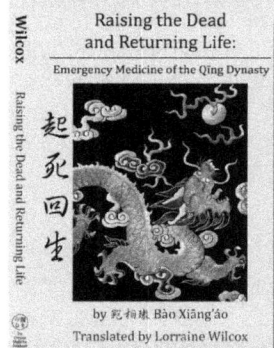

2014 Zhēn Jiǔ Zī Shēng Jīng 針灸資生經:
The Classic of Supporting Life with Acupuncture and Moxibustion Vol. I-III
by Wáng Zhízhōng 王執中
Translated by Yue Lu.
ISBN 978-0-9799552-1-1

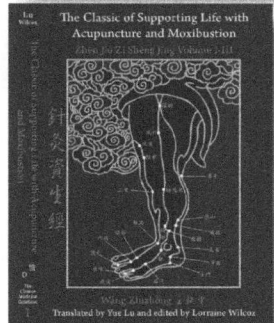

2014 Jīn Guì Fāng Gē Kuò 金匱方歌括:
Formulas from the Golden Cabinet with Songs
vol. IV - VI
by Chén Xiūyuán 陳修園
Translated by Eran Even.
ISBN 978-0-9799552-8-0

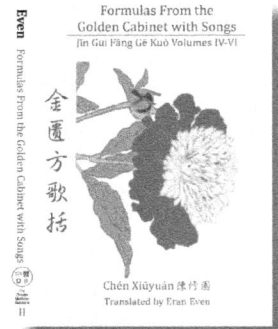

2015 Zhēn Jiǔ Zī Shēng Jīng 針灸資生經:
The Classic of Supporting Life with Acupuncture and Moxibustion Vol. IV-VII
by Wáng Zhízhōng 王執中
Translated by Yue Lu.
ISBN 978-0-9799552-9-7

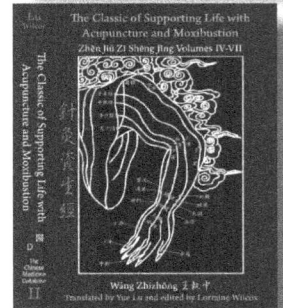

2015 Nǚ Yī Zá Yán 女醫雜言:
Miscellaneous Records of a Female Doctor
by Tán Yǔnxián 談允賢
Translated by Lorraine Wilcox.
ISBN 978-0-9906029-0-3

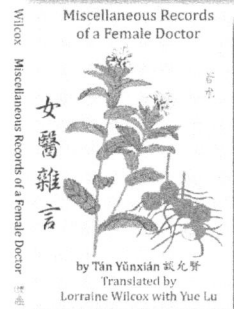

2016 Nǚ Kē Cuō Yào 女科撮要:
Outline of Female Medicine
by Xuē Jǐ 薛己
Translated by Lorraine Wilcox.
ISBN 978-0-9906029-1-0

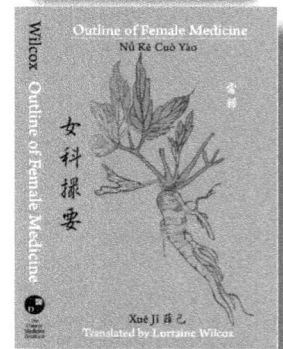

www.ingramcontent.com/pod-product-compliance
Lightning Source LLC
Chambersburg PA
CBHW061352210326
41598CB00035B/5959